Environmental Remediation Technologies, Regulations and Safety

nova
science publishers
www.novapublishers.com

Environmental Remediation Technologies, Regulations and Safety

Organophosphates: Detection, Exposure and Occurrence. Volume 2: Acute Exposure and Treatments
Tamara Lazarević-Pašti, PhD (Editor)
2022. ISBN: 978-1-68507-659-7 (Hardcover)
2022. ISBN: 978-1-68507-734-1 (eBook)

Investigations into the Decarbonisation of Railways
Inara Watson, PhD
2021. ISBN: 978-1-68507-250-6 (eBook)

Who Will Save Amazonia? World Heritage or Full Destruction
Marcílio de Freitas (Editor)
and Marilene Corrêa da Silva Freitas, PhD (Editor)
2021. ISBN: 978-1-53619-893-5 (Hardcover)
2021. ISBN: 978-1-53619-910-9 (eBook)

Modeling Forest Landscape Dynamics
Bharath Setturu, K.S. Rajan
and T. V. Ramachandra, FIE, FIEE (UK), FNIE
2021. ISBN: 978-1-53619-594-1 (Hardcover)
2021. ISBN: 978-1-53619-651-1 (eBook)

The Future of Phytoremediation
James C. Flores (Editor)
2021. ISBN: 978-1-53619-625-2 (Hardcover)
2021. ISBN: 978-1-53619-645-0 (eBook)

Müfide Aydoğan Ahbab
and Nurhayat Barlas
Editors

Phthalates

Environmental and Health Effects

nova
science publishers
www.novapublishers.com

DOI: https://doi.org/10.52305/UELB4255.

Library of Congress Cataloging-in-Publication Data

Names: Ahbab, Müfide Aydogan, editor. | Barlas, Nurhayat, editor.
Title: Phthalates : environmental and health effects / Müfide Aydodan Ahbab, PhD (editor), Associate Professor, Hamidiye Vocational School of Health Services, University of Health Sciences, İstanbul, Turkey, Nurhayat Barlas, PhD (editor), Professor, Science Faculty, Hacettepe University, Ankara, Turkey.
Description: New York : Nova Science Publishers, [2022] | Series: Environmental remediation technologies, regulations and safety | Includes bibliographical references and index. |
Identifiers: LCCN 2022027548 (print) | LCCN 2022027549 (ebook) | ISBN 9781685079703 (hardcover) | ISBN 9798886970388 (adobe pdf)
Subjects: LCSH: Phthalate esters--Toxicology. | Phthalate esters--Health aspects. | Phthalate esters--Physiological effect. | Phthalate esters--Environmental aspects.
Classification: LCC RA1242.P58 P484 2022 (print) | LCC RA1242.P58 (ebook) | DDC 615.9/5138--dc23/eng/20220628
LC record available at https://lccn.loc.gov/2022027548
LC ebook record available at https://lccn.loc.gov/2022027549

Published by Nova Science Publishers, Inc. † New York

Contents

Preface

Phthalates are esters of phthalic acid that are groups of chemicals used mainly in the production of plastics. Phthalates are also called plasticizers and they make solid plastics flexible and soft. Besides plastics, phthalates are also used as raw materials and/or auxiliary chemicals in many industrial activities.

Phthalates are classified as low molecular weight (C1-C6) and high molecular weight (C7-more) phthalates according to the carbon chain length of the subgroup in their chemical structure. Low molecular weight phthalates are used as raw materials or auxiliary chemicals in the production of cosmetics, detergents, shampoo, soap, paper, automotive, building materials, medical materials and paint. Diethyl phthalate (DEP), one of the low molecular weight phthalates, is used in cellulosic films as well as a stabilizer and carrier in perfumes and fragrances. High molecular weight phthalates are generally used as vinyl plasticizers in the production of polyvinylchloride (PVC).

Phthalates are lipophilic substances in terms of their chemical structure, and their solubility in water decreases inversely with the length of the subgroup carbon chain. Phthalates do not covalently bond to the plastics and release into their environment slowly over time. Because of their widespread use, phthalates are very common in nature and are classified as non-persistent pollutants. Their harmful effects have started to be shown by studies conducted in the last 20-30 years which revealed that phthalates have endocrine disrupting effects. For this reason, phthalates have begun to be classified as Endocrine Disruptive Chemicals. In addition, the use of certain phthalates has been restricted by the European Union and the United States at first. Diethylhexyl phthalate (DEHP), which is a widely used phthalate in the production of plastics, was the first phthalate to be restricted within the scope of the European Union REACH regulation in 1999 due to its effects on human health, especially infants and children. According to the restriction, DEHP should be less than 0.1% by mass in the manufacture of toys and materials related to children. Subsequently, Dibutyl phthlalate (DBP), butylbenzyl phthalate (BBP), di-iso-nonyl phthalate (DINP), di-iso-decyl phthalate (DIDP), dioctyl phthalate (DOP) and di-iso-butyl phthlalate (DIBP) were added to the restricted phthalates.

It has been determined that phthalates exert endocrine disrupting effects by changing the actions of some hormones in the body. Phthalates affect the endocrine system by mimicking or inhibiting endogenous hormones, interfering with hormone receptors, or inhibiting the synthesis of hormones. The effects of phthalates do not reflect the classical dose-response curve. Their harmful effects vary with dose, and they have a non-monotonic dose-response curve. In addition, harmful effects of phthalates are observed even at very low doses. Exposure to phthalates during developmental stages has been shown to cause greater effects. Therefore, it is necessary to monitor the exposure of these substances effectively in terms of human health. It is important to determine the concentrations of phthalates accurately and precisely, whose use is restricted, in various materials. As stated in ***Chapter I***, proper preparation and extraction of the samples are also an important issue that needs attention in order to determine the phthalate concentrations in the materials. Analysis of many phthalates is carried out by chromatographic methods. High-performance liquid chromatography, gas chromatography-mass spectrometry, liquid chromatography-tandem mass spectrometry and gas chromatography-tandem mass spectrometry are the most used analytical methods in phthalate analysis.

Exposure of human and natural life to phthalates occurs through inhalation, dietary and dermal routes. After phthalates are taken into the human body, they are metabolized by going through various detoxification stages. The primary and secondary metabolites of phthalates after detoxification stages are removed from the body by the kidneys. However, the metabolites of phthalates may exert more harmful effects than the parent chemical. Although phthalates have a short half-life in the body, they tend to accumulate in tissues such as adipose tissue, kidney and lung, due to their lipophilic properties. Especially during their developmental periods, the harmful effects of these accumulated phthalates may increase even more. Phthalates accumulated in the adipose tissue are released as energy needs of the body increase during pregnancy and cause adverse effects for both mother and child. Therefore, phthalates, which are known to pass through the placenta, impair the development of the fetus, especially the reproductive organs. Depending on the areas of usage, the effects of these substances may increase. DEHP, which is used especially in medical products, especially in tubes, serum and blood bags, causes more exposure of patients.

As mentioned in ***Chapter II***, phthalates have also been associated with cardiovascular diseases (CVDs) in recent studies. Heart failure, arrhythmias, stroke, atherosclerosis, hypertension and diabetes are some of the CVDs that have been associated with phthalates until now. DEHP and its metabolites have been found to be associated with heart failure and heart attack. In addition, *in vitro* and *in vivo* studies have shown that DEHP, DBP and DEP are associated with atherosclerosis. Nevertheless, there is little information about the effects of other phthalates on CVDs.

Recent studies reveal that phthalates can cause metabolic effects. Especially their interaction with PPARs has led to the investigation of the obesogenic properties of these substances. As noted in ***Chapter III***, phthalates interact with adipogenesis. It is suggested that phthalates increase adipose tissue mass, possibly by acting on PPARs. The metabolites of many phthalates, such as DEHP, DBP, BBP, and BBP, can bind to PPARg which leads to enhanced adipogenesis.

The genotoxic and mutagenic effects of phthalates have been studied much earlier. As mentioned in ***Chapter IV***, DEHP-induced single chromatid aberrations and sister chromatid exchange in human lymphocytes. Moreover, DEHP caused chromosome breaks in human lymphocyte cells. In mutagenicity tests with *Salmonella typhimurium*, DMP, DEP, DBP and DEHP metabolites were found to be mutagenic. MEHP was also found to have mutagenic activity in Rec-assay. Recent *in vitro* and *in vivo* studies showed that MEHP is genotoxic and causes DNA damage, as well as DBP, DHP and DCHP, in different type of cells.

It has been shown by both *in vivo*, *in vitro* and epidemiological studies that phthalates are also associated with metabolic diseases. Recent studies have shown that there is a relationship between phthalate exposure and diabetes, one of the most important metabolic diseases in the world. As noted in ***Chapter V***, phthalates are suggested to impair glucose metabolism and insulin production and signaling pathways, leading to diabetes-related conditions such as insulin resistance and high blood sugar. Moreover, they promote oxidative stress, inflammation and consequently beta cell loss through apoptosis. Phthalate metabolites associated with GDM have been identified.

Initially, phthalates were associated specifically with the reproductive system disorders. As mentioned in ***Chapter VI***, it has been shown that these substances reduce sperm quality and quantity, have anti-androgenic and estrogenic effects, impair the development of reproductive organs during development, shorten the anogenital distance and cause hypospadias, and all of these effects are called as "phthalate syndrome".

It is stated that phthalates, which are generally known for their endocrine disrupting properties, have harmful effects by affecting oxidative stress metabolism as well as these effects. As it is known, oxidative stress occurs with the deterioration of antioxidant defense and increase in ROS and is involved in the pathogenesis of many diseases (diabetes, cancer, obesity, metabolic syndrome, infertility, CVDs). As noted in ***Chapter VII***, phthalates can interfere with oxidative stress metabolism by disrupting detoxification pathways and altering antioxidant defense. Likewise, it is suggested that phthalates induce oxidative stress by binding and activating PPARs. In addition, it is also suggested that phthalates can interfere with the enzymes (glucose-6-phosphate dehydrogenase, 6-phosphogluconate dehydrogenase, glutathione s-transferase, glutathione reductase, superoxide dismutase, catalase, thioredoxin family, and glutathione peroxidase) responsible for antioxidant defense in cells and disrupt the redox balance.

As mentioned in ***Chapter VIII***, it is known that there is a relationship between epigenetic changes and diseases such as reproductive disorders, obesity, cancer, neurotoxicity, autoimmunity and diabetes. Among other effects, phthalates are also epigenetically toxic substances. Epigenetic mechanisms such as DNA methylation, histone modifications (acetylation, methylation, phosphorylation, ubiquitination, sumoylation and ADP ribosylation) and miRNAs play an important role in the disorders caused by phthalates. Especially in critical periods of development, epigenetic programming of gene expression becomes more crucial. *In vivo* and *in vitro* studies have shown that DEHP and its metabolite MEHP cause hypomethylation in DNA.

Considering the excessive use of these chemicals, the effects of phthalates, which are known and which this work tries to reveal, should be among the subjects that need further study. In addition to measuring phthalate exposure accurately and precisely, it is essential to develop methods that are rapid, reliable, selective, cost-effective, perform with smaller sample volume and detect any phthalates in a low concentration range. As stated in ***Chapter IX***, biosensor-based phthalate analysis methods including biological and/or engineered recognition elements and new sensor materials will provide a new approach in this regard. Especially in recent years, some biosensor-based detection techniques, notably electrochemical, optical and mass-sensitive biosensors, for the determination of phthalates from both aqueous and air samples are explained in the chapter.

In vitro, in vivo and epidemiological studies on phthalates are insufficient and inconsistent to fully understand the mechanisms of action of these chemicals. Epidemiological studies should be carried out to include a wider population and should also be supported by studies with human cell lines where the mechanism can be revealed.

Recent studies show that different endocrine disruptors and their metabolites can have a cumulative effect or create a synergistic effect on each other. Therefore, scientific studies should focus on examining the combined effect of multiple chemicals as well as the effect of a single substance. Therefore, it is of great importance to carry out ecotoxicological studies in which the distribution of endocrine disrupting chemicals in the environment is monitored and their effects on wildlife are investigated.

Müfide Aydoğan Ahbab
and Nurhayat Barlas,
Editors

Chapter 1

Analytical Aspects of Phthalate Exposure

Pelin Köseoğlu Yılmaz*
and Gamze Ergin Kızılçay
Department of Analytical Chemistry,
Faculty of Pharmacy, Istanbul University,
Istanbul, Turkey

Abstract

Phthalates are a group of ortho-phthalic acid diesters which are widely used to increase the flexibility of plastics or in common household products, cosmetics, detergents, flame retardants, adhesives, metal food can liners, and medical devices. Since phthalates are not chemically bounded to polymer matrices, they can easily migrate to foods, beverages, cosmetics, and pharmaceuticals, and may leach from polyvinyl chloride-based medical devices.

Some of the phthalates are considered as suspected endocrine disruptors by competing with 17β-estradiol for binding to the estrogen receptors and have significant adverse effects on male and female reproduction system. The lower molecular weight phthalates are irritating to eyes, nose, throat, and larger molecular weight phthalates are suspected carcinogens. Also they possess cardiotoxic, hepatotoxic and nephrotoxic effects.

The harmful impacts of phthalates have been known since the 1950s but they got more attention recently. From an analytical point of view, it is important to develop reliable and sensitive sample pre-treatment and analysis methods for the detection of phthalates considering the health hazards. Classical analytical procedures may be limited by their sensitivity and/or selectivity considering the low concentration levels and

* Corresponding Author's Email: pelink@istanbul.edu.tr.

In: Phthalates: Environmental and Health Effects
Editors: Müfide Aydoğan Ahbab and Nurhayat Barlas
ISBN: 978-1-68507-970-3

complex sample matrices such as biological materials, food, cosmetics, etc. Most of the phthalate analyses are perfomed by chromatographic techniques whereas the sample preparation procedure such as solid phase extraction, liquid-liquid extraction, solid phase microextraction, dispersive liquid-liquid microextraction, supercritical fluid extraction, pressurized solid phase extraction, microwave assisted extraction and etc. is selected regarding the nature of the sample. In this chapter, the analytical approaches to examine the phthalate exposure for human by personal care products, medical devices and food were discussed.

Keywords: Phthalate, medical device, food; personal care product, HPLC, GC; MS; GC-MS; LC-MS/MS; GC-MS/MS

Introduction

Phthalates are a group of dialkyl or alkyl aryl esters of 1,2-benzene-dicarboxylic acid (Figure 1). The variations in the side chains (R and R' in Figure 1) of the esters in length and structure specify the physical and chemical properties and as a result also the biological activities of phthalates (National Research Council Committee on the Health Risks of Phthalates 2008). A list of common phthalates and the abbreviations used in this chapter are given in Table 1 with their utilization areas.

Phthalates are used in a wide variety of consumer products, including food packaging materials, personal care products, medical devices, pharmaceuticals, children's toys, school supplies, household cleaners, glues, paints, automobile parts, home décor and building materials to improve the flexibility and elasticity, and to hold the color and the scent due to their properties and compatibility with polymeric materials. Phthalates with low molecular weights are generally used in cosmetics whereas phthalates with high molecular weights are utilized in tubing, food packaging and processing materials, containers, vinyl toys, vinyl floor coverings, and building products (Cao 2010, Ranjbari and Hadjmohammadi 2012).

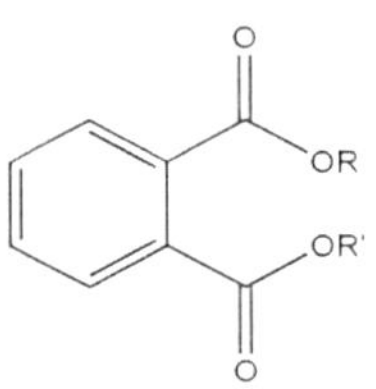

Figure 1. Chemical structure of phthalates.

Table 1. Common types of phthalates [partly adapted from Council (2008)]

Phthalate	Abbreviation used in this chapter	Molecular weight	Common use
Dimethyl phthalate	DMP	194	Insect repellent, plastic
Diethyl phthalate	DEP	222	Shampoo, scents, soap, lotion, cosmetics, industrial solvent, medications
Di(2-methoxyethyl) phthalate	DMEP	282	-
Diallyl phthalate	DAP	246	-
Dipropyl phthalate	DPP	250	-
Diisopropyl phthalate	DIPP	250	-
Di-n-butyl phthalate	DBP	278	Adhesives, caulk, cosmetics, industrial solvent, medications
Diisobutyl phthalate	DIBP	278	Adhesives, caulk, cosmetics, industrial solvent
Butyl benzyl phthalate	BBP	312	Vinyl flooring, adhesives, sealants, industrial solvent
n-pentyl-isopentyl phthalate	PnIPnP	306	-
Di-n-pentyl phthalate	DPnP	306	-
Diisopentyl phthalate	DIPnP	306	-
Dicyclohexyl phthalate	DCHP	330	Stabilizer in rubber, polymers
Di(2-ethylhexyl) phthalate	DEHP	390	Soft plastic, including tubing, toys, home products, food containers, food packaging
Di-n-octyl phthalate	DOP	390	Soft plastic
Diisononyl phthalate	DINP	419	Soft plastics, replacement for DEHP
Diisodecyl phthalate	DIDP	447	-
Di(2-propylheptyl) phthalate	DPHP	447	-

Unfortunately, phthalates used as plasticizers are not chemically bound to the polymers so that they may leach, migrate, or release to air, especially when the polymeric products are exposed to high temperatures. Because of that, exposure to phthalates may occur through different ways as ingestion, inhalation, dermal absorption, and parenteral administration (Council 2008). Many research on laboratory animals revealed several negative effects of phthalates caused by their carcinogenic and endocrine system disrupting activities by competing with 17β-estradiol for binding to the estrogen receptor. When the results of the toxicological studies were compared, it was determined that the low-molecular-weight phthalates were irritating to the eyes, nose, throat, and the high-molecular-weight phthalates were suspected carcinogens. They may also give rise to uterine damages. But the disturbances in the male reproductive system (infertility, decreased sperm count, cryptorchidism, hypospadias, etc.) are more serious which have led to a particular concern. Today, the adverse effects of phthalate exposure on human are still being investigated (Cao 2010, Ranjbari and Hadjmohammadi 2012, Council 2008).

The use and the presence of the phthalates in consumer products are strictly regulated in the European Union (EU). The restrictions of EU are explained especially under the regulations of the Registration, Evaluation, Authorization and Restriction of Chemicals (REACH) Regulation, the Toy Safety Directive and the Food Contact Materials Framework Regulation. The permitted concentrations are given in terms of concentration by weight, as lower than 0.1% by weight, or in terms of specific migration limits, as 1 mg/kg (especially for food). REACH Regulation sets restrictions on DBP, DMEP, DAP, BBP, DEHP, DPnP, PnIPnP and DIPnP which are in the list of carcinogenic, mutagenic or toxic to reproduction (CMR) substances under the Classification, Labelling and Packaging (CLP) Regulation. The maximum permitted limit for DBP, BBP and DEHP were stated as 0.1% by weight (individually or in combination) (Parliament 2008). For the cosmetic products DBP, DMEP, BBP, DEHP, DPnP, PnIPnP and DIPnP are banned by the Regulation (EC) 1223/2009 (UNION 2009). In toys for children under the age of 14, BBP, DBP and DEHP are restricted by a concentration lower than 0.1% by weight by Toy Safety Directive (Parliament and Union 2009). The maximum permitted phthalate contents of the polymeric food contact materials are stated in the Regulation (EC) 10/2011. DBP and DEHP can be used for non-fatty foods in repeated-use materials and articles. BBP, DIDP and DINP are allowed in repeated- and single-use food contact materials for non-fatty foods. These restrictions do not include infant and follow formulae. The specific maximum migration limits in Annex I of the regulation are 0.3 mg/kg for DBP, 30 mg/kg for BBP, 1.5 mg/kg for DEHP, 0.01 mg/kg for DAP and 9 mg/kg for the total of DIDP and DINP (Communities 2011).

When the hazardous effects and strict regulations of phthalates are considered, reliable analysis of these compounds become more of an issue. Development of accurate, precise, sensitive, and selective analytical methods is a challenge because of the complex samples which may contain interfering compounds or possess significant matrix effects. Another difficulty is the ubiquitous presence of phthalates in any laboratory. All of these problems may be solved or minimized by suitable procedures followed in the sample preparation and analysis steps (González-Sálamo et al. 2018). In the following part of the chapter, the strategies used for the determination of phthalates in potential exposure sources for human as personal care products, medical devices and food were discussed.

Analytical Methods for Phthalate Analysis

Phthalate Analysis in Personal Care Products

Personal care products may contain several types of phthalates in varying concentrations since the phthalates are included in different packaging materials as plasticizers. They can be transferred to these products during manufacturing or storage. Phthalates are also used as fixatives in perfumes and to form flexible films in hair sprays (Feng and Jiang 2012).

Sample preparation is a critical step in the analysis of phthalate contents of the personal care products. The procedure should be selected considering the complex matrices and varying concentration ranges. Although the traditional pretreatment methods like liquid-liquid extraction (LLE), solid phase extraction (SPE) are still found use, they have some drawbacks as requirement of large volumes of sample and extraction solvent and being time consuming. Today, generally the micro-scale sample treatment methods are applied to overcome these disadvantages and to obtain better extraction efficiency.

The extraction parameters have been generally optimized by one-variable-at a time trials. But nowadays experimental design for multivariate analysis is preferred. This approach provides determination of the effect of more than one variable on the extraction efficiency at a time. The effect of a variable may be different through different values of another. The best extraction conditions may be identified with a lower number of experiments.

Phthalate analysis in personal care products is mainly performed by chromatographic methods, especially by gas chromatography (GC) and high-performance liquid chromatography (HPLC). Mass spectroscopic (MS) detectors are common but also diode array (DAD) and ultraviolet (UV) detections are used in HPLC analysis (Feng and Jiang 2012, Gimeno et al. 2012, Yılmaz et al. 2014, Mostafa and Shaaban 2018, Shen et al. 2007, Kaur et al. 2016, Llompart et al. 2013, Wei et al. 2018, Hubinger 2010, Vinas et al. 2015, Kamarei et al. 2011, Su et al. 2010, Liu et al. 2018).

GC Analysis

GC is a common method for phthalate analysis in personal care products, mainly because of the volatile nature of the phthalates. The analysis procedures are generally distinguished from each other by means of the sample preparation techniques. In some of the studies, the traditional sample preparation methods have still found use. Gimeno et al. (2012) developed and validated a procedure including LLE and GC-MS for the analysis of 12 phthalates as DBP, DEHP, BBP, DMEP, DPnP, DIPnP, PnIPnP, DIBP, DCHP, DEP, DMP and DOP in cosmetics according to ISO 12787 international standard "Cosmetics - Analytical methods - Validation criteria for analytical results using chromatographic techniques." In the GC-MS analysis, the chromatographic separation was achieved on a cross-linked 5%-phenyl/95%-dimethylpolysiloxane capillary column (30 m x 0.25 mm, 0.25 μm) applying a temperature gradient. The temperature program was as follows: increasing from 100°C to 200°C at 30°C/min, then to 260°C at 3°C/min, and then to 320°C at 30°C/min and holding for 5 min. Split mode was used (1/20) with 1 μL injection. The injection port and transfer line temperatures were 300°C. The ion source temperature was set to 230°C. The rate of the carrier gas (He) was adjusted to 1.0 mL/min. Electron ionization (EI) was carried out at 70 eV. The acquisition was performed on full-scan (m/z = 40–350) and on selected-ion monitoring (SIM) mode. The quantifier ion m/z values were 163 for DMP, 149 for DEP, DIBP, DBP, DIPnP, PnIPnP, DPnP, BBP, DCHP, DEHP, DnOP and 59 for DMEP. The calibration curves were prepared by external calibration and the linear range was 0.5-5.0 μg/L for all of the analytes. LOQ of each phthalate was determined between 0.05 μg/mL and 0.25 μg/mL corresponding to an S/N ratio of ~10. Ready-to-inject cosmetic samples (i.e., perfumes) were directly analyzed after diluting with EtOH. Liquid/liquid extraction using tert-butyl methyl ether (TBME) was carried out for more complex sample matrices (i.e., milks and creams). Six perfumes, a shampoo, a cream, a body milk and a shower gel were analyzed using the proposed procedure. The results of the perfume analysis had RSD% around 5-10% (n = 3) and recoveries of the spiked sample ranged from 80% to 120%. Two samples were found to contain BBP and the others contained DEHP. For the other cosmetic products, the recoveries were between 80% and

130% with an RSD of <5%, except for DPnP in body milk and PnIPnP in shower gel, which were at RSD = 17% and RSD = 11%, respectively (Gimeno et al. 2012).

An enhanced LLE method, dispersive liquid-liquid micro extraction (DLLME), is based on the extraction of the analyte to an immiscible extracting solvent with the use of a disperser solvent. The disperser solvent is soluble in both of the liquid phases, so that it increases the contact between the two immiscible liquids, as the sample solution and the extracting solvent (Yılmaz et al. 2014). A DLLME coupled to GC-MS method was developed for the simultaneous determination of DMP, DEP, DBP, BBP and DEHP in perfumes. In the GC-MS analysis, the analytes were separated on Rxi-5MS capillary column (30 m x 0.25 mm, 1.00 μm). The carrier gas was He at a flow rate of 1 mL/min. A temperature program was applied starting from 90°C and holding for 0.5 min, which was increased to 220°C at 30°C/min. Then the temperature was risen to 280°C at 15°C/min and held for 10 min. The MS was operated in the EI mode (70 eV). For higher sensitivity and selectivity, SIM was selected. The analytes were confirmed by the retention times and the relative abundances of the monitored ions. The selected ions (m/z) for the phthalates were as follows (the first ones were used for quantitation): 163, 77, 194 for DMP; 149, 105,177 for DEP; 149, 104, 223 for DBP; 149, 91, 206 for BBP and 149, 113, 167 for DEHP. DLLME procedure was optimized considering the type and volume of extraction and dispersing solvents, the ionic strength, and the vortex time. Extraction efficiencies were evaluated by the extraction recovery and the enrichment factor. The final optimal conditions were obtained as 20.0 μL of C_6H_5Cl as the extractant, 0.5 mL acetone as the disperser solvent and vortex time of 30 s. The ionic strength had no significant effect on the extraction recovery. The proposed DLLME – GC-MS method was linear in the range of 0.0010-1.0 μg/mL (except BBP, 0.0015-1.0 μg/mL) with R^2 higher than 0.99. LODs were between $3x10^{-6}$-$7x10^{-6}$ μg/mL, whereas the LOQs were within $1.3x10^{-5}$ and 2.2×10^{-5}μg/mL. The precision was examined as intra- and inter-day studies with the RSD values of 1.36-3.66% and 2.75-4.12%, respectively. Recoveries were in the range of 85.6-95.8%. The proposed method was successfully applied to the analysis of perfume samples and satisfactory results were obtained. All of the phthalates were detected in most of the analyzed samples, with frequency rates of 12 out of 12 samples for DEP and DEHP, 11 out of 12 for BBP, 10 out of 12 for DBP and 6 out of 12 for DMP. The most common phthalate was DEP with varying concentrations between 0.22-4213 μg/mL (Mostafa and Shaaban 2018).

GC-MS analysis with SPE sample pre-treatment was also examined for the determination of phthalates in different kinds of personal care products. In a study, a SPE coupled to GC-MS method was used for the determination of 8 phthalates, as DEP, DPP, DIBP, DBP, BBP, DCHP, DEHP, DOP and 4 parabens, as methylparaben (MPB), ethylparaben (EPB), propyl paraben (PPB), and butyl paraben (BPB). The analytes were detected in EI mode using SIM for acquisition. The following ions were used for the quantification: m/z 121, 149, 177, 222 for DEP; m/z 149, 191, 209 for DPP; m/z 57, 149, 223 for DIBP m/z 104, 149 for DBP; m/z 91, 132, 149, 206 for BBP; m/z 55, 149, 167 for DCHP; m/z 113, 149, 167, 279 for DEHP; m/z 149, 279 for DOP; m/z 65, 93, 121, 152 for MPB; m/z 93, 121, 138, 166 for EPB; m/z 93, 121, 138, 180 for PPB; and m/z 93, 121, 138, 194 for BPB. The m/z 149 peak and the m/z 121 peak were used for the screening for phthalates and parabens, respectively. Personal care product samples including sprays, perfumes, deodorants, cream and lotion were analyzed. The analytes were extracted by sonication assisted extraction with methanol. Then the extracts were cleaned up by SPE using a LC-C18 column (3 mL). LODs were in the range of 0.1-5.0 μg/kg. Fourteen samples were found to contain at least 3 or more of these phthalates and/or parabens, commonly as MPB, PPB, DPP, DCHP and DEHP (Shen et al. 2007).

A method employing microextraction by packed sorbent (MEPS) coupled with GC-MS was developed for the determination of DEP, BBP, DCHP, DBP and DPP in cold drink and cosmetic (perfume and cream) samples. Before the MEPS process, the perfume sample was diluted with methanol, whereas the cream was mixed with methanol, centrifuged and then the clear supernatant was filtered. The solid phase sorbent (4 mg of solid phase silica-C18) was packed in a barrel insert and needle, which was inserted into a 250 μL gas-tight syringe. The sorbent was conditioned with 100 μL of methanol and 100 μL of water before the first use. To optimize the MEPS procedure, parameters as the pulling/pushing speed, number of extraction cycles, the composition of washing solution, the composition and the volume of the elution solution, pH, and carryover effects were examined. The best recoveries were obtained with 15 extraction cycles, water as the washing solvent (50 μL), ethyl acetate as the elution solvent (30 μL) and the pH of 4. A significant carryover effect was not observed. In the GC-MS analysis, the analytes were separated on a Rtx-1MS column (30 m x 0.25 mm, 0.25 μm). The injector was set to 250°C in the splitless mode. The carrier gas was He at a linear velocity of 35.9 cm/s. A temperature program was applied as setting the initial temperature of the column oven at 120°C for 0.5 min, increasing up to 240°C at 5°C/min and holding for 1 min, then increasing to 280°C at 6°C/min. The interface and ion source temperatures were 230°C and 200°C, respectively. The EI source was adjusted to 70 eV. A mass range of m/z 45–600 was recorded in the full-scan mode. The analytes were identified by the retention times and MS spectra of the standards. SIM mode was used for the quantification. Ions selected for GC-MS monitoring were 121, 149 and 177 for DEP; 91, 104 and 149 for DPP; 104, 132 and 149 for DBP; 91, 207 and 149 for BzBP; 55, 149 and 167 for DCHP. The ion with m/z 149 was the most abundant ion for all of the phthalates. The method was linear in the range of 0.5-500 ng/mL with R^2>0.9992. LODs were between 0.003-0.015 ng/mL, and LOQs ranged in 0.009-0.049 ng/mL. The recoveries were in the range of 92.35-98.90% for cold drink, 88.23-169.20% for perfume, and 88.90–184.40% for cream samples (Kaur et al. 2016).

Another analysis method consisting of matrix solid-phase dispersion (MSPD) followed by GC-MS allowed the determination of 18 plasticizers (phthalates: DMP, DEP, DIBP, DBP, DMEP, DIPnP, DPnP, BBP, diisoheptyl phthalate (DIHpP), DCHP, DEHP, diphenyl phthalate (DPhP), DOP, DINP and DIDP, adipates: dimethyl adipate (DMA), diethyl adipate (DEA) and bis(2-ethylhexyl) adipate (DEHA), 7 polycyclic musks and 5 nitromusks in rinse-off (hair conditioner, shampoo, liquid soap, body scrup) and leave-on (body milk, moisturizing lotion, moisturizing cream, sun block, hands cream, anti-aging cream, aftershave, deodorant, straightening cream, hair nutrition cream, hair foam, hair gel) cosmetic formulations. The GC-MS analysis was performed using a cross-linked 5%-phenyl/95%-dimethylpolysiloxane capillary column (30 m x 0.25 mm, 0.25 μm) and He was the carrier gas (1.0 mL/min). The temperatures of the transfer line, the quadrupole and the ion source were 290, 150 and 230°C, respectively. A temperature gradient was applied as holding at 80°C, then increasing to 290°C at 15°C/min and holding at the final temperature for 10 min. The detection was carried out with SIM mode by monitoring three ions per compound. The electron multiplier was adjusted to 1376 V. The quantification ions for DMP, DEP, DIBP, DBP, DMEP, DIPnP, DPnP, BBP, DIHpP, DCHP, DEHP, DPhP, DOP, DINP and DIDP were 163.3, 149.0, 149.0, 149.0, 59.1, 149.0, 149.0, 149.0, 265.1, 149.0, 149.0, 225.0, 149.0, 293.0 and 307.0, respectively. The linear range of the method was 2-500 ng/mL, except for DINP and DIDP (50-5000 ng/mL) with R > 0.997. RSD values ranged from 0.17 to 9.6% in the intra-day and were between 2.6 to 15% in the inter-day analyses with the standard solutions. The instrument detection limits (IDL) were lower than 1 ng/mL, which were higher for DIHpP, DINP and DIDP resulting from their complex isomer mixtures. In the MSPD procedure, the original and the spiked samples were blended with anhydrous Na_2SO_4 and dispersing sorbent, Florisil, in a porcelain pestle. The mixture was transferred into a glass Pasteur pipette (approximately 150 mm), with a small amount of glass wool at the bottom, containing 0.1 g of Florisil. The analytes were eluted by gravity flow. A volume of 1 mL of extract was collected in a volumetric flask and the extracts (diluted with ethyl acetate if necessary) were directly analyzed by GC-MS. The MSPD conditions were optimized using a multivariate experimental strategy, a factorial experimental design was carried out. The conditions of the final optimized procedure were as follows: 0.1 g of sample was mixed with 0.2 g of anhydrous Na_2SO_4 and 0.4 g of Florisil, Pasteur pipettes and glass wool plugs were used, and the elution solution was 1 mL of ethyl acetate. The analytical performance of the overall procedure was evaluated using real cosmetic samples. Recoveries from the spiked samples were higher than 87% for all the phthalates with RSD% values lower than 8%. LODs ranged from 1.4 to 17 ng/g except for DIHpP, DINP and DIDP which were 50 ng/g, 120 ng/g and 300 ng/g, respectively. The most frequently found target compounds were the musks as galaxolide and tonalide reaching concentrations above 0.1% (1000 μg/g), and DEP (between 0.7-357 μg/g). The presence of the banned substances such as the phthalates; DBP, DIBP, DMEP, BBP, DEHP, DIPP, DPP, and the musks; ambrette and tibetene, was confirmed in 16 of the 26 personal care products (Llompart et al. 2013).

HPLC Analysis

HPLC is also a common analysis method besides GC for the phthalate analysis in personal care products. Ten phthalates as DEHP, BBP, DAP, DBP, DCHP, DEP, DMP, DHP, DOP, DPP, which are forbidden by the hygenic standards for cosmetics in China (2007 edition) were determined in perfume samples by UHPLC– electrospray ionization (ESI)–MS/MS. The less complex nature of the samples made it possible to use a simple extraction method. Also, the use of a sophisticated instrument as UHPLC-ESI-MS/MS provided the analysis without the requirement of an enrichment step. Before the analysis, the samples were prepared by weighing 1 g of perfume into a 10 mL colorimetric tube and dilution with methanol. Then the solutions were vortexed for 5 min and filtered through a 0.2 μm PTFE membrane. UHPLC-ESI-MS/MS analysis was carried out with a stationary phase of C18 (150 x 2.0 mm, 3 μm) at 40°C. The elution gradient of the analytes from the column (with acetonitrile and water with formic acid, 0.1%) was determined based on theoretical prediction of the retention time of each. Five isocratic elution conditions and six gradients were designed for optimizing the chromatographic method. Protocols for estimation of the hold-up dwell time and optimizing the elution gradients were indicated. The optimized UHPLC gradients provided the separation of the analytes in a short time as 7 min and a reduced matrix effect which was important particularly for DMP and DCHP. The IDLs and instrument quantification limits (IQLs) were in the range of 0.03-27 μg/L and 0.12-89 μg/L, respectively. The linear ranges were 0.5-5000 μg/L for DPP and DAP, 50-5000 μg/L for DEHP and DBP, 5.0-5000 μg/L for the other phthalates with R^2 values higher than 0.99. The recoveries were in the range 88.82%-114.75%, whereas the intra- and inter-day RSDs were 14.5% and 13.9%, respectively. Twentysix perfume samples were analyzed and 23 of them were found to contain the analytes. DEP was detected with the measured concentrations in the range of 96.9 to 79787.6 μg/L in 22 perfumes and DEHP was found in 12 perfumes between 695.1-14214.7 μg/L. Nine of the samples were contaminated with DMP at lower concentrations (650.8-2980.9 μg/L). The contents of DCHP, DAP, and DBP were also high (up to 30429.3 μg/L, 1943.8 μg/L, and 9445.4 μg/L, respectively). DPP was detected in only 5 perfumes at 4.8 to 2651.1 μg/L. In none of the samples BBP, DHP, and DOP were present (Wei et al. 2018).

A simple extraction method applied in another study, a survey of 84 adult-use and baby-care cosmetic products for determination of DMP, DEP, BBP, DBP, DEHP, conducted by the U.S. Food and Drug Administration (FDA). In the sample preparation step, the phthalates were extracted just with hexane. The analysis was carried out with HPLC-UV. Chromatographic separation was achieved with a C18 column (250 mm x 4.6 mm, 5 μm) using a mobile phase consisted of a mixture of water/acetonitrile/2-propanol/methanol (50:34:12:2, v/v) with a gradient program. The detection wavelength was 230 nm. The recoveries were in the range of 88% to 104%. At least one phthalate was detected in 31 of the 60 adult-use cosmetic products. Twenty products contained DEP (80-36006 μg/g) and 11 nail products contained DBP (123-62607 μg/g). Five of the 24 baby-care products were contaminated with DEP at concentrations between 10-274 μg/g (Hubinger 2010).

A method consisting of ultrasound assisted extraction (UAE) and DLLME followed by LC–DAD-ESI-ion trap (IT)-MS/MS was developed and validated for the determination of DMP, DEP, BBP, DBP, DEHP, DOP in cleaning products, detergents and cosmetics (shampoo, gel, foot cream, deodorant, body milk, makeup and serum.). UAE step provided the advantage of less time and solvent volume requirement for the pretreatment. The chromatographic separation was performed by a C18 non-endcapped column (15 cm x 0.40 cm, 5 μm) with a mobile phase of acetonitrile and 10 mM ammonium acetate (pH 4) mixture. A gradient program was used as follows: an isocratic elution with a 55:45 acetonitrile: ammonium acetate (v/v) mixture for 3 min, then a linear gradient to 90:10 (v/v) in 0.5 min which was held for 4.5 min, then again a linear gradient to 100% acetonitrile in 0.5 min, which was held for 12 min. The flow rate was 0.4 mL/min and the injection volume was 20 μL. The wavelength of DAD was adjusted to 225 nm and the UV–visible spectra were recorded in the range of 200-600 nm. An IT mass spectrometer with an ESI source was used in multiple-reaction monitoring (MRM) mode. Data were collected in positive mode in a 50–500 m/z scanning range. The following settings were selected: The nebulizer gas pressure, 45 psi; drying gas flow, 10 L/min, drying gas temperature, 350°C. The parent ions for DMP, DEP, BBP, DBP, DEHP and DOP were the ions with m/z values of 195 (product ions as 163, 133, 89), 223 (product ions as 177, 149), 313 (product ions as 205, 149, 91), 279 (product ions as 205, 149, 91), 391 (product ions as 279, 167, 149) and 391 (product ions as 279, 177, 149) respectively. Before DLLME, the samples were homogenized by vigorous manual shaking. Then a volume 3 mL of acetonitrile was transferred to a centrifuge tube which contained 0.03 g sample. In the UAE step, the mixture was sonicated for 20 s (30% amplitude, 0.5 cycles per second), then, centrifuged for 5 min at 3000 rpm. The extracts were ready for DLLME after filtration through 0.45 μm PVDF filters. The extracting solvent was selected as carbon tetrachloride (CCl_4), whereas the disperser solvent was acetonitrile. The parameters of the DLLME procedure were optimized by a Taguchi design method. The factors that could affect the extration efficiency such as CCl_4 volume, acetonitrile volume, aqueous phase volume, pH, sodium chloride content and centrifugation time were selected as the variables. According to the results, the DLLME procedure was consisted of the following steps: 3 mL acetonitrile from the UAE of the sample was used as disperser solvent and 150 μL of CCl_4 was added. The mixture was then transferred into 10 mL of water. After centrifugation at 3000 rpm for 2 min, the extraction solvent sedimented at the bottom (volume recovered 100 ± 20 μL) was collected. CCl_4 was evaporated to dryness under Ar flow. The residue was desolved in 25 μL of acetonitrile before injection to LC–DAD-ESI-IT-MS/MS. The developed method was validated in terms of linearity, LOD, LOQ, selectivity, recovery, accuracy, and robustness. The linear range was 2 to 50 ng/mL (4-50 ng/mL for DMP) with LC-DAD and 0.4 to 50 ng/mL (2-50 ng/mL for DMP and DOP) with LC–ESI-IT-MS/MS with R^2> 0.99. The

LODs were in the range of 0.13-1.0 ng/mL and 0.042-0.45 ng/mL in the HPLC-DAD and LC–ESI-IT-MS/MS analysis, respectively. The repeatability and the reproducibility were found in the ranges of 3-10% and 5-14% in terms of RSD using ten replicate analyses of a sample spiked with all the analytes at 50 ng/g. The selectivity was confirmed both by the UV spectra and the mass spectra of the analytes. The accuracy was tested by fortified samples (detergent, cleaning product and body cream) with phthalates at 1.5 and 3 ng/g. The recoveries were in the range of 84-124%. The proposed method was applied for the determination of 32 samples successfully. The most commonly identified analyte was DEP (Vinas et al. 2015).

Ultrasound-assisted emulsification microextraction (USAEME) is an effective extraction method, in which a water-immiscible extraction solvent is dispersed into an aqueous solution without a dispersive solvent. As a disadvantage, USAEME requires high-density toxic extraction solvents (e.g., chloro- solvents), even though the volumes used are in micro levels. In another technique, called as liquid phase microextraction with solidification of floating organic droplet (LPME-SFO), an extraction solvent with low density and proper melting point (close to room temperature) is transferred on the surface of an aqueous sample while the sample solution is being agitated by a stirring bar. Following the extraction, the sample is cooled down and the extraction solvent is solidified which can be collected easily. But the extraction rate is slower in this procedure. In a study, these two extraction techniques were combined as USAEME-SFO and the efficiency was examined for the extraction of DMP, DEP, DAP, DIHP, DIBP and DBP in cosmetic products and water samples followed by HPLC-DAD analysis. To develop the sample preparation procedure, a factorial experimental design was employed. The variables (solvent volume, salt effect, extraction time and centrifugation time) which could be effective on the extraction efficiency were examined. The centrifugation time was found to be an insignificant factor. Therefore, the rest of them as extraction solvent volume, salt effect and extraction time were optimized by Box–Behnken design. The extraction conditions were determined as; extraction solvent volume, 30 μL; sodium chloride concentration, 20% (w/v); extraction time, 12 min; and centrifugation time, 5 min. Chromatographic separations were achieved by a C18 HPLC column (250 mm x 4.6 mm, 5 μm). Isocratic elution was carried out with the mobile phase as water/methanol (24:76) at a flow rate of 1 mL/min. The injection volume was 10 μL and the analytes were detected at 205 nm. Using the developed procedure preconcentration factors in the range of 355-409 were obtained. LODs were between 0.005-0.01 μg/L, whereas the linear ranges were 0.05-800 μg/L for DIBP and DBP, and 0.05-1000 μg/L for the other analytes. The procedure was applied for the determination of the phthalates in a shampoo, a after shave gel and a hair spray besides environmental samples. For the cosmetic products, the RSDs were ≤12.5% and the error values were between -5.0-8.5%. The shampoo sample was found to contain 28.6 μg/g DEP and 57.7 μg/g DBP. The after-gel sample had the DEP and DBP contents of 158.0 μg/g and 6.2 μg/g, respectively. DMP and DEP were detected in the hair spray sample at the concentrations of 4.2 μg/g and 11.8 μg/g (Kamarei, Ebrahimzadeh, and Yamini 2011).

Feng and Jiang (2012) compared the efficiencies of LLE, UAE, microwave-assisted extraction (MAE), DLLME, DLLME-SFO, and cloud point extraction (CPE) for the extraction of DMP, DEP, DPP, BBP, DBP, DPnP, DEHP, DCHP and DOP from cosmetics. The procedures of LLE, UAE and MAE consist of two immiscible phases, whereas there are three phases in DLLME and DLLME-SFO. Differently, surfactants are used in CPE, instead of organic solvents which provides a greener pretreatment procedure. After the extraction, the analytes were determined by a capillary liquid chromatography (CapLC) method with UV detection which had a linear range of 0.5 to 50 μg/mL, LODs in the range of 0.02-0.17 μg/mL, precision and bias lower than 5%. The extraction procedures were compared in terms of extraction time, solvent usage, instrumentation cost, ease of operation, labor intensiveness and enrichment factor. With the exception of DPP and DCHP, DLLME-SFO was suggested for the extraction with its low LOD and high extraction efficiency. If the major targets were DPP and DCHP, then DLLME was said to be more appropriate for sample preparation (Feng and Jiang 2012).

Solid phase microextraction (SPME) is another technique with significant advantages over traditional SPE including less use of toxic solvents, high enrichment factors, and integration of extraction and injection in a simple device. On the other hand, fibers used in SPME are fragile with limitted lifetime. Polymer monolith microextraction (PMME) is a kind of in-tube SPME technique, with features as frit-free construction, biocompatibility, easy preparation with good control of porosity and diverse surface chemistry. Moreover, it has advantages of the extraction devices, such as convenience, flexibility, and easy operation. A strategy was reported which was based on PMME followed by HPLC-UV for the determination of phthalates (DMP, DBP, DCHP, and DOP) in cosmetics. HPLC analysis was performed using a C18 column (4.6 x 250 mm, 5μm) and a mobile phase consisting of methanol/water (95:5, v/v) at a flow rate of 1.0 mL/min. Autosampler and column temperatures were 4°C and 35°C, respectively. The injection volume was adjusted to 5 μL. The detection wavelength was selected as 228 nm. A poly (methacrylic acid-co-ethylene glycoldimethacrylate) (MAA-EGDMA) monolith was used in the PMME procedure. The poly (MAA-EDGMA) monolithic capillary tube had the dimensions of 50 μm x 3 cm. The steps of the microextraction included preconditioning, sample loading, washing, and desorption. The PMME procedure was optimized by the parameters of sample flow rate, sample volume, sample pH, and eluent flow rate considering the peak area of the analyte. The optimized parameters were as follows: preconditioning with 0.2 mL of methanol at 0.057 mL/min for 3.5 min and then with 0.5 mL of Na_2HPO_4 (pH 4) at 0.16 mL/min for 3.2 min, sample loading with 1.0 mL of the sample solution at 0.20 mL/min for 5.0 min, washing with 0.2 mL of Na_2HPO_4 (pH 4) at 0.16 mL/min for 1.3 min, and desorption with 0.086 mL EtOH at 0.086 mL/min for 1.0 min. The proposed method was validated in terms of extraction efficiency, linear range, precision, LOD and LOQ. A good linear range was obtained between 3-5000 ng/mL (r>0.9992). LODs were in the range of 0.7-3.7 ng/mL and LOQs were between 2.3 and 12.3 ng/mL. RSDs in the intra-day and inter-day analysis were lower than 3.2% and 7.7%, respectively. The method was successfully applied for the determination of the analytes in 2 lacquer remover and 6 perfume samples with a recovery range of 81.2-108.8% (Su et al. 2010).

Analysis of total pthalate content may be useful to preliminarily screen the samples for the presence of the phthalates. In this purpose, phthalates are hydrolyzed to phthalic acid (PA) and the content of PA is determined. A simple sample preparation method for the determination of the total phthalate content in cosmetics was developed by Liu et al. (2018). PA, the hydrolysis product of phthalates, was determined by a LC-MS/MS method. The hydrolysis of phthalates and the removal of the interferences were performed in a three-phase system with an upper n-hexane phase, a middle ethanol phase, and a lower aqueous alkali solution. The nonpolar ingredients were extracted with n-hexane, the polar pigments accumulated in the ethanol phase, and PA remained in the hydrolysate. Thus, there was no requirement of an extra sample pretreatment step like SPE for colored cosmetic products. Samples were weighed (0.2 g) in a 25-mL glass vial and 1 mL n-hexane, 50 μL of 168 μM PA-d4 (internal standard), 1 mL of ethanol, and 8 mL of 8 M KOH were added. The mixture was heated at 80°C with magnetic stirring for 15 min at 800 rpm. Following cooling down, the upper n-hexane phase and colored middle layer were discarded. A volume of 10 mL of 6 M HCl was added, and the solution was mixed and allowed to cool to ambient temperature. The acid hydrolysate (8 mL) was transferred into a polypropylene tube containing 600 μL tributyl phosphate (TBP) and the tube was shaken for 2 min. The resulting cloudy solution was centrifuged and the upper TBP phase was transferred to a vial and mixed with an equal volume of methanol/water solution (4:1, v/v). Following filtration (0.45 μm), the sample was ready for the LC-MS/MS analysis. The chromatographic separations were carried out by a C18 column (150 x 3.0 mm, 2.2 μm) at 35°C. Gradient elution was applied with a mobile phase consisting of aqueous 0.1% formic acid and acetonitrile containing 0.1% formic acid. The flow rate was 0.3 mL/min. The injection volume was set to 10 μL. MS/MS instrument was equipped with an ESI source with declustering, and entrance potentials adjusted to -4500, -35, and -10 V, respectively. Analytes were detected in the MRM mode. The precursor ion for PA was m/z 164.9. The ion with m/z 77 was used for quantitation and m/z 120.9 was for qualification. The proposed method was applied to the total phthalate analysis of 57 cosmetic samples including skin toners, lotions, creams, perfumes, nail polishes and semi-solid or solid cosmetic products such as rouge, foundation, lipstick, and eyeliner. PA was detected in all the nail polish samples (25.0-110274.0 μmol/kg) and were detected in 66.7% of the perfumes (<LOQ-68377.3 μmol/kg). For solid or semi-solid cosmetics, the total phthalate contents were generally higher in oily samples, which were low in liquid skin care products (Liu et al. 2018).

Phthalate Analysis in Medical Devices

Polyvinyl chloride (PVC) polymers have been widely used to produce medical devices including tubing, intravenous bags, blood containers, etc. Phthalates, especially DEHP, are the plasticizers utilized to increase the flexibility and elasticity of PVC. Phthalates can be easily eluted into pharmaceuticals or biological fluids that come in contact with the PVC products and be migrated directly and/or indirectly into the human body since they are not chemically bound to the polymer (Haishima et al. 2005). Several parameters, like temperature, time, and lipophilicity of the solution, may affect the migration of the phthalates and other plasticizers.

The medical devices made up of PVC polymers are still commonly used although concerns about the heath hazards caused by the phthalates they contain, particularly DEHP, have been risen over recent years. DEHP is classified as a reprotoxic substance (CMR substance Category 1B). Moreover, it was recommended to replace DEHP in medical devices with other alternative plasticizers by a European Union regulation (Parliament 2008). In

France, incorporation of DEHP in medical devices for neonatology, pediatric and maternity wards was prohibited (Nakiwala 2020). Two approaches to prevent the use of DEHP in medical devices are based on the selection of another polymer (polypropylene or silicone) that does not require additional plasticizers, or substitution of the plasticizers. The common alternative plasticizers are diisononylcyclohexan-1,3-dicarboxylate (DINCH), tris(2-ethylhexyl)-trimellitate (TOTM), di(2-ethylhexyl)-terephthalate (DEHT) and some others with lower migration from PVC and lower toxicity compared to that of DEHP (Faessler et al. 2017).

Many studies were performed to analyze the plasticizer content of PVC polymer used in the production of the medical devices, or to analyze the migration of the plasticizers from PVC medical devices under conditions that are the same as or similar to those of medical use. The analytical methods with high sensitivity, accuracy, precision, and selectivity are required to determine these compounds especially for clinical assessment. The most common methods include GC-MS and LC-MS analysis followed by chromatographic techniques with other types of detectors, and methods like ^{1}H NMR and Raman spectroscopy (Haishima et al. 2005, Faessler et al. 2017, Haned et al. 2018, Kostic et al. 2016, Bourdeaux et al. 2016, Bernard et al. 2015a, Gimeno et al. 2014, Jeon et al. 2018, Bernard et al. 2015b, Veiga et al. 2012, Yılmaz 2019, Radaniel et al. 2014, Lecoeur et al. 2015, Al Salloum et al. 2016).

GC Analysis

A literature survey revealed that GC was the most widely preferred method for the phthalate analysis in medical devices. There are several studies carried out by GC with different types of detectors, particularly with MS detection, on both the phthalate content and the migration (or leaching) tests.

Haishima et al. (2005) performed DEHP analysis by GC-MS in a study for the determination of potential DEHP elution from medical devices made of PVC using the physicochemical properties of pharmaceutical preparations as the solubility of the lipophilic pigments, electrical conductivity, and static contact angle to PVC sheet. Two kinds of lipophilic injections (Sandimmun® and Prograf®) and three kinds of surfactants (HCO-60, Tween® 80, and SDS) were used as the test solutions for DEHP elution. After that, the relationship between the DEHP release from PVC tubing and physicochemical properties of 53 pharmaceutical injections used in gynecologic and obstetric fields were examined. To determine the total DEHP content of PVC sheet and tubing, 20 mg of each were dissolved in 20 mL of tetrahydrofuran (THF) overnight at room temperature. For elution tests the PVC tubing were cut to 10 cm length. Pharmaceuticals as Sandimmun® and Prograf® adjusted to the concentration used for medical treatment were enclosed in them for 1 h at room temperature by shaking. An aliquot of 0.1 mL of both of these solutions was taken and distilled water (2 mL), sodium chloride (10 mg), and 5 mL of diethyl ether were added. After shaking for 30 min and centrifugation at 3000 rpm for 10 min at room temperature, the organic phase was collected and dehydrated with anhydrous Na_2SO_4 before GC-MS analysis. The stationary phase of the GC-MS method was BPX-5 fused silica capillary column (25 m x 0.22 mm, 0.25 μm). The injector temperature was set to 260°C, and the flow rate of the carrier gas (He) was 1 mL/min. A temperature program was applied starting from 120°C for 2 min which was then increasing to 300°C at 10°C/min. EI-mass spectrum was recorded at 70 eV, and the ion of m/z 149.024 for DEHP was selected as the quantitative ion in the SIM mode. Before the analysis of the samples, the background contamination caused by the reagents and GC-MS instrument was checked. Considering the background value, the experimental LOD and LOQ were calculated as 1.85 and 4.01 ppb, respectively. The method was linear in the concentration range of 5-200 ppb ($r > 0.999$). Sandimmun® and Prograf®, lipophilic injections containing polyoxyethene castor oil or HCO-60, and ethanol as additives, were found to release DEHP in a concentration-dependent manner. The released DEHP concentrations were more significant when the test solution concentration was higher than 0.05 mg/mL, which reached to 22.19 ± 0.26 ppm by Sandimmun® (5 mg/mL) and 42.26 ± 1.64 ppm by Prograf® (0.5 mg/mL). The surfactants, HCO-60, Tween® 80, and SDS, also caused the release of DEHP from PVC concentration-dependently (Haishima et al. 2005).

In another study, the leaching of not only DEHP, but also some of the general alternative plasticizers as DEHT, TOTM and DINCH from PVC perfusion lines using different lipid emulsions under clinical conditions was examined. The plasticizers were analyzed by GC-MS with injector-internal thermal desorption. The PVC lines, from the producers; Fresenius kabi, CAIR LGL, BBraun and Dispomed, were perfused with the lipid emulsions: Intralipid® 20%, ClinOleic® 20% and SMOFlipid® 20%. The extraction of the plasticizers from the emulsion samples were performed by 10 mL of ethanol and 5 mL of TBME/hexane (20:80, v/v) solution. The mixture was shaken, 10 mL of distilled water was added and mixed. Finally, the organic phase was separated and injected to the GC-MS system. Injection conditions were optimized to retain the lipids in the injector and to vaporize and transfer the plasticizers into the GC column. The original plasticizer concentration in all of the lipid emulsions was below the LOQs. The highest DEHP leaching concentration was observed with the Fresenius PVC-line with a concentration of 48.3 µg/mL by ClinOleic® 20%, 47.6 µg/mL by Intra-lipid® 20% and 43.7 µg/mL by SMOFlipid®. Among all of the plasticizers DEHP showed the highest leaching as 18 and 9 times higher than those observed for DEHT and DINCH, respectively. The leaching concentration of TOTM was even lower. According to this study the leaching of DEHP by lipid emulsions under mimicking conditions of parenteral nutrition is much higher than the acceptable level and higher than the other plasticizers. No significant difference in the amounts of plasticizers was observed depending on to the type of the lipid emulsion, while the tube diameter was found to be an effective parameter on the leaching rate (Faessler et al. 2017).

The migration of plasticizers from PVC materials containing aqueous solutions instead of lipopilic solutions was also investigated. Haned et al. (2018) developed a procedure to determine the migration potential of nine plastic additives in infusion bags of NaCl (0.9%) and glucose (5%). Five phthalates (DMP, DEP, DBP, BBP, DEHP), one adipate (DEHA), two alkylphenols (nonylphenol (NP), and 4-tert-octylphenol (OP)) and benzophenone (BP) were analyzed in new and outdated plasticized PVC, and in trilaminate polyethylene-polyamide-polypropylene, a multilayer material which did not contain DEHP presumably. Also, the migration from PVC raw materials (film and grain) under controlled conditions were examined. SPE and LLE techniques were used in all tests. Oasis HLB 6 SPE cartridges (200 mg, 6 mL) were selected for the SPE process and LLE procedure was performed by hexane as the extraction solvent. The samples were analyzed with GC-MS. EI was set to 70 eV. A fused silica column DB-5MS (30 m x 0.25 mm, 0.25 µm) and a deactivated guard column were used for separation. A temperature program was applied starting from 70°C (holding for 2 min) to 135°C at 10°C/min, to 160°C at 3°C/min, to 175°C at 1°C/min, to 195°C at 3°C/min and finally to 310°C at 10°C/min, keeping the final temperature for 5 min. The injection volume was 2 µL in the splitless mode. The carrier gas (He) flow was 1.2 mL/min. Injector, GC interface and ion source temperatures were 280°C, 280°C and 200°C, respectively. SIM and scan mode (70-500 amu) were used to determine target compounds and to identify potential plasticizers. The phthalates analyzed were identified by the monitored ions with m/z values as 163, 77, 194 for DMP; 149, 177, 105 for DEP; 149, 150, 223 for DBP; 149, 91, 206 for BBP; and 149, 167, 279 for DEHP. Phthalates are generally present in the laboratory environment. Considering that, to prevent the external contamination any contact of samples with plastic materials were avoided, high-quality solvents were used, and glassware were rinsed with extran, then with distilled water and acetone, heated to 450°C overnight. The study was focused on the linearity, repeatability and reproducibility, the analysis of the blanks, and the evaluation of the extraction efficiency. The linear range was 0.01-1.5 μg/mL ($R > 0.99$, except for DBP). The repeatability was tested (at 0.3 μg/mL) in 5 injections, and the reproducibility by injecting the same concentration in 5 consecutive days. For the analytes present in blanks (phthalates and DEHA) because of external contamination, the method detection limits (MDL) (μg/L) were calculated. MDLs were evaluated with the concentration in NaCl or glucose blank solution plus 5 times of the standard deviation ($n = 3$). For the analytes which were not present in blanks (OP, BP, NP), the MDLs were calculated as the concentration with the signal to noise ratio of 5 using samples spiked at 1 μg/mL. The recovery was evaluated by the samples fortified at low and high concentrations (1 μg/L and 10 μg/L). The percentages of repeatability and reproducibility were lower than 15% and 28%, respectively. Both SPE and LLE procedures were found to be suitable in the migration study of plasticizers in infusion aqueous solutions. At lower concentrations, SPE was more accurate. In the analysis of the raw materials, the migration of DEHP in PVC grain was higher than the maximum permitted level (5000 μg/kg), which was much lower in PVC films. The concentration of DEHP in the outdated PVC bags were nearly 10 times of the one in new PVC bags. DEHP was the only compound detected in the new samples (4.31 ± 0.5 μg/L in NaCl and 4.29 ± 0.25 μg/L in glucose 5% serums). In multilayer bags, instead of DEHP, DBP and DEP were determined (0.7 ± 0.1μg/L and 4.14 ± 0.6 μg/L, respectively) which were not mentioned as additives allowed (Haned et al. 2018).

The presence of DEHP in dialysis and infusion sets for peritoneal dialysis and parenteral nutrition, which are made of PVC and other plastic polymeric materials, were investigated. Both the plastic material and the solutions (1.5% dextrose for peritoneal dialysis, 0.9% NaCl the physiological saline solution, and Ringer's solution, NaCl, KCl and $CaCl_2$) stored in PVC bags and LDPE bottles were analyzed. DEHP was extracted from the plastic materials which were cut into pieces (~1 cm^2) using 5 mL of n-hexane for a period of 3, 6, 15 and 30 days. The extraction procedure for the solutions was carried out with 5 mL of hexane for 500 mL of sample (mixed for 60 min and 24 h). The organic layer was analyzed by GC-MS after the addition of internal standard using a DB-5 MS capillary column (30 m x 0.25 mm, 0.25 μm). The temperature program was applied in the range of 60°C to 280°C. In the MS the operating temperature was 280°C with the EI at 70 eV. SIM mode at m/z 149 was used and the quantification ion was the one with m/z of 149 for DEHP. The calibration curve for DEHP was linear in the concentration range of 0.25-2.5 µg/mL. The peritoneal dialysis set made of PVC was found to contain high amount of DEHP, about 31-34%. The solution of peritoneal dialysis kept in the analyzed PVC bag, had a low concentration of DEHP (3.72 µg/L). The DEHP content of infusion bottle made of LDPE was lower than the amount in PVC bags. LDPE bottle of physiological saline solution contained higher amount of DEHP than LDPE bottle of Ringer's solution. On the other hand, the DEHP content of the solution stored in bottle with lower DEHP level (Ringer's solution) was about three times higher as 17.30 and 5.83 µg/L, respectively. Tukey's post-hoc test was performed to examine the effect of the extraction time on the release of DEHP and results changing with the type of the polymer and simulating solution were obtained (Kostic et al. 2016).

In some of the studies, a simulant solution instead of the pharmaceutical itself was used to examine the migration behavior of the phthalates from the PVC medical devices. Bourdeaux et al. (2016) developed a GC-MS method to identify and quantify DEHP, TOTM, DEHT, DINCH, DINP, DEHA, and acetyl tri-n-butyl citrate (ATBC) in medical devices with their migration abilities in a simulant solution. To determine the total content, the extraction of the plasticizers in the medical devices was made by soaking at least 10 mg of PVC to a 25 mL flask filled with chloroform at ambient temperature for one hour of contact. Then the solution was homogenized and 1 mL of it was injected into GC-MS. In the migration tests, a 50% v/v ethanol/water solution was used as the simulant solution. The lines were filled with the simulant solution and different contact times as 0, 1, 2, 4, 8, and 24 hours were examined. The released plasticizers were extracted from the ethanolic solution to chloroform and analyzed by GC-MS. GC-MS analysis were performed using EI tuned to 70 eV and a 5% diphenyl-95% dimethylpolysiloxane (30 m x 0.25 mm, 0.25 µm) capillary column. A temperature programming was applied starting at 200°C for 1 min, then increased to 300°C at a rate of 20°C/min which was remained for seven minutes. The carrier gas (He) flow rate was 1.20 mL/min. An experimental design was used to improve the GC-MS analysis with ten parameters as dilution solvent of the standard solutions, standard concentration, injection temperature, split, or splitless injection, micropipette type, injection volume, quantification m/z value, with or without chromatogram smooth for quantification, and injection speed. According to the results, chloroform was selected as the dilution solvent and the standard concentration was 0.5 µg/mL. The injector temperature was set to 300°C. Split injection mode was applied, and the ratio was 20 mL/split. An electronic micropipette was used and the injection volume was 1 μL. The quantification m/z value for TOTM was set to 305. Noise reduction was applied to smooth the chromatogram and normal injection speed was selected. But the analytes as DEHT, DINCH and DINP were found to be eluted together from the column. Instead of a longer analysis time, specific m/z values were determined to separate the plasticizers. Following a scan mode analysis, ions specific to each plasticizer were selected. For DEHP, the ions chosen for the SIM quantification were the ones with the m/z values of 149, 167, 279 and m/z 149 was used for quantification. For DINP, they were 149 and 293, and m/z 293 was used for quantification. Calibration ranged from 0.1 to 10 μg/mL for DEHP, DEHA, ATBC and DEHT; from 0.25 to 25 μg/mL for DINCH; 0.5-25 μg/mL for TOTM; and 1.5–25 μg/mL for DINP with R^2 above 0.997. LOQ values were the first level of calibration curves. The LODs were 0.03 μg/mL for DEHP, DEHA and ATBC; 0.05 μg/mL for DEHT and TOTM; 0.1 μg/mL for DINCH; and 0.45 μg/mL for DINP. The precision (in terms of RSD) and relative bias values (as percentage) for the quality control samples at 4 concentration levels were determined and all values were below 15%. Thirty-two medical devices including extracorporeal circulation circuit, enteral nutrition line, blood transfusion set, extension line, set for infusion were tested. TOTM was found to be the most frequently used plasticizer (45%) in the medical devices studied followed by DEHP (29%), DINCH (16%), DINP (7%), ATBC (3%), and DEHA (3%). In the migration tests, analysis of the plasticizers in the simulant solution showed the presence of TOTM and DEHA in quantifiable concentrations but also DEHT and DEHP at concentrations below the LOQ (0.1 μg/mL) (Bourdeaux et al. 2016).

Bernard et al. (2015b) examined the migration performance of DEHP, DEHT, DINCH and TOTM using a model adapted to the clinical use of the medical devices. Again, a mixture of ethanol/water (50/50 v/v) was selected as the simulant solution and migration tests were performed at 40°C for the time periods of 24 h, 72 h, and 10 days. The plasticizers in the PVC tubing after solvent extraction (before migration tests) and in the simulant solution after contact with the samples (specific migration) were analyzed by GC with flame ionization detector (FID). The mean linear regression equations obtained for each plasticizer gave good correlation coefficients (>0.998). The method had acceptable accuracy and precision, with the intra- and inter-assay coefficients of variation all lower than 10%. The results revealed that DEHP had the highest migration ability, increasing with contact time. The amount of TOTM and DEHT were much lower than DEHP. Only 0.2% of TOTM was migrated into the simulant solution and the migration did not continue with time unlike DEHP. On the other hand, DINCH had similar behavior to DEHP in terms of migration (Bernard et al. 2015b).

Some of the studies in the literature include only the quantification of the plasticizers in PVC products without the migration tests. Gimeno et al. (2014) developed a GC-MS method for the identification and quantification of 14 phthalates: 8 phthalates (DBP, DEHP, BBP, DMEP, DnPP, DiPP, DPP and DiBP) classified as H360 (may damage fertility or unborn child) according to EU regulations, 3 phthalates proposed to be forbidden in medical devices (DnOP, DiNP and DiDP) and 3 other none regulated phthalates (DMP, DCHP and DEP) which may interfere with hormone function. To identify and quantify other plasticizers that are commonly used in PVC medical devices instead of DEHP, 5 non-phthalate plasticizers (ATBC, DEHA, DEHT, TOTM, and DINCH) were included. Analyses were performed by a GC-MS system with EI using a cross-linked 5%-phenyl/95%-dimethylpolysiloxane capillary column (30 m x 0.25 mm, 0.25 μm) and a temperature gradient. The plasticizers were extracted by THF for dissolving the PVC followed by precipitation of the PVC by ethanol. Diluted supernatant is injected into the GC-MS system. Three different ions for each compound were monitored by SIM mode. The dilution solvent (ethanol) and each analyte were analyzed separately at the highest concentration to check the presence of any interferences or carryover. No interference was observed. DEHT, DnOP, DINCH, DiDP and DiNP were eluted together from the column. Thus, the analysis was performed by the ions specific to each of the analyte. The calibration range was 5.0-50.0 μg/mL for DINCH, DiDP and DiNP, whereas it was 0.5-5.0 μg/mL for the rest of them. LODs were in the range of 0.07-0.25 μg/mL for DINCH, DiDP and DiNP; and for the other analytes ranged in 0.01-0.06 μg/mL. For DINCH, DiDP and DiNP LOQs ranged from 0.1 μg/mL to 2.0 μg/mL and for the other compounds from 0.01 μg/mL to 0.1 μg/mL. Mean recoveries determined on spiked preparations ranged between 80% and 120% (RSD < 20.0%). The proposed method was used for the determination of the analytes in more than 60 PVC medical devices. Results showed that the use of TOTM was dominant. Also, it was reported that when the plasticizer used is TOTM, the content of DEHT as a contaminant was between 1000-3000 ppm although its concentration was below 100 ppm when a plasticizer other than TOTM was utilized. More than 65% of the samples were found to contain DEHP at a concentration level >0.01% where also TOTM was used as plasticizer. In the raw material analysis, TOTM seemed to contain the highest content of DEHP and DEHT (Gimeno et al. 2014).

A GC-MS/MS method for the quantitative determination of DBP, BBzP, DEHA, DEHP, DNOP, dioctyl terephthalate (DOTP), DINP, and DIDP in medical infusion sets (infusion tubing samples) was developed and validated in MRM mode. For sample preparation, solvent extraction with polymer dissolution was employed prior to analysis. The extraction of the plasticizers was carried out by sonication of 50 mg of small pieces from the tubing in 5 mL of THF at room temperature for 30 min in a glass tube. Then, 10 mL of hexane was added, and the solution was vortexed. An aliquot of 0.5 mL of the supernatant was transferred into a vial. After addition of the internal standard (benzyl benzoate), the solution was homogenized and filtered. Chromatographic separation was performed by a DB-5MS UI (5% diphenyl-95% dimethyl siloxane phase, 30 m x 0.25 mm, 0.25 μm) capillary column. The injector temperature was adjusted to 300°C and 1 μL of each solution was injected in the split mode (2:1). Flow rate of the carrier gas (He) was 1 mL/min. A temperature program was applied starting from the initial temperature of 150°C which was held for 3 min, then increased up to 300°C at 10°C/min and held for 12 min. The collision gas was N_2. The transfer line and ion source temperature were 250 and 230°C, respectively. The MS was tuned on EI at 70 eV in MRM mode. The calibration curves were in the range of 5–500 ng/g ($R^2 > 0.999$). Average recoveries were in the range of 91.8–122% with the relative standard deviations of 1.8–17.8%. LOQs were between of 54.1 and 76.3 ng/g (Jeon et al. 2018).

Bernard et al. (2015a) compared three different extraction methods as Soxhlet extraction in diethyl ether and ethyl acetate, polymer dissolution, and room temperature extraction in different solvents for TOTM, DINCH, DEHT, and DEHP using 0.1 g of plasticized PVC. The samples were analyzed by GC-FID system equipped with a fused silica capillary column coated with a 100% dimethyl polysiloxane stationary phase (30 m x 0.25 mm, 0.25 μm). The carrier gas (He) flow rate was 1.2 mL/min. The injection volume was adjusted to 5 μL. The oven temperature was increased from 200 to 290°C at a rate of 30°C/min and held at 290°C for 7 min. Injection was performed in split (1/10) mode and the detector temperature was set to 300°C. The GC-FID method was linear between 20-200 μg/mL for DEHP, 10-200 μg/mL for DEHT, and 100-800 μg/mL for TOTM and DINCH with good correlation coefficients over 0.998. The analytical performance of the method was examined by LOD, LOQ, precision, and accuracy. The method possessed suitable accuracy and precision, with the intra- and inter-assay coefficients of variation all below 10%. LODs were 5, 1, 20, and 0.2 μg/mL, and LOQs were 10, 8, 30, and 1 μg/mL for DEHP, DEHT, TOTM, and DINCH, respectively. The extraction trials showed that the simple room temperature chloroform extraction under optimized conditions (30 min, 50 mL) gave the highest extraction yields in the range of 92-100% for all the analytes, which was also confirmed by supplemented Fourier transform infrared spectroscopy-attenuated total reflection and gravimetric analyses. The proposed procedure was applied for 8 marketed PVC tubings and it was reported that the samples contained different amounts of plasticizers between 25 to 36% of the PVC weight (Bernard et al. 2015a).

HPLC Analysis

Veiga et al. (2012) investigated the presence of five plasticizer phthalates (DEHP, DMP, DEP, DBP, BBP) in bags and sets for intravenous administration and hemodialyzers made of PVC and of other polymeric materials by HPLC-UV. The samples analyzed were new and empty plastic infusion sets (PVC and ethylene vinyl acetate, EVA, bags and burette), hemodialyzers made of cellulose diacetate and polysulfone. Continuous ambulatory peritoneal dialysis (CAPD) bags were also analyzed, but in this case, the samples were collected from filled bags. Not only migration tests, but also analysis to determine the concentration of phthalates in the material itself was carried out. For the analysis of solid sample, 0.1 g of the material (cut into small pieces) was shaken with 2 mL hexane for 15 min in a horizontal shaker. Liquid samples were transferred into glass tubes and stored at 4°C until analysis. To 1 mL of each liquid sample, 1 mL hexane was added, and the mixture was vortexed for 10 min. Twenty (for DEHP) or 25 μL (for the other analytes) aliquot of the organic layer was injected into the HPLC-UV system. For the internal capillary of the hemodialyzers, the material was immersed in the pure dialysis solution and in the dialysis solution spiked with DEHP at 4.86 mg/L. Portions of the liquid were collected after 1 h and 5 days of the submersion. In the HPLC-UV analysis, the separation was performed on a C18 column (150 x 4.6 mm, 5μm). Two different chromatographic conditions were used: one for the determination of five of the phthalates and another for the determination of DEHP alone. The first one included the mobile phase of acetonitrile: water (94:6, v/v) with a gradient program. The detection wavelength was 202 nm. For the determination of DEHP alone, the mobile phase was acetonitrile: methanol (90:10, v/v). The detection wavelength was set to 220 nm. LOD was determined by the injection of a blank sample (hexane) 6 times. The calibration ranges were between 0.50-10.00 mg/L for

DEHP and 0.25-5.00 mg/L for the other phthalates. Repeatability and reproducibility values were between 0.7-1.6% and 2.1-4.1%, respectively. LODs were in the range of 0.01-0.05 mg/L. Only DEHP was found in the extracts of the bags. EVA bags also contained DEHP, but in low concentrations. On the other hand, DBP was detected in the tubing material coupled to the bags and the burette as well, but again in much lower concentrations. Hemodialyzers capillaries were found to contain both DEHP and DBP, whereas all other phthalates were present in the polysulfone capillary. A period of time of 1 year was examined for the migration tests of DEHP from PVC and EVA bags. Water and the solutions of NaCl, amino acids and glucose were used as the simulant. Leaching of DEHP from EVA bags and PVC bags were similar. Very low amounts migrated to water and saline solutions from both kinds of bags. Among amino acids, histidine and threonine caused the highest extraction rates with different kinetics of the migration for both kinds of polymers. While the extraction rate for PVC gradually increased over time, the extraction rate for EVA bags during the first 6 months was very low, but after that increased considerably. The concentration of phthalates in some commercial formulations were also analyzed and DEHP was the only phthalate found (Veiga et al. 2012).

Yılmaz et al. (2019) optimized a hydrophilic-lipophilic balance SPE method in terms of the type and the volume of the conditioning and the elution solvents for the extraction of seven phthalates as DMP, DPP, BBP, DBP, DCHP, DEHP and DOP from three types of liquid pharmaceutical preparations as an intravenous isotonic NaCl solution, an intravenous dextrose solution and an osmotic laxative preparation kept in polymeric packages. The phthalates were quantified by a validated HPLC-UV method. The optimized SPE conditions were as follows: 6 mL of conditioning solvent as methanol at pH 3.6 by phosphate buffer and 6 mL of elution solvent as acetonitrile containing 1% formic acid. The recovery values were higher than 80% for DMP, DPP, DBP, BBP and DCHP, whereas below 80% for DEHP and DOP since they have lower polarities. Only the intravenous isotonic NaCl solution was determined to be contaminated with DPP (13.2 ± 0.16 μg/L) (Yılmaz et al. 2019).

In another study an HPLC-UV method was developed to quantify the currently used alternative plasticizers to DEHP in tubing made of PVC. Five plasticizers as ATBC, DEHP, DEHT, DINCH, and TOTM, were separated on a C8 HPLC column (100 mm x 4.6 mm, 2.6 μm) using gradient elution with acetonitrile: water. The detection wavelength was 221 nm leading to a quantification threshold from 0.3 to 750 μg/mL as a function of the analyte.

Intra- and inter day precisions were below 0.9% and 18%, respectively. The linear ranges were 20-100, 1-40, 0.6-10, 90-750 and 0.3-40 µg/mL for ATBC, DEHP, DEHT, DINCH and TOTM, respectively. LODs and LOQs were between 0.1-17.4 and 0.2-52.8 µg/mL. Plasticizers were extracted from PVC-tubing by dissolving PVC in THF, then precipitating in methanol. Extraction yields were higher than 90% for all the analytes (Radaniel et al. 2014).

Instead of a reverse phase HPLC separation, Lecoeur et al. (2015) also discussed the quantitative performance of supercritical fluid chromatography (SFC) on the analysis of plasticizers. The study was focused on the comparison of SFC with evaporative light scattering detector (ELSD) to HPLC-ELSD for the determination of ATBC, DEHA, DEHT and TOTM in PVC tubing used as medical devices. The plasticizers were extracted from the tubing by sonication with chloroform for 1 h. The appropriately diluted samples were analyzed. Both methods were fast (<10 min). In the chromatographic analyses, while all compounds were separated with resolution values higher than 2.5 in HPLC, the resolution between DEHP and BBP was critical in SFC. When the quantitative performances were examined, it was determined that SFC allowed the quantitation of lower concentrations, while HPLC provided better accuracy and precision. Accuracy profiles of plasticizers draft in HPLC were in the ± 10% acceptance limits, whereas validation failed in SFC. SFC-ELSD could enable the quantification of the analytes in medical device tubing despite its low precision. However, neither HPLC-ELSD nor SFC-ELSD was powerful enough to quantify trace level of DEHP in such materials (Lecoeur et al. 2015).

Other Analysis Methods

A simple and sensitive procedure was developed to understand the diffusion of plasticizers from polymers into the surrounding media by using confocal Raman microscopy on a PVC sheet plasticized with around 40% DEHP. The results were correlated with standard measurements by UV spectroscopy. Water and ethanol were selected as the storage media. The lowest concentration of DEHP was observed at the surface in ethanol, which causes a less plasticized layer near the interface. When the PVC sheets were stored in water, a greater concentration of DEHP on the film surface was observed. This study showed differences in the concentration gradient observed due to the diffusion of the plasticizer inside a PVC sheet. Using the developed method, small variations in concentrations could be measured. It was reported that the storage in water did not significantly change the DEHP ratio in the material but promoted a DEHP exudation on the surface favoring leaching into the liquid. For the storage in ethanol, a concentration gradient from the core to the surface was clearly observed (Al Salloum et al. 2016).

In another study a new ^{1}H NMR spectroscopy method was proposed for the determination of DEHP, ATBC, DEHA, DEHT, DINCH, DINP and TOTM in PVC sheets, standard infusion tubing, and commercially available medical devices. Two techniques were compared: dissolution in deuterated THF and extraction by deuterated chloroform. ^{1}H NMR spectra were very similar in both deuterated solvents; dissolution and extraction provided similar results. Limits of detection and quantification were determined for each plasticizer: 40 and 201 μg/mL for ATBC, 37 and 185 μg/mL for DEHA, 58 and 195 μg/mL for DEHP, 39 and 195 μg/mL for DEHT, 42 and 212 μg/mL for DINCH, 42 and 210 μg/mL for DINP, and 54 and 273 μg/mL for TOTM, respectively. The sensitivity of the method provided the quantification of the minor plasticizers in PVC. In nine commercially available samples, the major plasticizer (different for different PVC tubing) was identified and quantified by ^{1}H NMR. In six samples, one, two, or three minor plasticizers were also identified and quantified. DEHP was detected in only one tubing as the major plasticizer. Only small quantities of solvent and sample were required for the analysis. It was not necessary to dilute samples to enter a quantification range, and the method was sufficiently sensitive to detect contaminants (Genay et al. 2017).

Phthalate Analysis in Food

Phthalates, which tend to migrate to natural resources and enter the food chain when absorbed by plants and animals, can migrate to food from illegally used food additives and food packaging materials. The analysis of phthalates, which are widely used as plasticizers in food processing and packaging, has become a popular topic of research in recent years due to their health effects. The extraction and cleaning methods for the analysis of phthalates in foods is very important because it is difficult to completely eliminate the matrix in food. Since phthalates are ubiquitous, contamination is likely to occur even during analysis and, traces of analytes tend to be lost during sample preparation. Phthalate contents of foods may be low, even lower than the LODs of the methods. For these reasons, it has become necessary to develop sample preparation and analysis methods for determination of phthalates in food samples with high accuracy and precision. The phthalate analysis strategies in food samples are developed considering the type of the sample. For the food materials with simple matrices, traditional extraction techniques may be useful. However, for the more complex samples, advanced pretreatment methods must be applied. Molecularly-imprinted polymer-solid phase extraction (MISPE), traditional SPME, stir-bar sorptive extraction (SBSE), magnetic solid-phase extraction (MSPE), DLLME, vortex-assisted liquid-liquid microextraction (VALLME) and quick, easy, cheap, effective, rugged and safe (QuEChERS) methods are among the most used extraction techniques in this purpose (Yang et al. 2015). Generally, chromatographic methods are used for quantitative analysis of phthalates in various types of foods. Among these, GC-MS, GC-MS/MS, LC-MS, LC-MS/MS are the most preferred ones. In these analyses, UV, DAD and FID are also used instead of the MS detector. Also, the enzyme-linked immunosorbent assay (ELISA), supercritical liquid chromatography (SFC) and sensors are other procedures used for phthalate analysis in foods.

GC Analysis

A GC-MS method allowed the analysis of phthalates in 78 foodstuffs purchased from the local market. Solid and liquid foodstuffs, which were examined in 6 categories as beverages (3), meat products (4), seafoods (3), cereal products (44), snacks (17), and condiments (7), were extracted with dichloromethane. The samples were cleaned-up by the gas purge microsyringe extraction method. In the chromatographic separation, a DB5 fused-silica capillary column (30 m x 0.25 mm, 0.25 μm) was used. The carrier gas was He at a flow rate of 0.9 mL/min. Column temperatures between 70-280°C were used and phthalate detection was performed in SIM mode. DMP, DEP, DBP, BBP, DEHP and DNOP were the analyzed phthalates in foodstuffs. The overall recoveries were calculated in the range of 85.7 to 102.6%, and the RSDs were found less than 10%. LODs ranged from 0.14 to 0.38 ng/g for solid samples and from 0.0021 to 0.0096 ng/mL for liquid samples. The method was linear between 5-1500 ng/mL. As a result of the examination, average total phthalate concentrations and median values were determined as 327 and 208 ng/g fresh weight in cereal, 175 and 154 ng/mL in beverages, 230 and 203 ng/g fresh weight in condiments, 1210 and 1380 ng/g fresh weight in seafood, 494 and 241 ng/g fresh weight in snacks, and 281 and 243 ng/g fresh weight in meat products. The highest concentrations (658-1610 ng/g) were detected in the seafood samples. The concentrations were in the order of DEHP > DBP > DEP ~ DMP > BBP ~ DNOP (He et al. 2015).

In another study, GC-MS method was used to examine the migration of monomers and plasticizers from packaged foods and microwave-heated foods. Three phthalates (DBP, BBP and DEHP), 4-tert-octylphenol (OP), 4-nonylphenol (NP), bisphenol A (BPA) and DEHA were analyzed using the QuEChERS sample preparation method in homemade courses and packaged liquid and solid foods. Two reagent products labeled as Reactive 1 and Reactive 2 (Agilent, Santa Clara, California) were used for QuEChERS extraction and purification. In GC-MS analysis the stationary phase was a DB-5MS column (30 m x 0.25 mm, 0.25 μm), and the carrier gas was He at 1.2 mL/min flow rate. The oven temperature was programmed ranging between 65°C-310°C. The QuEChERS extraction recoveries in the spiked cheese, cooked food and liquid food were calculated in the range of 36 ± 3%-106 ± 12%, while a similar trend was observed in spiked rice and eggs course, except for DEHP. For liquid foods, recoveries ranged from 63 ± 22% to 123 ± 1%. DEHP detection was not taken into account for the analysis of courses due to peak interference. LOD values were between 0.20 ng/g wet weight (DEHA) and 14.37 ng/g wet weight (NP) for solid foods, while it ranged from 0.02 ng/mL (DEHA) to 2.25 ng/mL (DEHP) for liquid foods. The analyte concentrations of the samples as meat, fish and vegetable broths were in mean ranges of 0.37 ± 0.03-9.61 ± 1.93 ng/mL, 0.40 ± 0.04-9.68 ± 1.75 ng/mL, <LOD of DEHP-7.30 ± 0.95 ng/mL, respectively. In the analysis of white and red wine, NP and DEHP concentrations were below LOD in white wine, while the DBP content was determined as the highest with an average of 6.67 ± 1.16 ng/mL. All of the mean phthalate concentrations in white wine samples were higher than the ones in red wine samples, except for DBP (8.72 ± 1.41 ng/mL) (Fasano et al. 2015).

Four major phthalates (DiBP, DBP, BBzP and DEHP) were analyzed by a newly developed and validated GC-MS/MS method in a wide variety of foodstuffs (n = 54). The food samples were selected from of various categories such as water, milk, oil, wine, soft drink, coffee, tea, cream, fruits, fish, crustacean, meat, ready cooked dishes, biscuits, chocolate, cheese, desserts. According to the matrix of the sample, one of the following 3 pretreatment procedures were applied with 10 g of freshly weighed sample. In the first procedure, the solid samples were freeze-dried and then ground into homogeneous form. The dried sample was weighed into a glass tube and spiked with deuterated internal standard. Analytes were extracted with acetonitrile. In the second procedure, liquid samples were directly weighed into glass tubes and likewise spiked with the internal standard. Ethyl acetate was used for extraction. The third method was for the fatty samples (e.g., butter, margarine, mayonnaise) which were placed in an oven at 80°C. When oil separation was not efficient enough, water was added to prepare samples. Then, liquid-liquid extraction was performed by acetonitrile. The GC-MS/MS analyses of the samples were carried out using a capillary column (30 m x 0.25 mm, 0.25 μm). A temperature program between 100-320°C was applied. EI was set to 70 eV in the MS detector. The method included both separation and detection by selected reaction monitoring (SRM); as well as quantification analysis according to the isotope dilution principle. The m/z 149 ion was not chosen as the precursor ion for DEHP, as the monitored transitions were selected for both their sensitivity and specificity. A full validation protocol was carried out with evaluating LOD and LOQ, specificity, linearity, precision, accuracy, and the relative combined uncertainty parameter. Also, attention was paid on background contamination at any stage of the work. Reporting limits were found to be 2.7, 0.53, 0.18 and 3.4 μg/kg for DiBP, DnBP, BBzP and DEHP, respectively and were statistically different from the identified background contamination. In the same order, relative combined uncertainties were calculated to be 7.6%, 12.2%, 12.0% and 14.1% (Cariou et al. 2016).

Different types of SPE techniques were applied for the extraction of phthalates from food matrices. Magnetic micro-solid phase extraction is one of them which was used for the analysis of phthalates in packaged foods followed by GC-FID analysis. In this purpose, a magnetic-MWCNTs-PVA cryogel-1-SPE sorbent was developed, which provided a good sorbent-to-sorbent reproducibility (RSD < 8%) and could be re-used for 30 times (RSD <6%). DBP and DEHP extracted from packaged foods with this sorbent were analyzed by GC-FID method, in which the separation was performed with a DB-5 fused silica capillary column (30 m x 0.25 mm, 0.25 μm). Detector and injector temperatures were set to 300°C and 270°C, respectively. The linear range was 0.025-10 μg/mL. LODs for DBP and DEHP were 36.4 ± 0.5 ng/mL and 26.3 ± 0.3 ng/mL, whereas LOQs were found as 121 ± 2 ng/mL and 88 ± 1 ng/mL, respectively. In hot water samples taken from plastic bags, DBP and DEHP were found in the range of 0.04-0.15 μg/mL and 0.03-0.20 μg/mL. In clear chicken soup samples, only DEHP was detected in the range of 0.02-0.07 μg/mL (Makkliang et al. 2015).

Another sorbent, a zeolitic imidazolate frame-based graphene oxide composite (ZIF-8 @ GO), was prepared to be used in the extraction of DEP, DPP, DIBP, BBP and DEHP from children's food samples as CiCi beverage, pear juice samples and jam samples. A hollow fiber stir bar was used in the extraction procedure showing high adsorption efficiency. In practice, the stir bar was filled with ZIF-8 @ GO. The trace level phthalate analysis was performed by GC-MS using a capillary column (30 m x 0.25 mm, 0.25 μm) for chromatographic separation and He with a flow rate of 2.0 mL/min as carrier gas. The injection port temperature was 240ºC and the injection was carried out in splitless mode. Column temperature was programmed between 120-280°C. The MS detector was set in EI mode and in full-scan mode from 50 to 500 m/z. For sample preparation, pear beverage and CiCi beverage samples were filtered directly, and jam samples were filtered after dilution with water, and then homogenized prior to sorbent extraction. The main experimental parameters that could impact the extraction efficiency were investigated. Under the determined analysis conditions, LOD values for DEP, DPP, DIBP, BBP and DEHP were found in the ranges of 0.15-0.6 μg/L for CiCi beverage and pear juice samples, and 0.75-2.2 μg/kg for jam samples. LOQ values were between 0.5-2.0 μg/L for CiCi beverage and pear juice samples, and 2.5-7.5 μg/kg for jam samples. The calibration range was studied over a wide range of 0.5-500.0 μg/L for CiCi beverage and pear juice samples, and 2.5-2000 μg/kg for jam. The proposed method had good repeatability (RSD < 11%) and high recovery (72%-100%). The data obtained showed that the ZIF-8 @ GO based hollow fiber stir bar could be re-used for 120 extraction cycles (Shen et al. 2019).

In another study, a method as SPME followed by GC-MS was used for the analysis of eight plasticizers (DEP, BBP, DEHA, DOP, DCHP, DIBP, DBP, DEHP) to examine the migration to roasted meat in plastic bags. The extraction of phthalates was carried out using a SPME fiber cooled with liquid nitrogen. In GC-MS analysis, the stationary phase was HP-5MS Agilent column (30 m x 0.25 mm, 0.25 μm) and the carrier gas was He (1.5 mL/min). Injector temperature was set to 250°C and splitless mode was used. The oven temperature was increased in the range of 120-280°C. The identification and quantification of compounds were carried out using SIM mode. The LOD and LOQ values of the developed method ranged from 0.01 to 0.18 μg/kg and from 0.07 to 0.26 μg/kg, respectively. Spices and roasted chicken meat were analyzed with the developed method. DIBP and DBP were determined in both samples. As a result of the analysis, the highest amount of plasticizer was determined in the spices used for cooking chicken meat (Moreira et al. 2015).

LLME is a widely used pre-treatment procedure in phthalate analysis. In a study, it was aimed to determine phthalates in baby food products. For this purpose, the analysis of DMP, DEP, DBP, isobutylcyclohexyl phthalate (iBcEP), BBP and DEHP in freeze-dried baby food was planned with a method based on ultrasound-vortex assisted LLME (UVALLME) combined with GC-IT/MS. The chromatographic separation was performed with a SE-54, 5% phenyl-95% dimethylpolysiloxane column (30 m × 250 μm, 0.25 μm). Helium was used as carrier gas at a flow rate of 0.3 mL/min. A temperature program between 100-300°C was applied. IT/MS system was used in EI mode at 70eV. Quantification of analytes was performed in SIM mode and identification in full scan mode (m/z 75-450). The linear range was between 10-5000 ng/g with $R^2 \geq 0.92$. The recoveries of the proposed method were found to be ranged from 96.2 to 109.2% with RSD ≤ 10.5%. The LOD and LOQ values of all phthalates (except iBcEP) were below 11 and 20 ng/g, respectively, which were 23 and 43 ng/g for iBcEP. With the optimized method, samples of commercial freeze-dried chicken and Turkey meats in the Italian pharmaceutical market were analyzed. Following dissolving the sample (0.1 g), anthracene was added as the internal standard. The analytes were extracted with n-heptane with a vortex time of 5 min and an ultrasonication time of 6 min at 100 W. These steps favor the solvent dispersion and as a result the extraction efficiency. After that, the mixture was centrifuged, 1 μL of n-heptane phase was injected in splitless mode into the GC-IT/MS system. As a result of the analysis, the preliminary defined three phthalates, DEP (14 ng/g), DBP (11 ng/g) and DEHP (64 ng/g), were quantified (Russo et al. 2016).

The phthalates, DnPP, DAP, BBP, DOP, in food-contacted plastics were detected with vortex-assisted liquid-liquid microextraction (VALLME) method followed by GC-FID. In this study, a novel class of eight low viscous hydrophobic deep eutectic solvents (DESs) were used for the extraction and preconcentration of phthalates from water samples. The advantages of DESs include being easily synthesized and low-cost, having a solubility that can be tailored for hydrophilic or hydrophobic organic analytes, and having lower toxicity. In the proposed work, DESs consisted of two types of quaternary ammonium salts and six types of water-insoluble fatty alcohol/acids. A hydrogen bond acceptor (HBA) (such as n-octyl alcohol) and a hydrogen bond donor (HBD) (such as decanoic-acid) were used for synthesizing DESs. Measured and uniformly mixed HBA and HBD were heated at 75°C. A clear liquid was obtained after 30 minutes. The synthesized DES was stored in a desiccator following cooling down to room temperature. In the GC-FID analysis, the chromatographic separation was performed on an Agilent HP-5 capillary column (30 m x 0.25 mm, 0.25 μm). A temperature program was applied between 80-280°C. Ultra-pure N_2 was used as the carrier gas. The FID and injection port temperatures were set at 300°C and 250°C, respectively.

MS conditions were set as; EI: 70 eV; triple quadrupole temperature: 150°C; interface temperature: 290°C; mass range: m/z 50–600. All the commercial food-contacted plastic products, including fresh-keeping film (0.8 g), plastic bag (0.8 g), instant-noodle packing bag (0.8 g), disposable PE glove (0.8 g) and mineral water bottle (3.0 g) were mixed with high purity water and heated to 90°C in water bath for 1 h. Then the samples were filtered. DES-enriched sample was prepared by mixing 5 mL of the spiked sample with DES. The DES phase was directly injected into GC system for analysis. A wide linear range of 5-1000 μg/L was obtained for all analytes in the proposed method and R^2s were higher than 0.997. The LOD and LOQ values for the target phthalates were about 1 μg/L and 5 μg/L, respectively. RSDs and recoveries were in the range of 3.6-5.6% and 86.4-103.2%, respectively. Phthalates from food contacted plastics were detected successfully with the proposed method which provided a green analysis by the utilization hydrophobic DESs as the extraction solvent (Li et al. 2020).

HPLC Analysis

HPLC with MS, MS-MS or DAD detector is a common method for phthalate analysis in food, in which various sample pre-treatment techniques are applied according to the sample type. In some of the studies, simple extraction procedures were preferred. In a migration study, the analytes were extracted only with acetonitrile. At first, a GC-MS scanning was performed to identify potential contaminants in materials to estimate exposure to different chemicals transferred from food packaging. The main plasticizer groups were determined as phthalates and citrates. Five different phthalates have been identified as DEP, DIBP, DEHP, BBP and DBP. DEP, DEHP and DIBP were detected in all samples. In addition, BBP and DBP were determined in 4 samples. Then, the study was applied to cereal-based foods packed with plastic packaging. An LC-MS/MS method was developed to analyze various chemicals such as ATBC, DEHA and DEP among others in the selected foodstuffs. In the developed method, separation was achieved in a reversed phase biphenyl column (100 mm x 3 mm, 2.6 μm). Methanol and water gradient system, both containing 0.1% formic acid, was used at a flow of 0.4 mL/min as the mobile phase. The samples were analyzed in the positive ESI mode on the MS detector. Recovery of the method was between 78% and 109%. Repeatability was good with the RSDs ranged between 4 and 18%, except octocyrylene. As a result of the study, it was found that the average ATBC migration in the analyzed foodstuffs was generally higher than those of phthalates and DEHA (Ibarra et al. 2019).

In another study, DMP, DEP, DiPP, DPP, DPhP, DBP, DPeP, DEHP, DnOP, DiNP, DiDP and BBP in Greek grape marc spirits were analyzed using a validated UHPLC-MS/MS method. 45 samples collected from Greece and Cyprus were analyzed directly without a pre-treatment. The analytes were separated on a C18 column (100 mm x 2.0 mm, 1.8 μm) by gradient elution. LODs and the recovery of the method ranged from 0.3 to 33.3 μg/L and from 81.6 to 109.6%, respectively. Calibration curves were prepared between 0.3-2500 μg/L by using standard addition method. All phthalates except DPhP and DiDP were proven to be present in at least one of the analyzed grape marc spirit samples. Only DEHP was measured above legal concentration limits (Diamantidou et al. 2019).

A procedure for the simultaneous determination of seven phthalates (DMP, DPP, DBP, BBP, DCHP, DEHP and DOP) in beverages using USVADLLME followed by HPLC-UV was developed by Yılmaz et al. (2014). The chromatographic separation was achieved by a C18 column (250 mm x 4.6 mm, 5.0 μm) and a gradient elution with a mobile phase consisting of methanol/acetonitrile (50:50) and 0.2 M KH_2PO_4 buffer. The detection wavelength was 230 nm. The linear range was 0.05-60.00 μg/L (except DEHP, 0.10-60.00 μg/L) with $R>0.99$. LODs were in the range of 0.019-0.208 μg/L and LOQs were between 0.072-0.483 μg/L. The intra- and inter-day RSDs were 0.03-3.93% and 0.02-4.74%, respectively. The accuracy was calculated in the range of -14.55 to 15.57% in terms of relative mean error. The USVADLLME parameters as type and volume of the extraction solvent, volume of the disperser solvent, concentration of NaCl, ultrasonication and vortex time were optimized to obtain good recoveries. Chloroform was the extraction solvent, and methanol was selected as the disperser. Seventeen different beverage samples in plastic bottles including lemon juice, ice tea, cherry juice, vinegar, turnip juice, lemon sauce, mineral water, coke, soda, and sports drink were successfully analyzed, and ten of them were found to be contaminated by different types of phthalates, mostly by DEHP (Yılmaz et al. 2014).

A procedure including the combination of DLLME with pressurized liquid extraction for the extraction and pre-concentration of endocrine disruptors DBP, DINP, DEHP, DEHA and BPA from cheese samples was developed by Pit-Bala et al. (2019). The HPLC-DAD analysis of the analytes was performed using a C18 (150 mm x 4.6 mm, 5 μm) column and a mobile phase of acetonitrile/water (60:40, v/v) mixture with isocratic elution at 1.0

mL/min. The wavelength was set to 235 nm for DBP, DINP, DEHP, and DEHA, and to 277 nm for BPA. The linear range was 2.8-100 ng/mL. LOD and LOQ values were calculated according to signal to noise ratios and found in the ranges of 0.82-3.1 ng/g and 2.8-10 ng/g, respectively. The extraction recoveries of the method were found between 78-96%. In extraction procedure, the analytes were first extracted under high pressure (1000 psi) and in the presence of CCl_4 at 70°C to a water-miscible extraction solvent (acetone). Then, the organic phase was removed, the cloudy solution dispersed in deionized water was centrifuged and the sedimented phase was analyzed in the HPLC system. As a result of the analysis, 46-62 ng/g DBP, 78-96 ng/g DEHP were detected in the cheese samples (Pil-Bala et al. 2019).

A new method based on ionic liquid enhanced magnetic solid phase extraction (MSPE) combined with HPLC was developed for the analysis of BBP, DEP, DBP, DNOP in food samples (instant noodles) with oleic acid coated-Fe_3O_4 nanoparticles (NP). The chromatographic separation was performed with reversed-phase C18 analytical column (150 mm x 4.6 mm), and the column temperature was set to 30°C. Acetonitrile and deionized water were used in gradient elution as the mobile phase with a flow rate of 1.0 mL/min. Analytes were detected at 226 nm. The linear range was 5-5000 ng/mL (R^2 = 0.9972-0.9998). Food samples containing instant noodles of different brands were powdered and extracted with methanol. MSPE procedure was applied to the supernatant obtained. Fe_3O_4 NPs were synthesized and stored at +4°C. Fe_3O_4 NP suspension and [C6MIM] [PF6] were added onto the sample according to the MSPE procedure. Then, the MNPs were separated with the aid of a magnet and the analytes were eluted with 1 mL of methanol. The eluate obtained was isolated again with the help of a magnet and 20 μL of the solution was injected into HPLC. LODs and RSDs were found to be 1.27-2.95 ng/mL and 3.9-5.3%, respectively. The proposed method had the advantages of having a very short extraction time, low LODs and satisfactory recovery with a small amount of adsorbent when compared with other methods reported (Liu et al. 2017).

Other Analysis Methods

SFC might be an alternative chromatographic method for the analysis of phthalates beside GC and HPLC. In a work, it was aimed to determine DEHP and five photoinitiators (PI) (2,2-diethoxyacetophenone, DEAP; o-methyl-benzoyl benzoate, OMBB; 2-methyl benzophenone, 2-MBP; 2-hydro-2-

methyl propiophenone; 4-methyl benzophenone, 4-MBP) simultaneously by combining SFC method and UAE. The chromatographic separation was performed with C18 analytical column (4.6 mm x 250 mm, 5 μm). CO_2 was used as the mobile phase and methanol (96:4, v/v) was used as the co-solvent with a flow rate of 1.4 mL/min. In the UV detector, the wavelengths of 245 nm (5 min) and 224 nm (5-7 min) were analyzed. The linear range was 0.1-20.0 μg/mL for PIs and 0.5-100.0 μg/mL for DEHP. LOD and LOQ values were determined between 0.021-0.150 μg/mL and 0.070-0.500 μg/mL, respectively. Absolute recoveries were evaluated by analyzing 3 different concentrations, low, medium, and high, and were found to be between the values of 91.2-108.3% and 95.2-101.2%, respectively. UAE conditions and SFC parameters were optimized. The analytes were simultaneously analyzed within 7 min. The proposed method was applied to real samples purchased from the market such as cans of chips, disposable cups, beverage bottles and instant noodle buckets. The samples were prepared by washing with deionized water and cutting into small pieces, then addition of acetonitrile and extraction in an ultrasonic bath at 40°C for 60 minutes. Then the extract was filtered and 5 μL of the solution was injected into SFC system. In the tows of the can of chips samples, OMBB was determined at 68.072 and 54.614 μg/g. In addition, DEAP was detected in low concentrations in one of the instant noodle buckets. In the rest of the samples, none of the six additives could be detected (<LOD) (Huang et al. 2020).

The amounts of DEHP and DBP in beverages stored in polypropylene containers were determined by ELISA. Generally, most of the foods have a neutral or medium pH. However, the pH of some fruits and fruit juices is as low as 2.2. A high pH may also be observed, such as the white of an egg with a pH of 9. Therefore, the pH range of 3-9 (3, 5, 7, 9) was chosen to represent most of the pHs found in the human diet. Each polypropylene beaker was filled with 200 mL of predetermined pH solutions. It was then heated by microwave for 1, 3 and 5 minutes, respectively. Control samples were not heated to examine storage conditions. The heated samples were cooled and stored at +4°C until the analysis. The samples were incubated with the enzyme (horseradish peroxidase, HRP) conjugate, at 37°C. DEHP and DBP levels were calculated by measuring the concentrations of HRP conjugates at 450 nm. The linear range of the method was 5-100 μg/L (R^2> 0.9998) and the LOD value was found to be 0.1 μg/L. As a result of the analysis, it was determined that DEHP and DBP had the highest migration at pH 3 with the highest cumulative concentrations of 159.8 and 104.9 mg/L, respectively. In addition, it was determined that the long heating time increased the migration. The concentration of 0.6 mg/kg was found as the highest DBP migration from the polypropylene food container, which exceeded the migration limit (Fang et al. 2017).

Zhu et al. (2018) designed a colorimetric immunosensor to detect DBP in environmental and food samples. To provide enough sensitivity to detect traces of DBP, the colorimetric immunosensor was composed of metal-organic frameworks (Cu-MOF) and HRP. The method was based on the labeling of Cu-MOFs on the second antibody (Cu MOFs@Ab2) for DBP detection in the sensor. When Cu-MOFs@Ab2 was captured by antigen-primary antibody complex, a high concentration Cu (II) was released from Cu-MOFs in the presence of nitric acid (HNO_3), and then reduced to Cu (I) by addition of sodium ascorbate, inhibiting the HRP to catalyze the colorless 3,3′,5,5′-tetramethylbenzidine (TMB) into blue oxidized TMB (ox TMB). In the analyses of DBP-spiked real samples, the accuracy and reproducibility of the method were determined in terms of recovery as 87.73-103.4% and in terms of coefficient of variation as 1.46-5.95%, respectively. The LOD as 1 μg/L was found to be almost 60 times lower compared to those using a conventional ELISA with the same antibody. The designed colorimetric immunosensor was used for the analysis of liquor, milk, red wine, and environmental water samples. The DBP concentrations obtained were 12.89 ± 0.44 μg/L, 10.65 ± 0.77 μg/L, 124.2 ± 4.2 μg/L, 14.93 ± 0.90 μg/L for Yudai River, Yunliang River, liquor, and milk samples, respectively. No DBP was detected in red wine (Zhu et al. 2018).

Conclusion

Phthalates are a group of ortho-phthalic acid diesters (dialkyl or alkylaryl esters of 1, 2-benzenedicarboxylic acid). In industry, they are used as plasticizer to soften the rough polymers such as polyvinyl chloride and to hold the scent and colour of consumer products.

Studies show that phthalates affected the endocrine system and consequently the activity of reproductive hormones. Some of the reasons of the exposure to phthalates for human include personal care products, medical devices and food contaminated by production conditions or packaging material. Considering the harmful effects development of high yielded extraction techniques followed by reliable analytical methods with high sensitivity and selectivity for phthalate analysis in various sample types has become of interest in recent years.

The procedure for analysis of phthalates generally consists of extraction, purification, separation, and instrumental detection steps. The physical state of the sample such as liquid, solid, semi-solid, phthalate concentration and type and interfering effects should be considered to develop an appropriate method for sample preparation, detection and quantification. The analysis of samples with simple matrices may be performed by traditional extraction procedures, but complex samples are required to be treated with more sophisticated techniques as SPE, SPME, LLME, DLLME and etc. Chromatographic methods are commonly used for detection and quantification. Among them GC and HPLC with MS detection provides excellent accuracy and precision with high sensitivity.

The issue of phthalate exposure ways for human is clear, but on the other hand there are various methods which could be used to determine the contamination sources in the literature. In addition, new developments in the pretreatment and analysis techniques provide more and more reliable results day by day.

References

Al Salloum, H., Saunier, J., Tfayli, A. and Yagoubi, N. 2016. "Studying DEHP migration in plasticized PVC used for blood bags by coupling Raman confocal microscopy to UV spectroscopy". *Materials Science & Engineering C-Materials for Biological Applications* 61: 56-62.

Bernard, L., Cueff, R., Bourdeaux, D., Breysse, C., Sautou, V. and Armed Study Grp. 2015a. "Analysis of plasticizers in poly(vinyl chloride) medical devices for infusion and artificial nutrition: comparison and optimization of the extraction procedures, a pre-migration test step." *Analytical and Bioanalytical Chemistry* 407 (6): 1651-1659.

Bernard, L., Cueff, R., Breysse, C., Decaudin, B., Sautou, V. and Armed Study Grp. 2015b. "Migrability of PVC plasticizers from medical devices into a simulant of infused solutions". *International Journal of Pharmaceutics* 485 (1-2): 341-347.

Bourdeaux, D., Yessaad, M., Chennell, P., Larbre, V., Eljezi, T., Bernard, L., Sautou V. and Armed study group. 2016. "Analysis of PVC plasticizers in medical devices and infused solutions by GC-MS." *Journal of Pharmaceutical and Biomedical Analysis* 118: 206-213.

Cao, X. L. 2010. "Phthalate esters in foods: sources, occurrence, and analytical methods." *Comprehensive Reviews in Food Science and Food Safety* 9 (1): 21-43.

Cariou, R., Larvor, F., Monteau, F., Marchand, P., Bichon, E., Dervilly-Pinel, G., Antignac, J. P. and B. Le Bizec. 2016. "Measurement of phthalates diesters in food using gas chromatography-tandem mass spectrometry." *Food Chemistry* 196: 211-219.

Communities, Commission of the European. 2011. "Commission Regulation (EU) No 10/2011 of 14 January 2011 on plastic materials and articles intended to come into contact with food." *The Official Journal of European Union L* 12: 1-89.

Diamantidou, D., Begou, O., Theodoridis, G., Gika, H., Tsochatzis, E., Kalogiannis, S., Kataiftsi, N., Soufleros, E. and Zotou, A. 2019. "Development and validation of an ultra high performance liquid chromatography-tandem mass spectrometry method for the determination of phthalate esters in Greek grape marc spirits." *Journal of Chromatography A* 1603: 165-178.

European Parliament. 2008. *Regulation (EC) No 1272/2008 of the European Parliament and of the Council of 16 December 2008 on Classification, Labelling and Packaging of Substances and Mixtures, Amending and Repealing Directives 67/548/EEC and 1999/45/EC, and Amending Regulation (EC) No 1907/2006.* Available from: https://eur-lex.europa.eu/eli/reg/2008/1272.

European Parliament and the Council of the European Union. 2009. "Directive 2009/48/EC of the European Parliament and of the Council of 18 June 2009 on the safety of toys." *The Official Journal of European Union.*

European Union. 2009. "Regulation (EC) No 1223/2009 of the European Parliament and of the Council." *Official Journal of the European Union L* 342: 59.

Faessler, D., McCombie, G., Biedermann, M., Felder, F. and Subotic, U. 2017. "Leaching of plasticizers from polyvinylchloride perfusion lines by different lipid emulsions for premature infants under clinical conditions." *International Journal of Pharmaceutics* 520 (1-2): 119-125.

Fang, H. Q., Wang, J. and Lynch, R. A. 2017. "Migration of di(2-ethylhexyl)phthalate (DEHP) and di-n-butylphthalate (DBP) from polypropylene food containers." *Food Control* 73: 1298-1302.

Fasano, E., Cirillo, T., Esposito, F. and Lacorte, S. 2015. "Migration of monomers and plasticizers from packed foods and heated microwave foods using QuEChERS sample preparation and gas chromatography/mass spectrometry." *Lwt-Food Science and Technology* 64 (2): 1015-1021.

Feng, C. H., and Jiang, S. R. 2012. "Micro-scale quantitation of ten phthalate esters in water samples and cosmetics using capillary liquid chromatography coupled to UV detection: effective strategies to reduce the production of organic waste." *Microchimica Acta* 177 (1-2): 167-175.

Genay, S., Feutry, F., Masse, M., Barthelemy, C., Sautou, V., Odou, P., Decaudin, B., Azaroual, N. and Armed Study Grp. 2017. "Identification and quantification by H-1 nuclear magnetic resonance spectroscopy of seven plasticizers in PVC medical devices." *Analytical and Bioanalytical Chemistry* 409 (5): 1271-1280.

Gimeno, P., Maggio, A. F., Bousquet, C., Quoirez, A., Civade, C. and Bonnet, P. A. 2012. "Analytical method for the identification and assay of 12 phthalates in cosmetic products: application of the ISO 12787 international standard "Cosmetics-analytical methods-Validation criteria for analytical results using chromatographic techniques." *Journal of Chromatography A* 1253: 144-53.

Gimeno, P., Thomas, S., Bousquet, C., Maggio, A. F., Civade, C., Brenier, C. and. Bonnet, P. A. 2014. "Identification and quantification of 14 phthalates and 5 non-phthalate plasticizers in PVC medical devices by GC-MS." *Journal of Chromatography B-Analytical Technologies in the Biomedical and Life Sciences* 949: 99-108.

González-Sálamo, J., Socas-Rodríguez, B. and Hernández-Borges, J. 2018. "Analytical methods for the determination of phthalates in food." *Current Opinion in Food Science* 22: 122-136.

Haishima, Y., Seshimo, F., Higuchi, T., Yamazaki, H., Hasegawa, C., Izumi, S. I., Makino, T., Nakahashi, K., Ito, R., Inoue, K., Yoshimura, Y., Saito, K., Yagami, T., Tsuchiya, T. and Nakazawa, H. 2005. "Development of a simple method for predicting the levels of di(2-ethylhexyl) phthalate migrated from PVC medical devices into pharmaceutical solutions." *International Journal of Pharmaceutics* 298 (1): 126-142.

Haned, Z., Moulay, S. and Lacorte, S. 2018. "Migration of plasticizers from poly(vinyl chloride) and multilayer infusion bags using selective extraction and GC-MS." *Journal of Pharmaceutical and Biomedical Analysis* 156: 80-87.

He, M., Yang, C., Geng, R. J., Zhao, X. G., Hong, L., Piao, X. F., Chen, T., Quinto, M. and Li, D. H. 2015. "Monitoring of phthalates in foodstuffs using gas purge microsyringe extraction coupled with GC-MS." *Analytica Chimica Acta* 879: 63-68.

Huang, L., Lou, C. Y., Chen, N., Wu, S. C., Gan, L., Chen, J. P., Shou, D. and Zhu, Y. 2020. "Simultaneous determination of di-(2-ethylhexyl) phthalate and five photoinitiators in food contact materials using ultrasonic-assisted extraction combined with supercritical fluid chromatography." *Analytical Methods* 12 (13): 1720-1727.

Hubinger, J. C. 2010. "A survey of phthalate esters in consumer cosmetic products." *Journal of Cosmetic Science* 61 (6): 457-465.

Ibarra, V. G., Sendón, R., Bustos, J., Losada, P. P. and Bernaldo de Quirós, A. R. 2019. "Estimates of dietary exposure of Spanish population to packaging contaminants from cereal based foods contained in plastic materials." *Food and Chemical Toxicology* 128: 180-192.

Jeon, S. H., Kim, Y. P., Kho, Y., Shin, J. H., Ji, W. H. and Ahn, Y. G. 2018. "Development and validation of gas chromatography-triple quadrupole mass spectrometric method for quantitative determination of regulated plasticizers in medical infusion sets." *Journal of Analytical Methods in Chemistry* 2018: 9470254.

Kamarei, F., Ebrahimzadeh, H. and Yamini, Y. 2011. "Optimization of ultrasound-assisted emulsification microextraction with solidification of floating organic droplet followed by high performance liquid chromatography for the analysis of phthalate esters in cosmetic and environmental water samples." *Microchemical Journal* 99 (1): 26-33.

Kaur, R., Heena, Kaur, R., Rani, S. and Malik, A. K. 2016. "Simple and rapid determination of phthalates using microextraction by packed sorbent and gas chromatography with mass spectrometry quantification in cold drink and cosmetic samples." *Journal of Separation Science* 39 (5): 923-931.

Kostic, I. S., Andelkovic, T. D., Andelkovic, D. H., Cvetkovic, T. P. and Pavlovic, D. D. 2016. "Determination of di(2-ethylhexyl) phthalate in plastic medical devices." *Hemijska Industrija* 70 (2): 159-164.

Lecoeur, M., Decaudin, B., Guillotin, Y., Sautou, V., Vaccher, C. and ARMED Study Grp. 2015. "Comparison of high-performance liquid chromatography and supercritical fluid chromatography using evaporative light scattering detection for the determination of plasticizers in medical devices." *Journal of Chromatography A* 1417: 104-115.

Li, T. M., Song, Y. F., Li, J. M., Zhang, M. N., Shi, Y. Y. and Fan, J. 2020. "New low viscous hydrophobic deep eutectic solvents in vortex-assisted liquid-liquid micro-extraction for the determination of phthalate esters from food-contacted plastics." *Food Chemistry* 309: 125752.

Liu, L. P., Wang, Z. M., Zhao, S. H., Duan, J. H., Tao, H., Wang, W. J. and Liu, S. H. 2018. "Determination of total phthalate in cosmetics using a simple three-phase sample preparation method." *Analytical and Bioanalytical Chemistry* 410 (4): 1323-1331.

Liu, R. Q., Liu, Y., Cheng, C. S. and Yang, Y. L. 2017. "Ionic liquid enhanced magnetic solid-phase extraction of phthalate esters in food samples with oleic acid coated-Fe3O4 nanoparticles prior to HPLC." *Separation Science and Technology* 52 (11): 1787-1795.

Llompart, M., Celeiro, M., Lamas, J. P., Sanchez-Prado, L., Lores, M. and Garcia-Jares, C. 2013. "Analysis of plasticizers and synthetic musks in cosmetic and personal care products by matrix solid-phase dispersion gas chromatography-mass spectrometry." *Journal of Chromatography A* 1293: 10-19.

Makkliang, F., Kanatharana, P., Thavarungkul, P. and Thammakhet, C. 2015. "Development of magnetic micro-solid phase extraction for analysis of phthalate esters in packaged food." *Food Chemistry* 166: 275-282.

Moreira, M. A., Andre, L. C. and Cardeal, Z. D. 2015. "Analysis of plasticiser migration to meat roasted in plastic bags by SPME-GC/MS." *Food Chemistry* 178: 195-200.

Mostafa, A., and Shaaban, H. 2018. "Development and validation of a dispersive liquid-liquid microextraction method for the determination of phthalate esters in perfumes using gas chromatography-mass spectrometry." *Rsc Advances* 8 (47): 26897-26905.

Nakiwala, D. 2020. "Prenatal exposure to phenols and phthalates, child neurodevelopment and the role of the thyroid hormones." *Université Grenoble Alpes.*

National Research Council Committee on the Health Risks of Phthalates. 2008. *Phthalates and Cumulative Risk Assessment: The Tasks Ahead.* Washington (DC): National Academies Press (US).

Pil-Bala, B., Khandaghi, J. and Mogaddam, M. R. A. 2019. "Analysis of endocrine-disrupting compounds from cheese samples using pressurized liquid extraction combined with dispersive liquid-liquid microextraction followed by high-performance liquid chromatography." *Food Analytical Methods* 12 (7): 1604-1611.

Radaniel, T., Genay, S., Simon, N., Feutry, F., Quagliozzi, F., Barthelemy, C., Lecoeur, M., Sautou, V., Decaudin, B., Odou, P. and ARMED Study Grp. 2014. "Quantification of five plasticizers used in PVC tubing through high performance liquid chromatographic-UV detection." *Journal of Chromatography B-Analytical Technologies in the Biomedical and Life Sciences* 965: 158-163.

Ranjbari, E., and Hadjmohammadi, M. R. 2012. "Magnetic stirring-assisted dispersive liquid-liquid microextraction followed by high performance liquid chromatography for determination of phthalate esters in drinking and environmental water samples." *Talanta* 100: 447-453.

Russo, M. V., Avino, P. and Notardonato, I. 2016. "Fast analysis of phthalates in freeze-dried baby foods by ultrasound-vortex-assisted liquid-liquid microextraction coupled with gas chromatography-ion trap/mass spectrometry." *Journal of Chromatography A* 1474: 1-7.

Shen, C., Wu, T. and Zang, X. H. 2019. "Hollow fiber stir bar sorptive extraction combined with gc-ms for the determination of phthalate esters from children's food." *Chromatographia* 82 (3): 683-693.

Shen, H. Y., Ying, L. Y., Cao, Y. F., Pan, G. and Zhou, L. 2007. "Simultaneous Determination of Phthalates and Parabens in Cosmetic Products by Gas Chromatography/Mass Spectrometry Coupled with Solid Phase Extraction." *Chinese Journal of Chromatography* 25 (2): 272-275.

Su, R. Y., Zhao, X. W., Li, Z. Y., Jia, Q. O., Liu, P. and Jia, J. B. 2010. "Poly(methacrylic acid-co-ethylene glycol dimethacrylate) monolith microextraction coupled with high performance liquid chromatography for the determination of phthalate esters in cosmetics." *Analytica Chimica Acta* 676 (1-2): 103-108.

Veiga, M., Bohrer, D., Nascimento, P. C., Ramirez, A. G., Carvalho, L. M. and Binotto, R. 2012. "Migration of phthalate-based plasticizers from PVC and non-PVC containers and medical devices." *Journal of the Brazilian Chemical Society* 23 (1): 72-77.

Vinas, P., Campillo, N., Pastor-Belda, M., Oller, A. and Hernandez-Cordoba, M. 2015. "Determination of phthalate esters in cleaning and personal care products by dispersive liquid-liquid microextraction and liquid chromatography-tandem mass spectrometry." *Journal of Chromatography A* 1376: 18-25.

Wei, X. B., Li, R. Q., Yu, H. and Wang, R. Q. 2018. "Fast and sensitive determination of 10 forbidden phthalates in perfumes by ultra-high performance liquid chromatography-electrospray ionization-tandem mass spectrometry." *Journal of Chromatography A* 1578: 45-52.

Yang, J. L., Li, Y. X., Wang, Y., Ruan, J., Zhang, J. and Sun, C. J. 2015. "Recent advances in analysis of phthalate esters in foods." *Trac-Trends in Analytical Chemistry* 72: 10-26.

Yılmaz, P. K. 2019. "Optimization of hydrophilic-lipophilic balance solid-phase extraction of phthalates in pharmaceutical preparations." *Journal of Turkish Chemical Society Section A: Chemistry* 6: 271-280.

Yılmaz, P. K., Ertas, A. and Kolak, U. 2014. "Simultaneous determination of seven phthalic acid esters in beverages using ultrasound and vortex-assisted dispersive liquid-liquid microextraction followed by high-performance liquid chromatography." *Journal of Separation Science* 37 (16): 2111-2117.

Zhu, N. F., Zou, Y. M., Huang, M. L., Dong, S. B., Wu, X. Y., Liang, G. X., Han, Z. X. and Zhang, Z. 2018. "A sensitive, colorimetric immunosensor based on Cu-MOFs and HRP for detection of dibutyl phthalate in environmental and food samples." *Talanta* 186: 104-109.

Chapter 2

Cardiovascular Consequences of Human Exposure to Phthalates

Melissa Mariana[1], Miguel Castelo-Branco[1,2], MD, PhD, Amadeu M. Soares[3], PhD and Elisa Cairrao[1,2,*], PhD

[1]Health Sciences Research Centre (CICS-UBI),
University of Beira Interior, Covilha, Portugal
[2]Faculty of Health Sciences (FCS-UBI),
University of Beira Interior, Covilha, Portugal
[3]Centre for Environmental and Marine Studies (CESAM),
University of Aveiro, Aveiro, Portugal

Abstract

In the last few years, there has been a growing concern about plastic and plastics consumption, and the constant human and environmental exposure to these materials has raised an alarm. As part of the composition of plastic, phthalates have caused a lot of controversy, with several studies implicating these compounds as harmful to human health. Studies have shown the presence of phthalates in 75–90% of the general population, which can be due to their ubiquity in the environment and to not being covalently attached to plastic, being easily released into the environment. These compounds, that are diesters of phthalic acid, are the most common plasticizers used in a variety of products, from polyvinyl chloride (PVC) to personal care products and even medical and pharmaceutical materials. Due to their endocrine-disrupting properties,

[*] Corresponding Author's Email: ecairrao@fcsaude.ubi.pt.

In: Phthalates: Environmental and Health Effects
Editors: Müfide Aydoğan Ahbab and Nurhayat Barlas
ISBN: 978-1-68507-970-3

phthalates have been associated with several diseases including cancer, diabetes, male reproduction and cardiovascular diseases. There are still few studies on the subject, but evidence shows the negative impact of phthalates on the cardiovascular system. From epidemiological and experimental studies, it has already been described the involvement of phthalates in the development heart failure, arrhythmias, stroke, atherosclerosis, hypertension and diabetes. Nevertheless the mechanisms by which phthalates induce these harmful effects are still unclear. In this chapter, we aim to elucidate and relate all the cardiovascular effects of phthalates described so far, and to suggest the following research approaches.

Keywords: plastic contaminants, phthalates, human exposure, cardiovascular diseases

Introduction

In recent years, there has been a huge increase in the incidence of several diseases, including cancer and cardiovascular diseases, and one of the possible causes is the great increase in human exposure to environmental contaminants. This hypothesis has generated an increased concern, since many of these compounds are ubiquitous in the environment, and the human being is continuously exposed to them. In addition, another worrying factor is that maternal exposure can impair the health of the offspring. Phthalates are one of the many contaminants, and due to its ubiquity in the environment, they have already been detected in 75–90% of the general population (Ramadan et al. 2020). These compounds are mostly used in plastics to increase flexibility, pliability and elasticity, and in a great variety of products, including cosmetics, building materials, medical devices and daily life products (Lin et al. 2020b). The most commonly used plasticizer worldwide is di-(2-ethylhexyl) phthalate (DEHP), used in polyvinyl chloride (PVC) and several medical devices (blood storage bags, tubing circuits, enteral feeding tubes, endotracheal tubes and catheters) (Lin et al. 2020b, Jaimes et al. 2019). Due to their chemical properties, phthalates are easily absorbed when in contact with blood, plasma and other lipophilic solutions, and thus affecting human and animal health as well as the environment (Jaimes et al. 2019, Mu et al. 2020). They can also bind to molecular targets in the body and interfere with hormonal function, thus they are considered as endocrine-disrupting compounds (EDCs), being confirmed their antiandrogenic and estrogenic activities (Mariana et al. 2016).

Despite not being the most studied, phthalate exposure has been associated with several cardiovascular diseases (CVDs). These include a diversity of diseases affecting the heart or blood vessels, and their incidence has increased over the years, with a 30% increase in CVD related death between 1990 and 2010, being one of the leading causes of global death (Piepoli 2017, Vinceti et al. 2012, Fu et al. 2020). Until now, phthalates have been related with heart failure, arrhythmias, stroke, atherosclerosis, hypertension and diabetes (Rahmani et al. 2016, Trasande and Attina 2015, Trasande et al. 2013, Lind and Lind 2011, Lind et al. 2012, Jaimes et al. 2019, Shiue 2013). Therefore, with this chapter we aim to present and list the most recent studies regarding the implications of phthalates effects on the cardiovascular system, both in animals and in humans.

Properties of Phthalates

The reaction of phthalic anhydride with oxo alcohols results in diesters of phthalic anhydride, also known as phthalates. There is a variety of phthalates, depending on the nature and length of the origin oxo alcohols (C1 to C13) (Huang et al. 2013, Mariana et al. 2016), and they can be classified as high molecular weight (HMW) and low molecular weight (LMW) phthalates. The LMW phthalates have a higher bioaccumulation than the HMW and are mainly excreted in urine and faeces as monoesters (Kim and Park 2014, Mankidy et al. 2013, Wittassek et al. 2011). This type of phthalates includes di-n-butyl phthalate (DBP) - the most studied so far, dimethyl phthalate (DMP), diethyl phthalate (DEP) and di-isobutyl phthalate (DiBP), and are mainly used in paints, solvents, fixatives, personal care products and cosmetics, components of food and pharmaceutical packaging (Mariana et al. 2016, Mariana and Cairrao 2020). With a lower bioaccumulation, HMW phthalates monoesters are further metabolized through hydroxylation or oxidation resulting in oxidative metabolites, that will suffer conjugation and form easily excreted hydrophilic glucuronide conjugates (Hauser et al. 2004, Kim and Park 2014, Ventrice et al. 2013). Belonging to HMW phthalates are DEHP - the most commonly used phthalate plasticizer for polyvinyl chloride (PVC) (Talsness et al. 2009, Wetherill et al. 2007), butylbenzyl phthalate (BBzP), diisononyl phthalate (DiNP), di-n-octyl phthalate (DnOP), diisodecyl phthalate (DiDP), dicyclohexyl phthalate (DCHP) and di-n-hexyl phthalate (DnHP). These plasticizers are mostly used in PVC, building materials, cables and wires, toys and food packaging, and DEHP is also used in medical devices

(Johns et al. 2015, Zota et al. 2014, Mariana et al. 2016). Phthalates are not covalently bound to the plastic, so they can be released during their manufacture, use, or disposal into the environment and enter the human body through the main routes of exposure, including ingestion of contaminated food and medications, dermal contact, parenteral and environmental exposure (Kim and Park 2014). They have already been found in human blood, urine, saliva, amniotic fluid, breastmilk and cord blood (Latini et al. 2003, Main et al. 2006, Mankidy et al. 2013, Silva et al. 2004a, Silva et al. 2004b, Silva et al. 2005). Once in the human body, these chemicals can bind to molecular targets and interfere with hormone homeostasis, being considered as endocrine-disrupting compounds (EDCs). According to the Endocrine Society, EDCs are defined as "chemicals, or mixtures of chemicals, that interfere with any aspect of hormone action" (Zoeller et al. 2012). These compounds have the ability to compete with endogenous steroid hormones for the receptors and transport proteins, and to interfere with metabolism or synthesis of endogenous hormones (Casals-Casas and Desvergne 2011, Tabb and Blumberg 2006, Talsness et al. 2009, Wetherill et al. 2007). Another particular characteristic of EDCs, including phthalates, is that they do not present a typical dose-response curve, instead they have a non-monotonic one, so, most of the phthalates relating studies include different types and times of exposure and a larger concentration range (Gore et al. 2015, Mariana et al. 2016).

Cardiovascular Effects of Phthalates

Heart Failure and Myocardial Infarction

Since we spend a large part of our life at home, we are continuously exposed to the conditions and materials of each house. In fact, some researchers have been investigating if different housing types have adverse effects on human health, demonstrating a positive association, mainly in children (Jacobs et al. 2009, Shiue and Shiue 2013, Shiue and Bramley 2015). Thus, gathering information on demographics, housing built and health status, Shiue et al. (2015) conducted a study to relate the chemicals released in old houses with adult health. The authors concluded that people living in houses built before 1990 had several health issues, like stroke, heart failure and diabetes, and had higher urinary levels of environmental chemicals, including mono-cyclohexyl phthalate (MCHP) and mono-isobutyl phthalate (MiBP) (Shiue and Bramley 2015). In experimental studies, heart failure has been indirectly associated with exposure to environmental toxicants. Knowing from toxicological studies that the high mobility group transcription factor SOX9 and sox9b were downregulated in tetrapod and zebrafish after exposure to DEHP and that SOX9 is important in the development of the heart, Gawdzik et al. conducted a study to analyse how sox9b and toxicant-induced inhibition of sox9b affected the zebrafish cardiomyocyte development and function. The authors concluded that, besides decreasing the expression of some cardiac development genes (nkx2.5, nkx2.7, myl7, c-fos), the inhibition of sox9b function led to a decrease and an increase of ventricular and atrial cardiomyocytes, respectively, hypoplastic endothelial cushions and impaired epicardial development, leading to heart failure (Gawdzik et al. 2018). Using a mouse model as human physiological relevant perinatal exposure, Svoboda and co-workers demonstrated that long-term perinatal DEHP exposure affects the DNA methylation in the hearts of adult offspring mice (Svoboda et al. 2020). The authors also found that this DNA methylation changes are sex-specific, in which pathway analysis of differentially methylated cytosines showed an enhancement of insulin signalling, regulation of histone methylation and tyrosine phosphatase activity for female mice, while in male mice it was glucose transport, energy generation and developmental programs. In addition, the expression of several genes associated with differentially methylated cytosines and regions upon DEHP exposure were also differentially methylated in heart tissue collected from human heart failure patients. For example, SMAD7, a protein that has a protective role in cardiac fibrosis induced by myocardial infarction or hyperglycaemia, was differentially methylated in male mice exposed to DEHP and in the heart failure samples, and epsilon isoform of protein kinase C (PKCε), which may give low susceptibility to myocardial infarction effects, was increased in female hearts compared to males (Svoboda et al. 2020).

The occurrence of heart attack, also known as myocardial infarction, has also been associated with exposure to phthalates. In 2019, Shang et al. measured phthalate metabolites concentration in urine samples from Canadian men before and after a cardiac surgery, demonstrating that metabolites of DEHP, BBzP, DiDP and DBP were significantly increased 12h after the surgery. It was demonstrated that DEHP was the main phthalate released from the medical devices after surgery, this being the most likely to cause adverse effects. Besides, the authors used a mouse model of cardiac surgery to replicate the phthalates exposure in men. A myocardial infarction was surgery-induced to C57bl/6N male mice and then treated with a mixture of bisphenol A (BPA) and phthalates during the recovering time, and the results showed a reduction in the mice survival and cardiac function, an increase in the cardiac dilation and expression of pro-inflammatory markers. These findings suggest that there is an increased phthalates release from medical devices used in surgery that can lead to a delayed patient recovery (Shang et al. 2019). However, only one study has promoted and concluded this association, so further investigations are needed to prove whether phthalates may actually be involved in the occurrence of a heart attack.

Arrhythmia

One of the first studies relating phthalates with the occurrence of arrhythmia was performed in 1989 by Barry et al. In this study, the levels of DEHP and its main metabolite mono(2-ethylhexyl) phthalate (MEHP) were measured in adult and infant patients who have been through different cardiac surgical interventions. The results showed that, at the end of some of the procedures, the levels of DEHP and MEHP were increased and these compounds could be detected even 120h after surgery. However, in these patients, the levels of MEHP in circulation were 20-35-fold lower than the levels that reduce in 50% the contractile force and arrhythmias in a human atrial trabecular preparation (Barry et al. 1989). Due to the already established exposure of MEHP in patients subject to medical interventions, Jaimes et al. analysed its cardiac safety and biocompatibility in a clinically relevant concentration (60 μM) through a perfusion system. Using isolated and intact hearts from Langendorff rats, several cardiac parameters were measured at baseline and after MEHP treatment. It was demonstrated that an acute MEHP exposure lead to slowed atrioventricular conduction and epicardial conduction velocity, increased atrioventricular and ventricular refractory periods. Besides, MEHP-treated hearts exhibited a triangulated action potential and a steeper electrical restitution curve, which are indicators of increased arrhythmic risk (Jaimes et al. 2019). In order to analyse if DEHP caused changes in gene expression related to cardiac arrhythmias, isolated rat cardiac muscle cells were exposed to DEHP. Through microarray analysis, the authors showed that calsequestrin and calponin (calcium binding proteins) were downregulated, which has been demonstrated to trigger arrhythmia via calcium leak, besides, there was an increased expression of some calcium handling genes, including ryanodine receptor and triadin, which have been associated with cardiac myocytes arrhythmia (Posnack et al. 2011). Nonetheless, new studies are needed to understand if phthalates are involved with the development of arrhythmias since the data is scarce and inconsistent, with experimental studies suggesting a risk of arrhythmia by DEHP while the study performed by Barry et al. (1989) showed the opposite.

Stroke

Besides the study performed by Shiue et al. in 2015, where chemicals, including phthalates, released in old houses were related with stroke (Shiue and Bramley 2015), a previous study from the same authors also investigated that relationship. The risk of stroke was assessed based on a cross-sectional study from the National Health and Nutrition Examination Surveys (NHANES), from 2001-2004. The responses to the questionnaires, that included demographics, medical conditions (stroke status) were compared to the phthalates' concentrations found in urine samples. The authors found a positive association between mono-n-butyl phthalate (MnBP) and mono-(3-carboxypropyl) phthalate (MCPP) – a BBzP metabolite – concentrations and the risk of stroke (Shiue 2013). However, new studies are needed to understand the mechanisms by which phthalates can lead to stroke in humans, but until today they have not been carried out.

Atherosclerosis

Several CVDs have been associated with phthalates, and the relationship between phthalate exposure and atherosclerosis has been one of the most studied. An experimental study showed that DEP had a pro-atherogenic and pro-senescence activity in human cells and caused impairment of embryonic development and several lipidic parameters (Kim et al. 2015). Upon absorption, DEP is released into blood and, since it is a high hydrophobic compound, binds to serum lipoproteins, being able to modify them. So, the authors analysed the DEP (50 μM) effects on human lipoproteins that led to a degradation, oxidation and aggregation of high-density lipoproteins (HDL) and low-density lipoproteins (LDL). When macrophages were treated with DEP and lipoproteins, there was foam cell formation via accelerated phagocytosis of LDL, and in human dermal fibroblasts DEP led to cellular senescence. Besides, in vivo assays were performed using zebra fish, where injection of 5 μM and 10 μM of DEP and exposure to water containing DEP caused embryonic death and impairment of skeletal development, and, in adults exposed to water containing DEP for 4 weeks, the total cholesterol levels were reduced and hepatic inflammation enzymes were increased. These lipidic and hepatic alterations can lead to atherosclerosis (Kim et al. 2015). Matrix metalloproteinases (MMP)-2 and MMP-9 have also been associated with the occurrence of atherosclerosis. So, Shih et al. (2015) went to analyse the effect of a range concentrations of DEHP (2-17.5 ppm) at different exposure times in several proteins that have been related to atherosclerosis. The results showed an increase of MMP-2 and MMP-9 expression and an increase in the most common MMP-regulatory pathways (p38 mitogen-activated protein kinase (MAPK), extracellular signal regulated kinase 1 and 2 (ERK1/2), protein kinase B (Akt) and nuclear factor-kappaB (NF-κB)), confirming the atherosclerotic effect of DEHP in rat thoracic aorta smooth muscle cells (Shih et al. 2015). Since the deregulation of lipid profile is involved in the development of atherosclerosis, the effects of DBP on the lipid metabolism of human macrophages were analysed. THP-1 macrophages were exposed to different concentrations of DBP (0.01-100 μM) or DMSO as control. At 0.1 μM of DBP there was an increase of lipid accumulation in the cells due to inhibition of cholesterol efflux through miR200c-5p-ABCA1 cascade. These events can potentiate the development of atherosclerosis, a worrisome fact, since 0.1 μM of DBP is lower than the concentrations found in human blood, meaning that DBP exerts its effects at concentrations the humans are exposed to (Wang et al. 2020).

Two different *in vivo* studies have resorted to apolipoprotein E-deficient (ApoE-/-) mice (an animal model of atherosclerosis) to study the effects of DEHP in the development of atherosclerosis, however, had contradictory results (Zhou et al. 2015, Zhao et al. 2016). The first one was performed in 2015, and six-week-old female mice were exposed to DEHP in drinking water (100 mg/kg/day) for 12 weeks. The atherosclerotic lesions in the aortic root were measured through histological analysis, however, the mice exposed to DEHP had no significant differences for atherosclerotic lesions compared to the control (Zhou et al. 2015). On the contrary, DEHP showed significant effects on five-month-old apoE-/- male mice. In this study, mice were exposed to DEHP through intraperitoneal administration (500 mg/kg/day) for 4 weeks and then serum, heart, aorta, liver and adipose tissues were collected for histological analysis and evaluation of several lipid and inflammatory parameters. The demonstration of an inflammatory response and cholesterol homeostasis deregulation caused by exposure to DEHP led the authors to conclude pro-atherogenic properties of DEHP (Zhao et al. 2016). The differences between the results of these studies may be due to the DEHP dose administered (being 5 times higher in the second study), the age and the sex of the animals. With the intention to analyse oxidative cardiac effects of phthalates in mice, Amara et al. (2019) analysed the biochemical profile, parameters related to myocardial oxidative stress, antioxidant status and acetylcholinesterase (AChE) activity. Six-week-old BALB/c male mice were exposed intraperitoneally to different doses of DEHP (5, 50 and 200 mg/kg/day) for 30 days. Besides increasing serum marker enzymes involved in the onset of myocardial damage, DEHP also led to a decrease in HDL-cholesterol and increased levels of total cholesterol, triglycerides and LDL-cholesterol, increasing the atherogenic index (Amara et al. 2019).

The ultrasound measure of carotid intima-media thickness is the most widely used imaging technique for atherosclerosis, being an indicator for CVD events in adult and young populations (Hodis et al. 1998, Kim et al. 2015, Lin et al. 2020a, Lin et al. 2019, Lin et al. 2020b). The first epidemiological study relating phthalates with atherosclerosis was performed by Lind and Lind (2011). In this study, blood samples were collected and blood pressure was measured from 1016 men and women (70 years old) from the Prospective Investigation of the Vasculature in Uppsala Seniors (PIVUS), in Sweden. The prevalence of overt plaques and echogenicity of carotid artery plaques were recorded, thickness and echogenicity of the intima-media complex, glucose and lipid profile were measured and 10 phthalate metabolites were quantified in serum. The results demonstrated an association between monomethyl phthalate (MMP – DMP metabolite) and atherosclerotic plaques, independently of CV risk factors (Lind and Lind 2011). Using the same prospective study, MBzP (monobenzyl phthalate - main metabolite of BBzP) was quantified in serum and related to atherosclerosis in the carotid arteries. The levels of MBzP measured in the serum of 1003 participants were associated with the prevalence of carotid atherosclerotic plaques, intima-media thickness and echogenicity of the intima-media complex, suggesting that exposure to MBzP containing products contribute to the development of atherosclerosis (Wiberg et al. 2014). Due to the widespread use of phthalate containing products, it became necessary to develop a comparative study between the exposure to these compounds and CVD in a younger population. Thus, urine and blood samples from 787 young participants (mean age of 21 years old) of the YOung TAiwanese Cohort (YOTA) Study were collected and clinical atherosclerosis assessed through the measurement of carotid intima-media thickness. Urinary DEHP and DiBP metabolites were associated with carotid intima-media thickness and, consequently, with increased risk subclinical atherosclerosis (Su et al. 2019). A more recent study also resorted to YOTA

Study to investigate the association between DNA methylation, DEHP exposure and atherosclerosis (Lin et al. 2020b). Urine samples were collected from 793 young participants and DEHP metabolites concentrations were measured, and leukocyte global methylation levels were analysed for 569 participants. The carotid intima-media thickness and 5mdC/dG (global DNA methylation marker) levels were positively associated with MEHP in urine, mainly for higher levels of 5mdC/dG. These results confirm that DEHP is associated with atherosclerosis and that the mechanism may involve DNA methylation (Lin et al. 2020b). In another study, 697 participants were recruited from the YOTA Study and again exposures to DEHP and DBP were compared to circulating endothelial and platelet microparticles (EMPs and PMPs). A dose-response association was found for urinary ΣDEHP (sum of DEHP metabolites) and MnBP levels and microparticles formation, with female and overweight participants presenting higher levels of MnBP. This can lead to endothelial dysfunction that can manifest in the form of vascular diseases related to atherosclerosis (Chu et al. 2021).

Fortunately, some studies have been investigating the protective effects of some compounds and molecules against DEHP exposure. It has been proved that β-thujaplicin (a compound purified from a Taiwanese tree) can reduce pro-inflammatory cytokine-induced adhesion molecules and block DEHP-induced MMP-2 and MMP-9 expression (Shih et al. 2018), and that glucagon-like peptide-1 receptor (GLP1R) agonist (used as treatment for diabetes) inhibited tissue remodelling and adhesion factors and atherosclerotic Akt and ERK1/2 pathways of vascular smooth muscle cells exposed to DEHP (Kim 2020). These compounds counteract the adverse effects of phthalates preventing the initiation or development of atherosclerosis.

Hypertension

Hypertension is defined as either a systolic blood pressure ≥ 140 mmHg, a diastolic blood pressure ≥ 90 mmHg, or both (Sutton et al. 2018). The connection between phthalates exposure and hypertension has been studied, with the effect on blood pressure (BP) being dependent on the type of phthalates, LMW and HMW phthalates.

In animals, most of the studies related phthalate effects with changes in angiotensin-converting enzyme (ACE) and angiotensin II receptor type 1 (AT1R) levels and the bradykinin-nitric oxide (NO) pathway, as it is stated below, but the mechanisms are still to be clarified. It has been shown that maternal exposure to DEHP (0.25 and 6.25 mg/kg/day - from gestational day 0 to postnatal day 21) resulted impaired renal development and increased systolic and diastolic BP in rat offspring, through inhibition of renin and angiotensin II levels (Wei et al. 2012). On the other hand, Martinez-Arguelles et al. (2013) detected a decrease in systolic and diastolic BP after maternal DEHP exposure. In this study, Sprague-Dawley pregnant rats were exposed to a much higher concentration of DEHP (300 mg DEHP/kg/day) from gestational day 14 to birth day, and systemic arterial BP were analysed in the offspring, in two time points (2 and 6.5 months-old). These results may be explained by long-lasting effects on aldosterone levels (Martinez-Arguelles et al. 2013). In a different study, DEHP oral administration (30 mg/kg/day) to female mice begun 4 weeks before copulation and lasted up to 8 weeks of the offspring life (Lee et al. 2016). Besides analysing serum levels of cholesterol, triglycerides and glucose of the offspring, BP was measured using tail-cuff plethysmography and expression of different proteins was studied. Maternal DEHP exposure led to impaired endothelial nitric oxide synthase (eNOS) phosphorylation and increased angiotensin II–AT1R signalling in offspring, that in turn can lead to vasoconstriction increasing the BP, that is in accordance with the 20% increase in BP of mice offspring (Lee et al. 2016). In agreement with these results, Jaimes et al. (2017) also found a non-significant increase in systolic BP and a significant increase in endothelin-1, ACE and NO synthase gene expression in male mice (12 weeks old) treated with DEHP (1 μg-4 mg/mL) for 6 weeks. These results can lead to vasoconstriction and increased vascular resistance (Jaimes et al. 2017). Besides analysing the relationship between DEHP exposure and BP, Deng and co-workers (2019) also investigated the mechanism involved in this connection. 5-6 weeks old male mice were exposed to different doses of DEHP (0.1, 1, 10 mg/kg/day) for 42 days and then systolic BP was measured. There was a dose dependent increase of BP, with a 22% increase after 10 mg/kg/day DEHP exposure, similar results to the previous findings of Lee et al. (Lee et al. 2016). It was also demonstrated a significantly increase in ACE levels and a decrease in bradykinin levels, concluding that DEHP can induce an increase in BP through increasing ACE levels and inhibiting the bradykinin-NO pathway (Deng et al. 2019a). A study performed by the same research group investigated the differences in BP induced by DEHP and DBP exposure (Xie et al. 2019). Intragastric administration of DEHP and DBP (0.1, 1, 10 mg/kg/day) was performed to male mice (6-7 weeks old) for six weeks. Exposure to increasing DEHP, but not DBP, concentrations, led to increased BP through activation of renin-angiotensin-aldosterone system. However, exposure to DBP significantly increased oestradiol levels. Besides being phthalates with different molecular weights, this difference might be due to different levels of oestradiol induced by DEHP and DBP exposure, since oestrogen reduces AT1R expression, altering angiotensin signalling (Xie et al. 2019). Resorting to an identical experimental design, dexamethasone (DEXA) was used to build the hypertension model and the effects of DiNP exposure (0.15, 1.5, 15 mg/kg/day) on blood pressure were analysed (Deng et al. 2019b). There was an increase in systolic, diastolic and mean BP, with an increase of 17.7% in systolic BP for the highest dose administered. DiNP exposure also resulted in increased ACE expression and AT1R activation, leading to decreased eNOS expression and NO production, culminating in elevated BP. When ACE inhibitor was added these results were inverted, alleviating the elevated BP that was induced by DiNP exposure (Deng et al. 2019b). In a different perspective, the direct effects of DEHP (0.001-100 μM) were analysed in rat aorta through contractility and electrophysiology experiments. At higher concentrations DEHP inhibited the L-type calcium channels and led to vasorelaxation of rat aortic rings (Mariana et al. 2018). These results are in accordance with the sex hormones effects in vascular beds but differ from those obtained for oestradiol in vivo. Thus, more studies are needed to further explore the underlying phthalates mechanism.

Regarding human studies, the majority of the epidemiological ones have been performed in pregnant women and children, however, in a Chinese population aged between 18-55 years old, a relation between phthalates and BP was found (Zhang et al. 2018). BP, lipid profile and phthalates concentration were measured in the serum of 474 participants, and the results showed that DBP was the dominant phthalate in all samples and only DEHP was significantly associated with increased systolic BP (Zhang et al. 2018).

Hypertension is the most prevalent maternal complication worldwide, having been reported to affect 7-10% of all pregnancies and is associated with a high rate of maternal and foetal morbidity and mortality (Peres et al. 2018, Say et al. 2014). The hypertensive disorders in pregnancy (HDP) include gestational and chronic hypertension, preeclampsia, eclampsia and HELLP syndrome (Sutton et al. 2018, Werner et al. 2015), and phthalates have been associated with the occurrence of HDP, mainly gestational hypertension and preeclampsia. Resorting to data from the Health Outcomes and Measures of the Environment Study, urine samples were collected from 369 American pregnant women (16- and 26-weeks' gestation) and phthalates concentrations were measured (Werner et al. 2015). Only MBzP concentrations were found to be significantly associated with higher diastolic BP and an increased risk of developing HDP, an alarming conclusion since BBzP is ubiquitous among American women (Werner et al. 2015). In a population of 152 pregnant women from three different European countries (Spain, France and Norway), phthalate metabolites were measured in urine samples in the second and third trimesters of pregnancy (collected 3 times/day for 2 weeks) and BP measurement was performed at the end of each week (Warembourg et al. 2019a). Monoethyl phthalate (MEP – DEP metabolite) was associated with decreased diastolic BP, while MiBP was related to decreased diastolic and systolic BP, particularly in the 2nd trimester (Warembourg et al. 2019a). However, opposite results were observed in the study conducted by Han et al. (2020), where increased MiBP exposure in the 1st trimester was associated with increased systolic and diastolic BP in the 2nd trimester in pregnant women with male foetuses. In this study, urinary phthalate metabolite and BP measurements were carried out in each of the three trimesters for 633 participants, to cover the whole pregnancy (Han et al. 2020). A small American case-control study analysed phthalate metabolites concentration in four urine samples collected during pregnancy of 50 preeclamptic women. There was an association between DEHP metabolites and preeclampsia throughout pregnancy, with a higher risk at the end of pregnancy (Cantonwine et al. 2016). In a different study, 1233 Dutch pregnant women (median gestational age 13.1 weeks) provided urine samples for phthalate metabolites measurement and blood samples to investigate placental angiogenic markers and hemodynamic function (Philips et al. 2019). There was no association between urinary phthalate levels in early pregnancy and maternal blood pressure or HDP, on the other hand, HMW phthalate metabolite concentrations were associated with increased placental angiogenic markers (soluble fms-like tyrosine kinase-1 and placental growth factor ratio - sFlt-1/PlGF), that are related with the onset of preeclampsia (Philips et al. 2019). The results from most of these studies show that phthalates are associated with increased BP in pregnancy, however, further studies are needed to understand whether this increase can contribute to the development of HDP.

The increased BP during pregnancy can also have serious consequences for the offspring hypertension later in life. In a Spanish population-based birth cohort, 391 mother-child pairs were recruited to enter a study to evaluate prenatal phthalate exposure with childhood growth and BP. Phthalate metabolites were measured in two spot urine samples, provided in the first and third trimesters of pregnancy, and the pairs were followed at delivery and at different ages of the children (6 months, 1, 4 and 7 years). At 4 and 7 years, the children's BP was measured and compared to pregnancy phthalate concentrations, with DEHP metabolites and MEP being associated with decreased systolic BP in girls only (Valvi et al. 2015). A different study also evaluated gestational exposure to phthalates with cardiometabolic risks (including BP) in childhood (Vafeiadi et al. 2018). Spot urine samples were collected from 500 Greek pregnant women in the 1st trimester and then from their children at 4 years. Children's BP was measured at 4 and 6 years, with negative associations between phthalate metabolite concentrations and systolic and diastolic BP at the two time points, both in girls and boys (Vafeiadi et al. 2018). An observational study gathered 1277 children, from 6-11 years old, assembling data from six cohorts from different countries (United Kingdom, France, Spain, Lithuania, Norway, and Greece) (Warembourg et al. 2019b). Aiming to evaluate the connection between pre- and postnatal environmental exposures and BP in children, pregnancy blood and urine samples were collected and compared to children systolic and diastolic BP. Only MBzP was associated with a decrease in BP (Warembourg et al. 2019b). Similarly, to investigate if foetal exposure to phthalates is related to BP later in childhood, Sol and co-workers (2020) resorted to the Generation R Study (a Dutch prospective cohort study from early foetal life onwards). Urinary phthalate levels were measured in 1064 mothers in each trimester of pregnancy and compared to the offspring BP at 10 years old. There was a sex-specific difference, with higher levels of DEHP and DnOP in the third trimester associated with decreased systolic and diastolic BP only in girls (Sol et al. 2020). This study is in agreement with the one from Valvi et al. since exposure to phthalates have been associated with BP only in girls (Valvi et al. 2015, Sol et al. 2020).

Children and adolescents are more exposed to phthalate containing products, mainly young children, due to hand-to-mouth activity (Kim and Park 2014) and, therefore, become more vulnerable to these chemicals (Frederiksen et al. 2007, Wormuth et al. 2006, Mariana et al. 2016). Besides, it has been reported that children with high BP are more likely to develop hypertension later in life (Lurbe et al. 2009, Mariana and Cairrao 2020). With the aim to explore the associations between exposure to phthalates and BP in children and adolescents, Trasande and Attina (2015) developed a cross-sectional study that included 1619 US children and adolescents (6-19 years old). Urinary phthalates metabolites were measured and compared to BP, triglycerides and lipoproteins, where a significant association was found only between DiNP and DiDP metabolites with higher systolic BP (Trasande and Attina 2015). Similarly, urine and blood samples were collected from a smaller population (242 children and adolescents aged between 6-18 years) to investigate the association between phthalates exposure and obesity indices and BP (Amin et al. 2018). The results showed an association between phthalate metabolites with increased obesity and BP in this Iranian population, with MBzP, MnBP and MMP found in all the participants and MEHP, mono(2-ethyl-5-oxohexyl) phthalate (MEOHP) and mono(2-ethyl-5-hydroxyhexyl) phthalate (MEHHP) in 99.6%, 87.85% and 29.26% of them, respectively (Amin et al. 2018). Due to lack of studies in Chinese children, Yao et al. (2020) investigated if high BP was related to exposure to phthalates. 1044 children (6-8 years old) provided urine samples to correlate phthalate exposure with systolic/diastolic BP, pulse pressure, mean arterial pressure and the risk of high BP. Associated with increased systolic/diastolic BP z-scores, pulse pressure and mean arterial pressure were MMP, MiBP, MnBP, mono(2-ethyl-5-carboxypentyl) phthalate (MECPP), mono-[2-(carboxymethyl)hexyl] phthalate (MCMHP), ΣLMW and the sum of all nine phthalate metabolites, and the risk of high BP was only related with MMP concentration (Yao et al. 2020). In a different perspective, DEHP exposure and systolic BP were investigated in 20 premature infants at two medical centres (Jenkins et al. 2019). Infants were followed from birth to 8 months old and a single urine sample was collected for phthalate metabolites measure that was compared between hypertensive and normotensive premature infants and related to BP in the overall cohort. The results showed that DEHP exposure is increased in hypertensive infants and intravenous exposure is predictive of systolic BP, due to evaluation of the medical equipment for the presence of DEHP. Activation of the mineralocorticoid receptor through inhibition of 11β-Hydroxysteroid dehydrogenase 2 may be a possible mechanism associated with idiopathic low-renin hypertension in premature infants (Jenkins et al. 2019). These studies confirm the risk of phthalate exposure (during pre- and postnatal period) for cardiovascular health in children, a very concerning issue since they are still growing and developing, and this early exposure to environmental contaminants may affect their health in the future. Overall, besides most of these studies, either in animal and human, show an association between exposure to phthalates and increased BP, the mechanisms by which this increase occurs are still unknown.

Diabetes

Diabetes is a complex metabolic disorder that results from insulin production and/or action impairment (Ruiz et al. 2018), and epidemiological studies have been associating this disease and insulin resistance with exposure to phthalates

(Zhou et al. 2015). In a study performed by Zhou et al. (2015), six-week-old apoE-/- female mice (C57BL/6 genetic background) were exposed to DEHP in drinking water (100 mg/kg/day) for 12 weeks. This animal model of atherosclerosis was used due to hyperglycaemia and type 2 diabetes mellitus (T2DM) development after fed with a Western diet. Then body weight, glucose and insulin tolerance, plasma glucose and triglyceride levels were analysed, with DEHP affecting glucose homeostasis and tolerance in the first weeks of exposure (2-3 weeks), having no significant effects on body weight and T2DM at the end of exposure time (12 weeks) (Zhou et al. 2015). In a different perspective, exposure to DEHP was investigated in adolescents with T2DM. Normal and T2DM (established with high-sugar and high-fat diet) ICR male mice (3 weeks old) were orally administered with different concentrations of DEHP for 3 weeks (Ding et al. 2019). The results showed that adolescent T2DM mice were more susceptible to DEHP exposure than normal mice, with increased levels of fasting blood glucose and glycated haemoglobin, besides DEHP had negative effects on glucose, lipid and protein metabolism, causing more adverse effects on cardiovascular functions. The authors hypothesised a potential mechanism, with DEHP interfering with the insulin signalling transduction pathway to inhibit the glucose intake and synthesis of glycogen, fat and protein in T2DM mice (Ding et al. 2019). Similarly, the same research group studied the effects of DEHP but this time in adolescent T2DM female mice (Ding et al. 2021). The same way, normal and T2DM female mice were orally administered with DEHP for 3 weeks, and they were shown to be more sensitive to DEHP exposure when compared to normal and male mice. Metabolic toxicity of DEHP was investigated for T2DM male and female mice, with an increased risk to suffer T2DM, metabolic disorders, cardiovascular events and hepatotoxicity for female mice. The possible mechanism may involve activation of Jun-N-terminal kinase (JNK) by DEHP, that will lead to apoptosis and inhibit insulin sensitivity, culminating in hepatic dysfunction and metabolic disorders (Ding et al. 2021). These two reports came to confirm the sex differences caused by exposure to DEHP, with increased suffering for female T2DM mice.

Besides the in vivo studies presented, epidemiological studies have also linked exposure to phthalates with diabetes. In 2015, Attina and Trasande investigated the link between DEHP alternatives and increased insulin resistance in adolescents. DiNP, DiDP and DEHP metabolite concentrations were measured in the urine of 356 fasting adolescents (12-19 years old). Increased insulin resistance was showed to be associated with urinary levels of DEHP and, for the first time, with DiNP (Attina and Trasande 2015). In an older population (mean age of 51.2 years for males and 65 years for females), 24 hours urine was collected and levels of phthalate metabolites were analysed in 168 patients with metabolic syndrome from Prague (Piecha et al. 2016). The sample population was classified dyslipidaemic (n = 87), hypertensive (n = 96) and T2DM (n = 58), and four phthalate metabolites (MnBP, MEHHP, MEOHP, and MECPP) were significantly increased in T2DM patients compared to those without T2DM (Piecha et al. 2016). 2330 Shanghai adults (median age of 53 years) participated in a cross-sectional study to investigate phthalates' contribution to diabetes and CVD (Dong et al. 2017). The participants entered the 2012 Shanghai Food Consumption Survey so, besides collecting urine samples, they also responded to a questionnaire to collect the seasonal data of food consumption for four times. Urinary levels of MEOHP, MEHHP and MECPP were associated with T2DM, MMP and MCMHP were associated with increased odds of hyperlipidaemia and MEHP was inversely related to hyperlipidaemia. These results show that oxidative metabolites of DEHP may be considered as biomarkers for phthalates toxicity. In addition, a sex difference was also found, with T2DM males, but not females, being associated with the oxidative metabolites of DEHP (Dong et al. 2017). In a study performed by the same research group (Dong et al. 2018), the authors deepened the study and explored the role of oxidative stress in the cardiometabolic risk induced by phthalates exposure. An elderly diabetic population (mean age of 69 years) from Shanghai entered the study, blood and urine samples were collected, and 10 phthalate metabolites and biomarkers of oxidative stress were measured from all 300 participants. It was found that phthalate metabolites were associated with higher insulin resistance and oxidative stress, being mediated by γ-glutamiltransferase effect. These results show that phthalates exposure and oxidative stress may be risk factors for insulin resistance in diabetic patients (Dong et al. 2018). Two different studies confirmed once more the connection between exposure to phthalates and the development of diabetes and obesity (Nam et al. 2020, Lee et al. 2021). Resorting to data from Korean National Environmental Health Survey (KoNEHS), 3781 adults (1648 men and 2133 women) aged between 19 and >70 years old participated in the study (Nam et al. 2020). After urine samples analysis, the authors concluded a positive association between phthalate concentrations and the prevalence of diabetes, with no sex differences found (Nam et al. 2020). On the other hand, Lee et al. (2021) demonstrated the importance of the urinary dilution adjustment method since the direction of the association vary with the method chosen, for this population. Besides, from the urinary samples analysed, DEHP and BBzP levels were positive associated with obesity (Lee et al. 2021). Not all of the studies mentioned have related gender differences, however, distinct results found between male and female may be due to the hormonal differences and due to endocrine disrupting properties of each phthalate, with DEHP displaying anti-androgenic and -estrogenic activities. Also, in menopausal women, there is a decrease in oestrogen and an increase in androgen levels, associated with alterations in the metabolic risk profile (Dong et al. 2017).

Three studies have related phthalates with T2DM only in women, considering that they are more susceptible to these EDC due to a higher use of personal care products. In a population of 221 Mexican women, the ones that had diabetes were found to have higher levels of DEHP metabolites (MEHHP, MEOHP, MECPP) in urine (Svensson et al. 2011). These results were in accordance with those from the James-Todd et al. study, where MnBP, MiBP, MBzP, MCPP and ΣDEHP urinary levels were associated with diabetes in women. In this study, 2350 American women (aged between 20 and 79 years) were included in the primary analysis (to relate phthalates exposure with diabetes), and for the secondary analysis (to relate phthalates exposure with factors preceding the onset of diabetes) 985, 971 and 2092 women without diabetes were included for fasting blood glucose, homeostasis model assessment-estimated insulin resistance (HOMA-IR) and glycosylated haemoglobin A1c, respectively. The findings suggested an association between ΣDEHP and insulin resistance in women without diabetes, concluding that DEHP can lead to T2DM (James-Todd et al. 2012). In order to compare phthalates with the risk of T2DM in different ages, women from the Nurses' Health Study (NHS) (53–79 years old) and the younger counterpart NHSII cohort (32–52 years old) were enrolled in the study (Sun et al. 2014). There was a positive association between butyl phthalates concentration in urine and incident diabetes for middle-aged U.S. female nurses but not in older counterparts. This difference may be attributed, in part, to the menopausal status (Sun et al. 2014). Women with gestational diabetes mellitus (GDM) are at higher risk to develop T2DM later in life. Since phthalates have been associated with risk factors for diabetes, James-Todd et al. (2016) conducted a study to evaluate phthalates and GDM risk factors (James-Todd et al. 2016). 350 pregnant women from Boston, USA, were recruited for the Lifecodes pregnancy cohort and, besides pregnancy urinary phthalate metabolite levels, 1st trimester body mass index (BMI), gestational weight gain (GWG) and 2nd trimester glucose levels were also evaluated. There was a positive correlation between urinary MEP concentration in the 2nd trimester and increased GWG and impaired glucose tolerance, and MnBP,

MCPP and ΣDEHP were inversely related to excessive GWG, continuous blood glucose and impaired glucose tolerance, respectively (James-Todd et al. 2016). In a different perspective, 40 pregnant Mexican women (24-45 years old) in the second trimester of pregnancy were recruited for the study and blood and urine samples were collected. There is a correlation between dysregulation of microRNA expression and obesity, T2DM and GDM (Guarino et al. 2018, Sliwinska et al. 2017, Martínez-Ibarra et al. 2019), so microRNAs related to GDM were measured in serum and compared to urinary phthalate metabolites, for all the participants (18 women with GDM and 22 women without GDM – control group). The results reflect the exposure of Mexican pregnant women to DEHP, showing increased levels of phthalates in the urine of both study groups, women with and without GDM, with MEHP being the most abundant metabolite; also, there was a correlation between phthalates concentration and miRNA expression levels in the control group compared to GDM patients (Martínez-Ibarra et al. 2019). Although there are several studies relating the influence of phthalates on the development of diabetes, the results are still inconsistent, being influenced by age and gender.

Conclusion

With this chapter we aimed to describe the implications of phthalates effects on the cardiovascular system, including heart failure, arrhythmias, stroke, atherosclerosis, hypertension and diabetes, both in animals and humans. Most of the data relating phthalates with CVDs comes from epidemiological studies, and in a less extent from experimental studies. The purpose of epidemiological studies is to identify the extent of chemical exposure and their association with adverse health outcomes, while resorting to experimental studies will enlighten the causation and potential mechanisms (Ramadan et al. 2020). So, the combination of these two types of studies is essential to better understand the adverse health effects of phthalates.

Regarding heart failure and myocardial infarction, there is no consistency on the studies, with different animals and different parameters analysed, making it difficult to compare the results. Nevertheless, the studies presented point to a connection between phthalates exposure, mainly DEHP and its metabolites, with the risk of heart failure and heart attack. In an old epidemiological study, MEHP was found at lower levels than those causing arrhythmias in adults and infants, contradicting the experimental ones, that suggested that DEHP and MEHP promoted some parameters associated with the risk of arrhythmia. In addition, only one epidemiological study related increased phthalate levels (MnBP and MCPP) with the risk of stroke. Data is still very limited, and new longitudinal and experimental studies are needed to understand if and how phthalates are associated with these diseases.

With more studies carried out, phthalates have been associated with the occurrence of atherosclerosis, both in animals and humans. In experimental studies, both in vitro and in vivo, DEHP, DBP and DEP were positive related to atherosclerosis, with oxidative stress, modifications in cholesterol homeostasis and deregulation of the inflammatory response pointed out as possible mechanisms. In accordance, MMP, MBzP, DEHP and DiDP were also associated with this disease in different age groups. Nevertheless, a deeper investigation on this subject is needed to validate these results and the mechanisms involved.

Blood pressure, as a risk factor or a CVD, has been the most studied regarding phthalates implications. Most studies that analysed the effects of DEHP in animals, showed that this contaminant can induce an increase in BP, both in pre and postnatal exposure. It was hypothesised that increased levels of ACE and AT1R and inhibition of the bradykinin-NO pathway are responsible for the BP increase. The same way, DiNP, used as DEHP substitute, also leads to an increase in BP, unlike DBP, that led to a decrease in BP. Regarding epidemiological studies, children and pregnant women have been the most studied populations, with several phthalates and their metabolites inducing an increase in BP; however, when phthalate levels in the mother's urine were compared with the children's BP, the results revealed a decrease in BP. In addition, oxidative stress has been associated with pregnant women exposed to phthalates, that, in turn, can lead to the release of the circulating angiogenic factors, increasing the risk of preeclampsia (Ferguson et al. 2015, Burton et al. 2009, Han et al. 2020). Most of these studies show an association between phthalates and elevated blood pressure, and, although some mechanisms have been proposed, they remain to be unveiled.

There are several studies relating phthalates exposure with the incidence of insulin resistance and diabetes. In animals, DEHP has been found to affect glucose homeostasis, and that diabetic female mice are more sensitive to this contaminant than diabetic and normal males. Epidemiological studies have shown that there is an increase in insulin resistance in adolescents exposed to DEHP and DiNP, and several phthalate metabolites are associated with diabetes and its risk factors, however, the results are not consistent with the age and gender of the participants from the several studies.

Hormonal differences may be the cause for the distinct results found between male and female, as well as between women from different ages, since menopausal women have a decrease in oestrogen and an increase in androgen levels, that are associated with alterations in the metabolic risk profile (Dong et al. 2017). Besides, each phthalate has specific endocrine disrupting properties, with DEHP displaying anti-androgenic and -estrogenic activities. Other discrepancies between the studies may be due to differences in sources and levels of exposure, race/ethnicity, genetic variability, population size, sample collection and lifestyle. Therefore, more epidemiological studies to understand these discrepancies, and experimental research to explore the mechanisms involved, are needed to fill the gap between phthalates exposure and cardiovascular health.

References

Amara, I., R. Timoumi, E. Annabi, F. Neffati, M. F. Najjar, C. Bouaziz, and S. Abid-Essefi. 2019. "Di (2-ethylhexyl) phthalate induces cardiac disorders in BALB/c mice." *Environ Sci Pollut Res Int* 26 (8):7540-7549. doi: 10.1007/s11356-019-04219-w.

Amin, M. M., K. Ebrahimpour, S. Parastar, B. Shoshtari-Yeganeh, M. Hashemi, M. Mansourian, P. Poursafa, Z. Fallah, N. Rafiei, and R. Kelishadi. 2018. "Association of urinary concentrations of phthalate metabolites with cardiometabolic risk factors and obesity in children and adolescents." *Chemosphere* 211:547-556. doi: 10.1016/j.chemosphere.2018.07.172.

Attina, T. M., and L. Trasande. 2015. "Association of exposure to Di-2-Ethylhexylphthalate replacements with increased insulin resistance in adolescents from NHANES 2009-2012." *J Clin Endocrinol Metab* 100 (7):2640-50. doi: 10.1210/jc.2015-1686.

Barry, Y. A., R. S. Labow, W. J. Keon, M. Tocchi, and G. Rock. 1989. "Perioperative exposure to plasticizers in patients undergoing cardiopulmonary bypass." *J Thorac Cardiovasc Surg* 97 (6):900-5.

Burton, G. J., H. W. Yung, T. Cindrova-Davies, and D. S. Charnock-Jones. 2009. "Placental endoplasmic reticulum stress and oxidative stress in the pathophysiology of unexplained intrauterine growth restriction and early onset preeclampsia." *Placenta* 30 Suppl A:S43-8. doi: 10.1016/j.placenta.2008.11.003.

Cantonwine, D. E., J. D. Meeker, K. K. Ferguson, B. Mukherjee, R. Hauser, and T. F. McElrath. 2016. "urinary concentrations of bisphenol a and phthalate metabolites measured during pregnancy and risk of preeclampsia." *Environ Health Perspect* 124 (10):1651-1655. doi: 10.1289/EHP188.

Casals-Casas, C., and B. Desvergne. 2011. "Endocrine disruptors: from endocrine to metabolic disruption." *Annu Rev Physiol* 73:135-62. doi: 10.1146/annurev-physiol-012110-142200.

Chu, P. C., C. Wu, and T. C. Su. 2021. "Association between urinary phthalate metabolites and markers of endothelial dysfunction in adolescents and young Adults." *Toxics* 9 (2). doi:10.3390/toxics9020033.

Deng, T., X. Xie, J. Duan, and M. Chen. 2019a. "Di-(2-ethylhexyl) phthalate induced an increase in blood pressure via activation of ACE and inhibition of the bradykinin-NO pathway." *Environ Pollut* 247:927-934. doi: 10.1016/j.envpol.2019.01.099.

Deng, T., X. Xie, J. Duan, and M. Chen. 2019b. "Exposure to diisononyl phthalate induced an increase in blood pressure through activation of the ACE/ AT1R axis and inhibition of NO production." *Toxicol Lett* 309:42-50. doi: 10.1016/j.toxlet.2019.03.011.

Ding, Y., K. Gao, Y. Liu, G. Mao, K. Chen, X. Qiu, T. Zhao, L. Yang, W. Feng, and X. Wu. 2019. "Transcriptome analysis revealed the mechanism of the metabolic toxicity and susceptibility of di-(2-ethylhexyl)phthalate on adolescent male ICR mice with type 2 diabetes mellitus." *Arch Toxicol* 93 (11):3183-3206. doi: 10.1007/s00204-019-02590-8.

Ding, Y., T. Xu, G. Mao, Y. Chen, X. Qiu, L. Yang, T. Zhao, X. Xu, W. Feng, and X. Wu. 2021. "Di-(2-ethylhexyl) phthalate-induced hepatotoxicity exacerbated type 2 diabetes mellitus (T2DM) in female pubertal T2DM mice." *Food Chem Toxicol* 149:112003. doi: 10.1016/j.fct.2021.112003.

Dong, R., J. Chen, J. Zheng, M. Zhang, H. Zhang, M. Wu, S. Li, and B. Chen. 2018. "The role of oxidative stress in cardiometabolic risk related to phthalate exposure in elderly diabetic patients from Shanghai." *Environ Int* 121 (Pt 1):340-348. doi: 10.1016/j.env int.2018.09.028.

Dong, R., S. Zhao, H. Zhang, J. Chen, M. Zhang, M. Wang, M. Wu, S. Li, and B. Chen. 2017. "sex differences in the association of urinary concentrations of phthalates metabolites with self-reported diabetes and cardiovascular diseases in shanghai adults." *Int J Environ Res Public Health* 14 (6). doi: 10.3390/ijerph14060598.

Ferguson, K. K., T. F. McElrath, D. E. Cantonwine, B. Mukherjee, and J. D. Meeker. 2015. "Phthalate metabolites and bisphenol-A in association with circulating angiogenic biomarkers across pregnancy." *Placenta* 36 (6):699-703. doi: 10.1016/j.placenta.20 15.04.002.

Frederiksen, H., N. E. Skakkebaek, and A. M. Andersson. 2007. "Metabolism of phthalates in humans." *Mol Nutr Food Res* 51 (7):899-911. doi: 10.1002/mnfr.200600243.

Fu, X., J. Xu, R. Zhang, and J. Yu. 2020. "The association between environmental endocrine disruptors and cardiovascular diseases: A systematic review and meta-analysis." *Environ Res* 187:109464. doi: 10.1016/j.envres.2020.109464.

Gawdzik, J. C., M. S. Yue, N. R. Martin, L. M. H. Elemans, K. A. Lanham, W. Heideman, R. Rezendes, T. R. Baker, M. R. Taylor, and J. S. Plavicki. 2018. "sox9b is required in cardiomyocytes for cardiac morphogenesis and function." *Sci Rep* 8 (1):13906. doi: 10.1038/s41598-018-32125-7.

Gore, A. C., V. A. Chappell, S. E. Fenton, J. A. Flaws, A. Nadal, G. S. Prins, J. Toppari, and R. T. Zoeller. 2015. "Executive summary to EDC-2: The Endocrine Society's second scientific statement on endocrine-disrupting chemicals." *Endocr Rev* 36 (6):593-602. doi: 10.1210/er.2015-1093.

Guarino, E., C. Delli Poggi, G. E. Grieco, V. Cenci, E. Ceccarelli, I. Crisci, G. Sebastiani, and F. Dotta. 2018. "Circulating MicroRNAs as biomarkers of gestational diabetes mellitus: updates and perspectives." *Int J Endocrinol* 2018:6380463. doi: 10.1155/2018/6380463.

Han, X., J. Li, Y. Wang, S. Xu, Y. Li, H. Liu, Y. Zhou, H. Zhao, J. Fang, Z. Cai, and W. Xia. 2020. "Association between phthalate exposure and blood pressure during pregnancy." *Ecotoxicol Environ Saf* 189:109944. doi: 10.1016/j.ecoenv.2019.109944.

Hauser, R., J. D. Meeker, S. Park, M. J. Silva, and A. M. Calafat. 2004. "Temporal variability of urinary phthalate metabolite levels in men of reproductive age." *Environ Health Perspect* 112 (17):1734-40.

Hodis, H. N., W. J. Mack, L. LaBree, R. H. Selzer, C. R. Liu, C. H. Liu, and S. P. Azen. 1998. "The role of carotid arterial intima-media thickness in predicting clinical coronary events." *Ann Intern Med* 128 (4):262-9. doi: 10.7326/0003-4819-128-4-199802150-00002.

Huang, J., P. N. Nkrumah, Y. Li, and G. Appiah-Sefah. 2013. "Chemical behavior of phthalates under abiotic conditions in landfills." *Rev Environ Contam Toxicol* 224:39-52. doi: 10.1007/978-1-4614-5882-1_2.

Jacobs, D. E., J. Wilson, S. L. Dixon, J. Smith, and A. Evens. 2009. "The relationship of housing and population health: a 30-year retrospective analysis." *Environ Health Perspect* 117 (4):597-604. doi: 10.1289/ehp.0800086.

Jaimes, R., 3rd, A. Swiercz, M. Sherman, N. Muselimyan, P. J. Marvar, and N. G. Posnack. 2017. "Plastics and cardiovascular health: phthalates may disrupt heart rate variability and cardiovascular reactivity." *Am J Physiol Heart Circ Physiol* 313 (5):H1044-H1053. doi: 10.1152/ajpheart.00364.2017.

Jaimes, R., 3rd, D. McCullough, B. Siegel, L. Swift, D. McInerney, J. Hiebert, E. A. Perez-Alday, B. Trenor, J. Sheng, J. Saiz, L. G. Tereshchenko, and N. G. Posnack. 2019. "plasticizer interaction with the heart: chemicals used in plastic medical devices can interfere with cardiac electrophysiology." *Circ Arrhythm Electrophysiol* 12 (7):e007294. doi: 10.1161/CIRCEP.119.007294.

James-Todd, T. M., J. D. Meeker, T. Huang, R. Hauser, K. K. Ferguson, J. W. Rich-Edwards, T. F. McElrath, and E. W. Seely. 2016. "Pregnancy urinary phthalate metabolite concentrations and gestational diabetes risk factors." *Environ Int* 96:118-126. doi: 10.1016/j.envint.2016.09.009.

James-Todd, T., R. Stahlhut, J. D. Meeker, S. G. Powell, R. Hauser, T. Huang, and J. Rich-Edwards. 2012. "Urinary phthalate metabolite concentrations and diabetes among women in the National Health and Nutrition Examination Survey (NHANES) 2001-2008." *Environ Health Perspect* 120 (9):1307-13. doi: 10.1289/ehp.1104717.

Jenkins, R., S. Tackitt, L. Gievers, S. Iragorri, K. Sage, T. Cornwall, D. O'Riordan, J. Merchant, and D. Rozansky. 2019. "Phthalate-associated hypertension in premature infants: a prospective mechanistic cohort study." *Pediatr Nephrol* 34 (8):1413-1424. doi: 10.1007/s00467-019-04244-4.

Johns, L. E., G. S. Cooper, A. Galizia, and J. D. Meeker. 2015. "Exposure assessment issues in epidemiology studies of phthalates." *Environ Int* 85:27-39. doi: 10.1016/j.envint.2015.08.005.

Kim, J. H. 2020. "Glucagon-like peptide-1 receptor agonist reduces di(2-ethylhexyl) phthalate-induced atherosclerotic processes in vascular smooth muscle cells." *Physiol Res* 69 (6):1095-1102. doi: 10.33549/physiolres.934480.

Kim, S. H., and M. J. Park. 2014. "Phthalate exposure and childhood obesity." *Ann Pediatr Endocrinol Metab* 19 (2):69-75. doi: 10.6065/apem.2014.19.2.69.

Kim, S. M., J. A. Yoo, J. M. Baek, and K. H. Cho. 2015. "Diethyl phthalate exposure is associated with embryonic toxicity, fatty liver changes, and hypolipidemia via impairment of lipoprotein functions." *Toxicol In Vitro* 30 (1 Pt B):383-93. doi: 10.1016/j.tiv.2015.09.026.

Latini, G., C. De Felice, G. Presta, A. Del Vecchio, I. Paris, F. Ruggieri, and P. Mazzeo. 2003. "In utero exposure to di-(2-ethylhexyl)phthalate and duration of human pregnancy." *Environ Health Perspect* 111 (14):1783-5.

Lee, I., Y. J. Park, M. J. Kim, S. Kim, S. Choi, J. Park, Y. H. Cho, S. Hong, J. Yoo, H. Park, G. J. Cheon, K. Choi, and M. K. Moon. 2021. "Associations of urinary concentrations of phthalate metabolites, bisphenol A, and parabens with obesity and diabetes mellitus in a Korean adult population: Korean National Environmental Health Survey (KoNEHS) 2015-2017." *Environ Int* 146:106227. doi: 10.1016/j.envint.2020.106227.

Lee, K. I., C. W. Chiang, H. C. Lin, J. F. Zhao, C. T. Li, S. K. Shyue, and T. S. Lee. 2016. "Maternal exposure to di-(2-ethylhexyl) phthalate exposure deregulates blood pressure, adiposity, cholesterol metabolism and social interaction in mouse offspring." *Arch Toxicol* 90 (5):1211-24. doi: 10.1007/s00204-015-1539-0.

Lin, C. Y., P. C. Huang, C. Wu, F. C. Sung, and T. C. Su. 2020a. "Association between urine lead levels and cardiovascular disease risk factors, carotid intima-media thickness and metabolic syndrome in adolescents and young adults." *Int J Hyg Environ Health* 223 (1):248-255. doi: 10.1016/j.ijheh.2019.08.005.

Lin, C. Y., Y. T. Hwang, P. C. Chen, F. C. Sung, and T. C. Su. 2019. "Association of serum levels of 4-tertiary-octylphenol with cardiovascular risk factors and carotid intima-media thickness in adolescents and young adults." *Environ Pollut* 246:107-113. doi: 10.1016/j.envpol.2018.11.110.

Lin, C. Y., H. L. Lee, Y. T. Hwang, C. Wang, C. J. Hsieh, C. Wu, F. C. Sung, and T. C. Su. 2020b. "The association between urine di-(2-ethylhexyl) phthalate metabolites, global DNA methylation, and subclinical atherosclerosis in a young Taiwanese population." *Environ Pollut* 265 (Pt B):114912. doi: 10.1016/j.envpol.2020.114912.

Lind, P. M., B. Zethelius, and L. Lind. 2012. "Circulating levels of phthalate metabolites are associated with prevalent diabetes in the elderly." *Diabetes Care* 35 (7):1519-24. doi: 10.2337/dc11-2396.

Lind, P. M., and L. Lind. 2011. "Circulating levels of bisphenol A and phthalates are related to carotid atherosclerosis in the elderly." *Atherosclerosis* 218 (1):207-13. doi: 10.1016/j.atherosclerosis.2011.05.001.

Lurbe, E., R. Cifkova, J. K. Cruickshank, M. J. Dillon, I. Ferreira, C. Invitti, T. Kuznetsova, S. Laurent, G. Mancia, F. Morales-Olivas, W. Rascher, J. Redon, F. Schaefer, T. Seeman, G. Stergiou, E. Wuhl, and A. Zanchetti. 2009. "Management of high blood pressure in children and adolescents: recommendations of the European Society of Hypertension." *J Hypertens* 27 (9):1719-42. doi: 10.1097/HJH.0b013e32832f4f6b.

Main, K. M., G. K. Mortensen, M. M. Kaleva, K. A. Boisen, I. N. Damgaard, M. Chellakooty, I. M. Schmidt, A. M. Suomi, H. E. Virtanen, D. V. Petersen, A. M. Andersson, J. Toppari, and N. E. Skakkebaek. 2006. "Human breast milk contamination with phthalates and alterations of endogenous reproductive hormones in infants three months of age." *Environ Health Perspect* 114 (2):270-6.

Mankidy, R., S. Wiseman, H. Ma, and J. P. Giesy. 2013. "Biological impact of phthalates." *Toxicol Lett* 217 (1):50-8. doi: 10.1016/j.toxlet.2012.11.025.

Mariana, M., and E. Cairrao. 2020. "phthalates implications in the cardiovascular system." *J Cardiovasc Dev Dis* 7 (3). doi: 10.3390/jcdd7030026.

Mariana, M., J. Feiteiro, and E. Cairrao. 2018. "Cardiovascular response of rat aorta to Di-(2-ethylhexyl) Phthalate (DEHP) exposure." *Cardiovasc Toxicol* 18 (4):356-364. doi: 10.1007/s12012-017-9439-6.

Mariana, M., J. Feiteiro, I. Verde, and E. Cairrao. 2016. "The effects of phthalates in the cardiovascular and reproductive systems: A review." *Environ Int* 94:758-76. doi:10. 1016/j.envint.2016.07.004.

Martinez-Arguelles, D. B., M. McIntosh, C. V. Rohlicek, M. Culty, B. R. Zirkin, and V. Papadopoulos. 2013. "Maternal in utero exposure to the endocrine disruptor di-(2-ethylhexyl) phthalate affects the blood pressure of adult male offspring." *Toxicol Appl Pharmacol* 266 (1):95-100. doi: 10.1016/j.taap.2012.10.027.

Martínez-Ibarra, A., L. D. Martínez-Razo, E. R. Vázquez-Martínez, N. Martínez-Cruz, R. Flores-Ramírez, E. García-Gómez, M. López-López, C. Ortega-González, I. Camacho-Arroyo, and M. Cerbón. 2019. "Unhealthy levels of phthalates and bisphenol A in Mexican pregnant women with gestational diabetes and its association to altered expression of miRNAs involved with metabolic disease." *Int J Mol Sci* 20 (13). doi: 10.3390/ijms20133343.

Mu, X., X. Chen, J. Liu, L. Yuan, D. Wang, L. Qian, Y. Qian, G. Shen, Y. Huang, X. Li, Y. Li, and X. Lin. 2020. "A multi-omics approach reveals molecular mechanisms by which phthalates induce cardiac defects in zebrafish (Danio rerio)." *Environ Pollut* 265 (Pt B):113876. doi: 10.1016/j.envpol.2019.113876.

Nam, D. J., Y. Kim, E. H. Yang, H. C. Lee, and J. H. Ryoo. 2020. "Relationship between urinary phthalate metabolites and diabetes: Korean National Environmental Health Survey (KoNEHS) cycle 3 (2015-2017)." *Ann Occup Environ Med* 32:e34. doi: 10.35371/aoem.2020.32.e34.

Peres, G. M., M. Mariana, and E. Cairrao. 2018. "Pre-eclampsia and eclampsia: an update on the pharmacological treatment applied in Portugal." *J Cardiovasc Dev Dis* 5 (1). doi: 10.3390/jcdd5010003.

Philips, E. M., L. Trasande, L. G. Kahn, R. Gaillard, E. A. P. Steegers, and V. W. V. Jaddoe. 2019. "Early pregnancy bisphenol and phthalate metabolite levels, maternal hemodynamics and gestational hypertensive disorders." *Hum Reprod* 34 (2):365-373. doi: 10.1093/humrep/dey364.

Piecha, R., S. Svacina, M. Maly, K. Vrbik, Z. Lacinova, M. Haluzik, J. Pavlouskova, A. Vavrous, D. Matejkova, D. Mullerova, M. Mraz, and M. Matoulek. 2016. "Urine levels of phthalate metabolites and bisphenol a in relation to main metabolic syndrome components: dyslipidemia, hypertension and type 2 diabetes. a pilot study." *Cent Eur J Public Health* 24 (4):297-301. doi: 10.21101/cejph.a4704.

Piepoli, M. F. 2017. "2016 European Guidelines on cardiovascular disease prevention in clinical practice : The Sixth Joint Task Force of the European Society of Cardiology and Other Societies on Cardiovascular Disease prevention in clinical practice (constituted by representatives of 10 societies and by invited experts)." *Int J Behav Med* 24 (3):321-419. doi: 10.1007/s12529-016-9583-6.

Posnack, N. G., N. H. Lee, R. Brown, and N. Sarvazyan. 2011. "Gene expression profiling of DEHP-treated cardiomyocytes reveals potential causes of phthalate arrhythmogenicity." *Toxicology* 279 (1-3):54-64. doi: 10.1016/j.tox.2010.09.007.

Rahmani, A., K. Soleimannejad, M. R. Hafezi Ahmadi, K. Asadollahi, and Z. Khalighi. 2016. "prenatal exposure to phthalic acid induces increased blood pressure, oxidative stress, and markers of endothelial dysfunction in rat offspring." *Cardiovasc Toxicol* 16 (4):307-15. doi: 10.1007/s12012-015-9337-8.

Ramadan, M., B. Cooper, and N. G. Posnack. 2020. "Bisphenols and phthalates: Plastic chemical exposures can contribute to adverse cardiovascular health outcomes." *Birth Defects Res* 112 (17):1362-1385. doi: 10.1002/bdr2.1752.

Ruiz, D., M. Becerra, J. S. Jagai, K. Ard, and R. M. Sargis. 2018. "Disparities in environmental exposures to endocrine-disrupting chemicals and diabetes risk in vulnerable populations." *Diabetes Care* 41 (1):193-205. doi: 10.2337/dc16-2765.

Say, L., D. Chou, A. Gemmill, O. Tuncalp, A. B. Moller, J. Daniels, A. M. Gulmezoglu, M. Temmerman, and L. Alkema. 2014. "Global causes of maternal death: a WHO systematic analysis." *Lancet Glob Health* 2 (6):e323-33. doi: 10.1016/S2214-109X (14)70227-X.

Shang, J., J. Corriveau, A. Champoux-Jenane, J. Gagnon, E. Moss, P. Dumas, E. Gaudreau, J. Chevrier, and L. E. Chalifour. 2019. "Recovery from a myocardial infarction is impaired in male C57bl/6 N mice acutely exposed to the bisphenols and phthalates that escape from medical devices used in cardiac surgery." *Toxicol Sci* 168 (1):78-94. doi: 10.1093/toxsci/kfy276.

Shih, M. F., K. H. Pan, C. C. Liu, C. R. Shen, and J. Y. Cherng. 2018. "Treatment of beta-thujaplicin counteracts di(2-ethylhexyl)phthalate (DEHP)-exposed vascular smooth muscle activation, inflammation and atherosclerosis progression." *Regul Toxicol Pharmacol* 92:333-337. doi: 10.1016/j.yrtph.2017.12.021.

Shih, M. F., K. H. Pan, and J. Y. Cherng. 2015. "Possible mechanisms of Di(2-ethylhexyl) phthalate-induced MMP-2 and MMP-9 expression in A7r5 rat vascular smooth muscle cells." *Int J Mol Sci* 16 (12):28800-11. doi: 10.3390/ijms161226131.

Shiue, I. 2013. "Urine phthalate concentrations are higher in people with stroke: United States National Health and Nutrition Examination Surveys (NHANES), 2001-2004." *Eur J Neurol* 20 (4):728-31. doi: 10.1111/j.1468-1331.2012.03862.x.

Shiue, I., and G. Bramley. 2015. "Environmental chemicals mediated the effect of old housing on adult health problems: US NHANES, 2009-2010." *Environ Sci Pollut Res Int* 22 (2):1299-308. doi: 10.1007/s11356-014-3468-5.

Shiue, I., and Y. Y. Shiue. 2013. "The role of housing characteristics in biomarkers: US NHANES, 2003-2006." *Int J Cardiol* 168 (5):5069-71. doi: 10.1016/j.ijcard.2013.07.200.

Silva, M. J., J. A. Reidy, A. R. Herbert, J. L. Preau, Jr., L. L. Needham, and A. M. Calafat. 2004a. "Detection of phthalate metabolites in human amniotic fluid." *Bull Environ Contam Toxicol* 72 (6):1226-31.

Silva, M. J., A. R. Slakman, J. A. Reidy, J. L. Preau, Jr., A. R. Herbert, E. Samandar, L. L. Needham, and A. M. Calafat. 2004b. "Analysis of human urine for fifteen phthalate metabolites using automated solid-phase extraction." *J Chromatogr B Analyt Technol Biomed Life Sci* 805 (1):161-7. doi: 10.1016/j.jchromb.2004.02.038.

Silva, M. J., J. A. Reidy, E. Samandar, A. R. Herbert, L. L. Needham, and A. M. Calafat. 2005. "Detection of phthalate metabolites in human saliva." *Arch Toxicol* 79 (11):647-52. doi: 10.1007/s00204-005-0674-4.

Sliwinska, A., M. A. Kasinska, and J. Drzewoski. 2017. "MicroRNAs and metabolic disorders - where are we heading?" *Arch Med Sci* 13 (4):885-896. doi: 10.5114/aoms.2017.65229.

Sol, C. M., S. Santos, A. G. Asimakopoulos, M. P. Martinez-Moral, L. Duijts, K. Kannan, L. Trasande, and V. W. V. Jaddoe. 2020. "Associations of maternal phthalate and bisphenol urine concentrations during pregnancy with childhood blood pressure in a population-based prospective cohort study." *Environ Int* 138:105677. doi: 10.1016/j.envint.2020.105677.

Su, T. C., J. S. Hwang, P. L. Torng, C. Wu, C. Y. Lin, and F. C. Sung. 2019. "Phthalate exposure increases subclinical atherosclerosis in young population." *Environ Pollut* 250:586-593. doi: 10.1016/j.envpol.2019.04.006.

Sun, Q., M. C. Cornelis, M. K. Townsend, D. K. Tobias, A. H. Eliassen, A. A. Franke, R. Hauser, and F. B. Hu. 2014. "Association of urinary concentrations of bisphenol A and phthalate metabolites with risk of type 2 diabetes: a prospective investigation in the Nurses' Health Study (NHS) and NHSII cohorts." *Environ Health Perspect* 122 (6):616-23. doi: 10.1289/ehp.1307201.

Sutton, A. L. M., L. M. Harper, and A. T. N. Tita. 2018. "Hypertensive Disorders in Pregnancy." *Obstet Gynecol Clin North Am* 45 (2):333-347. doi: 10.1016/j.ogc.2018.01.012.

Svensson, K., R. U. Hernández-Ramírez, A. Burguete-García, M. E. Cebrián, A. M. Calafat, L. L. Needham, L. Claudio, and L. López-Carrillo. 2011. "Phthalate exposure associated with self-reported diabetes among Mexican women." *Environ Res* 111 (6):792-6. doi: 10.1016/j.envres.2011.05.015.

Svoboda, L. K., K. Wang, R. G. Cavalcante, K. Neier, J. A. Colacino, M. A. Sartor, and D. C. Dolinoy. 2020. "Sex-specific programming of cardiac DNA methylation by developmental phthalate exposure." *Epigenet Insights* 13:2516865720939971. doi: 10.1177/2516865720939971.

Tabb, M. M., and B. Blumberg. 2006. "New modes of action for endocrine-disrupting chemicals." *Mol Endocrinol* 20 (3):475-82. doi: 10.1210/me.2004-0513.

Talsness, C. E., A. J. Andrade, S. N. Kuriyama, J. A. Taylor, and F. S. vom Saal. 2009. "Components of plastic: experimental studies in animals and relevance for human health." *Philos Trans R Soc Lond B Biol Sci* 364 (1526):2079-96. doi: 10.1098/rstb.2008.0281.

Trasande, L., S. Sathyanarayana, A. J. Spanier, H. Trachtman, T. M. Attina, and E. M. Urbina. 2013. "Urinary phthalates are associated with higher blood pressure in childhood." *J Pediatr* 163 (3):747-53 e1. doi: 10.1016/j.jpeds.2013.03.072.

Trasande, L., and T. M. Attina. 2015. "Association of exposure to di-2-ethylhexylphthalate replacements with increased blood pressure in children and adolescents." *Hypertension* 66 (2):301-8. doi: 10.1161/HYPERTENSIONAHA.115.05603.

Vafeiadi, M., A. Myridakis, T. Roumeliotaki, K. Margetaki, G. Chalkiadaki, E. Dermitzaki, M. Venihaki, K. Sarri, M. Vassilaki, V. Leventakou, E. G. Stephanou, M. Kogevinas, and L. Chatzi. 2018. "association of early life exposure to phthalates with obesity and cardiometabolic traits in childhood: sex specific associations." *Front Public Health* 6:327. doi: 10.3389/fpubh.2018.00327.

Valvi, D., M. Casas, D. Romaguera, N. Monfort, R. Ventura, D. Martinez, J. Sunyer, and M. Vrijheid. 2015. "Prenatal phthalate exposure and childhood growth and blood pressure: evidence from the Spanish INMA-Sabadell birth cohort study." *Environ Health Perspect* 123 (10):1022-9. doi: 10.1289/ehp.1408887.

Ventrice, P., D. Ventrice, E. Russo, and G. De Sarro. 2013. "Phthalates: European regulation, chemistry, pharmacokinetic and related toxicity." *Environ Toxicol Pharmacol* 36 (1):88-96. doi: 10.1016/j.etap.2013.03.014.

Vinceti, M., I. Bottecchi, A. Fan, Y. Finkelstein, and J. Mandrioli. 2012. "Are environmental exposures to selenium, heavy metals, and pesticides risk factors for amyotrophic lateral sclerosis?" *Rev Environ Health* 27 (1):19-41. doi: 10.1515/reveh-2012-0002.

Wang, Y., Y. Wen, P. Xiao, J. Sun, M. Chen, C. Gu, Y. Kong, A. Gu, and J. Zhang. 2020. "Di-n-butyl phthalate promotes lipid accumulation via the miR200c-5p-ABCA1 pathway in THP-1 macrophages." *Environ Pollut* 264:114723. doi: 10.1016/j.envpol.2020.114723.

Warembourg, C., X. Basagana, C. Seminati, J. de Bont, B. Granum, S. Lyon-Caen, C. B. Manzano-Salgado, I. Pin, A. K. Sakhi, V. Siroux, R. Slama, J. Urquiza, M. Vrijheid, C. Thomsen, and M. Casas. 2019a. "Exposure to phthalate metabolites, phenols and organophosphate pesticide metabolites and blood pressure during pregnancy." *Int J Hyg Environ Health* 222 (3):446-454. doi: 10.1016/j.ijheh.2018.12.011.

Warembourg, C., L. Maitre, I. Tamayo-Uria, S. Fossati, T. Roumeliotaki, G. M. Aasvang, S. Andrusaityte, M. Casas, E. Cequier, L. Chatzi, A. Dedele, J. R. Gonzalez, R. Grazuleviciene, L. S. Haug, C. Hernandez-Ferrer, B. Heude, M. Karachaliou, N. H. Krog, R. McEachan, M. Nieuwenhuijsen, I. Petraviciene, J. Quentin, O. Robinson, A. K. Sakhi, R. Slama, C. Thomsen, J. Urquiza, M. Vafeiadi, J. West, J. Wright, M. Vrijheid, and X. Basagana. 2019b. "Early-life environmental exposures and blood pressure in children." *J Am Coll Cardiol* 74 (10):1317-1328. doi:10.1016/j.jacc.2019.06.069.

Wei, Z., L. Song, J. Wei, T. Chen, J. Chen, Y. Lin, W. Xia, B. Xu, X. Li, X. Chen, Y. Li, and S. Xu. 2012. "Maternal exposure to di-(2-ethylhexyl)phthalate alters kidney development through the renin-angiotensin system in offspring." *Toxicol Lett* 212 (2):212-21. doi: 10.1016/j.toxlet.2012.05.023.

Werner, E. F., J. M. Braun, K. Yolton, J. C. Khoury, and B. P. Lanphear. 2015. "The association between maternal urinary phthalate concentrations and blood pressure in pregnancy: The HOME Study." *Environ Health* 14:75. doi: 10.1186/s12940-015-0062-3.

Wetherill, Y. B., B. T. Akingbemi, J. Kanno, J. A. McLachlan, A. Nadal, C. Sonnenschein, C. S. Watson, R. T. Zoeller, and S. M. Belcher. 2007. "In vitro molecular mechanisms of bisphenol A action." *Reprod Toxicol* 24 (2):178-98. doi: 10.1016/j.reprotox.2007.05.010.

Wiberg, B., P. M. Lind, and L. Lind. 2014. "Serum levels of monobenzylphthalate (MBzP) is related to carotid atherosclerosis in the elderly." *Environ Res* 133:348-52. doi: 10.1016/j.envres.2014.06.009.

Wittassek, M., H. M. Koch, J. Angerer, and T. Bruning. 2011. "Assessing exposure to phthalates - the human biomonitoring approach." *Mol Nutr Food Res* 55 (1):7-31. doi: 10.1002/mnfr.201000121.

Wormuth, M., M. Scheringer, M. Vollenweider, and K. Hungerbuhler. 2006. "What are the sources of exposure to eight frequently used phthalic acid esters in Europeans?" *Risk Anal* 26 (3):803-24. doi: 10.1111/j.1539-6924.2006.00770.x.

Xie, X., T. Deng, J. Duan, S. Ding, J. Yuan, and M. Chen. 2019. "Comparing the effects of diethylhexyl phthalate and dibutyl phthalate exposure on hypertension in mice." *Ecotoxicol Environ Saf* 174:75-82. doi: 10.1016/j.ecoenv.2019.02.067.

Yao, Y., D. Y. Chen, J. W. Yin, L. Zhou, J. Q. Cheng, S. Y. Lu, H. H. Li, Y. Wen, and Y. Wu. 2020. "Phthalate exposure linked to high blood pressure in Chinese children." *Environ Int* 143:105958. doi: 10.1016/j.envint.2020.105958.

Zhang, S. H., Y. X. Shen, L. Li, T. T. Fan, Y. Wang, and N. Wei. 2018. "Phthalate exposure and high blood pressure in adults: a cross-sectional study in China." *Environ Sci Pollut Res Int* 25 (16):15934-15942. doi: 10.1007/s11356-018-1845-1.

Zhao, J. F., S. H. Hsiao, M. H. Hsu, K. C. Pao, Y. R. Kou, S. K. Shyue, and T. S. Lee. 2016. "Di-(2-ethylhexyl) phthalate accelerates atherosclerosis in apolipoprotein E-deficient mice." *Arch Toxicol* 90 (1):181-90. doi: 10.1007/s00204-014-1377-5.

Zhou, W., M. H. Chen, and W. Shi. 2015. "Influence of phthalates on glucose homeostasis and atherosclerosis in hyperlipidemic mice." *BMC Endocr Disord* 15:13. doi: 10.1186/s12902-015-0015-4.

Zoeller, R. T., T. R. Brown, L. L. Doan, A. C. Gore, N. E. Skakkebaek, A. M. Soto, T. J. Woodruff, and F. S. Vom Saal. 2012. "Endocrine-disrupting chemicals and public health protection: a statement of principles from The Endocrine Society." *Endocrinology* 153 (9):4097-110. doi: 10.1210/en.2012-1422.

Zota, A. R., A. M. Calafat, and T. J. Woodruff. 2014. "Temporal trends in phthalate exposures: findings from the National Health and Nutrition Examination Survey, 2001-2010." *Environ Health Perspect* 122 (3):235-41. doi: 10.1289/ehp.1306681.

Chapter 3

Role of Phthalates on Adiposity: Epidemiological Evidence

Cláudia Ribeiro, Joana Araújo and Elisabete Ramos*

EPIUnit - Institute of Public Health,
University of Porto, Porto, Portugal
Laboratory for Integrative and Translational Research
in Population Health (ITR), Porto, Portugal and
Department of Public Health and Forensic Sciences, and Medical Education,
Faculty of Medicine of the University of Porto, Porto, Portugal

Abstract

Overweight and obesity in adults have become a priority many decades ago, however, it remains one of the critical problems in public health around the world. It is also increasingly prevalent in children and adolescents and in the last three decades child obesity rates have tripled to approximately 17% in children aged between 2 to 19 years, and to 32% of overweight and obesity combined.

Phthalates are classified as endocrine-disrupting compounds (EDCs). The EDCs compounds interfere with the endocrine system, and their potential to interfere in metabolic processes regulating and promoting adipogenesis has been described. However, most of the information regarding EDCs potential to promote obesity is based on *in vitro* or animal models and the knowledge regarding their impact on human samples is inconsistent.

Although there are concerns regarding the use of phthalates, its use is highly widespread in products used in daily life such as adhesives,

* Corresponding Author's Email: eliramos@med.up.pt.

In: Phthalates: Environmental and Health Effects
Editors: Müfide Aydoğan Ahbab and Nurhayat Barlas
ISBN: 978-1-68507-970-3

detergents, food packaging, plastic bottles, children's toys, flame retardants, and personal care products including perfume, hair gels, hair sprays, body lotion, deodorant, and nail polish. The concerns over the potential adverse health effects related to phthalates exposure had led to the implementation of legislative procedures to minimize the risks, namely in children's products. These procedures drive the search for alternative compounds such as 1,2-Cyclohexane dicarboxylic acid diisononyl ester (DINCH), however, its impacts on health are still largely uncharacterized.

Therefore, this chapter aims to discuss current developments in phthalates exposures and metabolic health in children and adults. We aimed to summarize the available epidemiological data on this topic, presenting the results through a critical approach to clarify the possible causal relationship between exposure to phthalates and adiposity and its consequences. The five following topics are addressed: Phthalates' chemical structure; Phthalates as endocrine disruptors; Sources of phthalate exposure in human populations; Association between phthalates exposure and obesity; and Association between phthalates exposure and other metabolic alterations.

Keywords: phthalates, adiposity, metabolic alterations

Introduction

Phthalate's Chemical Structure

Phthalates are short-lived pollutants abundantly detected in the environment. They are diesters of 1,2-benzenedicarboxylic acid (phthalic acid) containing one benzene ring and two ester functional groups linked with two consecutive carbons on the ring. They are synthetically produced by the reaction between phthalic acid with different alcohols. Depending on the alcohols used in their production, molecules with different physicochemical properties are obtained (Katsikantami et al. 2016, Giuliani et al. 2020). Phthalate esters (PEs) are classified into two distinct groups, according to the length of their carbon chain: high molecular weight (HMW) phthalates that include those with 5 or more carbon atoms, and low molecular weight (LMW) with 1–4 carbon atoms in their carbon chain (Wang, Zhu, and Kannan 2019).

The water-soluble properties of these compounds decrease with the increasing length of the side chain. As a result, LMW phthalates are more soluble than HMW phthalates (Giuliani et al. 2020). In contrast, fat solubility (lipophilic) increases with the number of carbon atoms in the molecule

(Giuliani et al. 2020, Larsen and Nielsen 2008). Thus, adipose tissue could act as a reservoir for the accumulation of phthalates and their metabolites, especially for HMW phthalates (Larsen and Nielsen 2008, Chiang et al. 2016).

The most common HMW phthalates are diisodecyl phthalate (DiDP), diisononyl phthalate (DiNP), di2-propylheptyl phthalate (DPHP), diisoundecyl phthalate (DiUP), diisotridecyl phthalate (DTDP) and di 2-ethylhexyl phthalate (DEHP). DEHP is among the most abundantly used phthalate ester (Feige et al. 2007) and they are widely used in industry as plasticizers to increase the softness, flexibility, elongation, and durability of rigid polymers such as polyvinyl chloride (PVC) (Katsikantami et al. 2016). LMW phthalates include dibutyl phthalate (DBP), diisobutyl phthalate (DiBP), butyl benzyl phthalate (BBzP), dimethyl phthalate (DMP), and diethyl phthalate (DEP). LMW phthalates are used in PVC products, in medical devices, adhesives, paints, and enteric-coated tablets (Katsikantami et al. 2016). In addition, some of these LMW compounds can also be used in personal care products because of their ability to hold color, denature alcohol, and fix fragrance (Parlett, Calafat, and Swan 2013). These products include fragrances, hair care products (hair sprays, mousses, and gels), deodorants (including antiperspirants), nail polishes, lotions (body lotions, and body creams), skin cleansers, and baby products (oils, lotions, shampoos, and diaper creams) (Koniecki et al. 2011). They are particularly important since they are present in our daily routine.

Phthalates as Endocrine Disruptors

The endocrine system is essential for the regulation of several functions, including growth, development, reproduction, energy balance, metabolism, and body weight regulation (La Merrill et al. 2020). It is part of a complex communication system mostly based on the interaction of hormones with specific receptors. These interactions can be disrupted by exogenous compounds leading to adverse health effects that may impact, not only the individual directly exposed but also the offspring and future generations - a process known as transgenerational inheritance (Lauretta et al. 2019, Kahn et al. 2020). Endocrine-disrupting chemicals (EDCs) are one of those exogenous compounds that may interfere with the synthesis, secretion, transport, metabolism, receptor binding, or elimination of endogenous hormones, altering the endocrine and homeostatic systems (Lauretta et al. 2019). EDCs are now identified as serious and urgent threats to public health since it has been shown that some EDCs exert effects on human health even at lower concentrations (Bateman et al. 2016, Lauretta et al. 2019).

Several studies have pointed out the role of EDCs in the development of obesity and diabetes (Stojanoska et al. 2017, Lauretta et al. 2019). The hormonal activity of EDCs occurs through a variety of mechanisms (Elobeid and Allison 2008). The most commonly proposed mechanism is by direct binding to nuclear receptors like estrogen receptors (ER), androgen receptors (AR), thyroid receptors (TR), progesterone receptors (PR), mineralocorticoid receptors (MR), glucocorticoid receptors (GR), and peroxisome proliferator-activated receptors (PPAR).

Phthalates are among those EDCs with the potential to interfere with adipogenesis and are widely used (Maresca et al. 2016, Stojanoska et al. 2017). A recent paper from Anika Engel et al. (2017) examined the impact of a broad set of phthalates, and their metabolites, on the human steroid receptors ERα, ERβ, and AR by using reporter gene assays. The authors showed that phthalates, but not their metabolites, affect the activity of these receptors, by either stimulating or inhibiting ERα and ERβ activity and inhibiting AR activity (Engel et al. 2017).

Exposure to phthalates during intrauterine life leads to an increased number of adipocytes. There are a variety of data using animal models showing that phthalates can increase adipose tissue mass both during early development and in adulthood (Heindel, Newbold, and Schug 2015). The mode of action is not clear, but the potential of phthalates to act as endocrine receptors binding to nuclear receptors, and, in particular, PPAR receptors is one of the proposed mechanisms (Hao et al. 2012, Huo, Lyons, and Magliano 2016). The PPAR family is composed of three isotypes (PPARα, -β, and -γ), which play important roles in the control of cellular differentiation programs and the transcriptional control of lipid and carbohydrate metabolism (Casals-Casas, Feige, and Desvergne 2008). PPARs are implicated in metabolic disorders, and pharmaceutical compounds have been developed as agonists for PPAR-α (hypolipidemic fibrates) and -γ (insulin-sensitizing thiazolidinediones) to modulate their action through the binding of specific synthetic agonists. It shows how EDCs with the potential to interfere with those receptors may impact adiposity. Moreover, PPAR-γ antagonists are used for the treatment of type 2 diabetes based on the knowledge of their influence on glucose homeostasis via reduction of insulin resistance (Casals-Casas, Feige, and Desvergne 2008, Lind, Zethelius, and Lind 2012).

PPARs are lipid sensors that cooperate in different organs to adapt gene expression to a given metabolic status. Exposure to DEHP promoted fat accumulation and exacerbated obesity in mice expressing human PPARα. Additionally, fetal exposure to MEHP significantly increased the bodyweight of male offspring at postnatal day 60, while these effects were not observed in female offspring (Hao et al. 2012). The metabolites of DEHP such as MEHP, stimulated transactivation of the human PPARα and PPARγ in analogous reporter gene assays, although DEHP itself did not activate these nuclear receptors (Engel et al. 2017).

Phthalates do not interact with androgen receptors directly; their anti-androgenic effects are mediated through PPARα (Corton and Lapinskas 2005, Foster et al. 2001). As decreased androgen activity induces obesity, the anti-androgen effect through PPARα may be a possible mechanism of phthalate-induced obesity (Kim and Park 2014).

The main mechanism of phthalates involved in adipogenesis acts through PPAR-γ function (Elobeid and Allison 2008). PPARγ is a receptor highly expressed in selected extrahepatic human tissues, including adipose tissue, where lipophilic foreign chemicals tend to accumulate (Maloney and Waxman 1999). It is a master regulator of adipocyte differentiation and metabolism, required for adipocyte differentiation, regulation of insulin sensitivity, lipogenesis, and adipocyte survival and function (Lefterova et al. 2014). Therefore, PPARγ controls fat storage in the adipose tissue by promoting the differentiation and the survival of adipocytes (Feige et al. 2007). Many phthalate metabolites such as DEHP, MEHP, DBP, BBP, and MBzP target PPARγ by binding to it directly to activate downstream cascades that lead to enhanced adipogenesis or by increasing PPARγ expression to allow for a lower threshold for activation (Kim and Park 2014, Sonkar, Powell, and Choudhury 2016, Desvergne, Feige, and Casals-Casas 2009, Pereira-Fernandes et al. 2013, Bateman et al. 2016).

The phthalate metabolite MEHP has been found to directly activate PPAR-γ *in vivo* models (Maloney and Waxman 1999) by induction a selective activation of different PPARγ target genes (Feige et al. 2007).

Benzyl butyl phthalate treatment has also been reported to activate PPARγ (Pereira-Fernandes et al. 2014). Yin et al. (2016) showed that BBP promoted the differentiation of *in vitro* 3T3-L1 murine preadipocyte model, through the activation of the adipogenic pathway and metabolic disturbances (Yin et al. 2016). In particular, BBP significantly induced the expression of transcriptional factors C/EBPα and PPARγ, their downstream genes, and several adipogenic proteins in a dose and time-dependent manner (Yin et al. 2016). Moreover, the metabolomic analysis showed that BBP exposure leads to perturbation of metabolites that are associated with glyceroneogenesis and fatty acid synthesis (Yin et al. 2016, Muscogiuri et al. 2017).

Sources of Phthalate Exposure in Human Populations

Phthalates are among the most common synthetic chemicals to which humans are exposed (Stojanoska et al. 2017), due to their diverse applications in plastic-based consumer products, such as building materials (flooring and wall coverings, and electric cables), baby toys, clothing, printing inks, packaging materials, pesticides, personal care and cosmetics products (phthalates are added as fixatives and solvents in perfumes, deodorants, hair sprays, and other products for personal care), pharmaceuticals, as well as medical devices (Giuliani et al. 2020).

Phthalates can enter through several routes such as oral, nasal, and transdermal (Giuliani et al. 2020). Approximately 60% of the ingested phthalates are metabolized within 24 h and their residues are in less than 48 h. The maximum amount of metabolites is excreted with the urine, and may be present in the blood, saliva, feces, amniotic fluid and breast milk (Frederiksen, Skakkebaek, and Andersson 2007, Stojanoska et al. 2017). Due to their lipophilic capacity, they can be stored in adipose tissue and lead to later exposure after adiposity mobilization such as during lactation or weight loss (Regnier and Sargis 2014, Jackson et al. 2017).

Oral exposure by ingestion of contaminated foods or dust is considered to be the main route of exposure, accounting for more than 67% (Giuliani et al. 2020). It is estimated that the total dietary DEHP intake is highest in children followed by adolescents. Katsikantami et al. recently published a cross-sectional study that evaluated seven phthalate metabolites in the hair of 100 pregnant women and showed that the frequent use of plastics for food storage was strongly associated with MEHP exposure (Katsikantami et al. 2020). Although phthalates are physically bound to the plastics, they are not covalently bound to the plastic matrix and they can leak out of products (Cao et al. 2017). So, in addition to dietary exposure, oral intake of phthalates also occurs when children suck, chew or otherwise placed in the mouth toys containing phthalates (Bouma and Schakel 2002, Lyche 2011). Therefore, in 1999 the European Union (EU) restricted the use of certain phthalates (DEHP, DBP, BBP and DiDP) in children's toys and child-care items. In the USA, the use of DiNP in toys is still allowed, which leads to considerable levels of DiNP in children because of mouthing (Kavlock et al. 2002, Lyche 2011).

Consumer and building products made of plastics may also release phthalates into the indoor environment, thereby contributing to the overall exposure (Boberg et al. 2018), mainly from inhalation, and dermal absorption (Wang, Zhu, and Kannan 2019). There are several phthalates present in indoor air, such as DEHP, butyl benzyl phthalate (BBzP) di-n-butyl phthalate (DnBP), di-isobutyl phthalate (DiBP) and DEP (Bornehag and Nanberg 2010). DEHP is the most common phthalate found indoors (Lyche 2011).

Human exposure can also occur through direct dermal contact with clothes, bags, or toys, but also by using cosmetics (Boberg et al. 2018). Dermal exposure may also be an important route of exposure to phthalates, namely DEP and DBP, which are used in many cosmetics. A study in the USA found significantly higher urinary levels of DBP metabolites in women of reproductive age compared with concentrations in males or other age groups (Blount et al. 2000, Lyche 2011), probably due to higher use of beauty products containing DBP. Baby-care products such as lotions, powder and shampoo also represent a relevant dermal route of phthalate exposure for infants (Sathyanarayana et al. 2008, Lyche 2011). A Canadian study that determined phthalate levels in cosmetic and personal care products found that of the 18 investigated phthalates, DEP, DMP, DiBP, DnBP and DEHP were detected (Koniecki et al. 2011). DEP and, to a lesser extent, DnBP were detected more often and at higher concentrations than the other phthalates. DEP was detected in almost all types of products with the highest levels found in fragrances. DnBP was largely present with the highest concentration in nail polish products, however, DnBP was also found in other products such as hair sprays, hair mousses, skin cleansers and baby shampoos at lower concentrations (Koniecki et al. 2011).

Despite its widespread use, information on the labels of products about the presence of phthalates is very scarce, making it virtually impossible for a person to protect themselves. Children are among those with the highest exposure to phthalates, and infants in neonatal intensive care units that are treated with PVC plastic medical devices containing DEHP can be significantly exposed (Boberg et al. 2018).

Results/Discussion

Association between Phthalates Exposures and Obesity

The increasing prevalence of obesity over the last decades is a major concernsince it may potentially compromise the gains in life expectancy achieved in recent years (Heindel and Blumberg 2019). Childhood obesity requires additional attention because of its tracking into adulthood, increasing the risk of a wide range of diseases that despite being diagnosed its adulthood, have their onset during childhood (Hruby and Hu 2015). This effect can be attributed to a complex interaction between genetic and environmental factors (Gruss et al. 2019).

Among the environmental factors, EDCs with the potential to interfere in adipogenesis, such as phthalates, have been considered as one of the potential risk factors. In the last years, three systematic reviews and meta-analyses were published regarding this topic (Ribeiro et al. 2019, Ribeiro et al. 2020, Radke et al. 2019). A study addressing the association between exposure to EDCs and anthropometric measures suggested that phthalates had an overall positive association with obesity, defined by body mass index (BMI) and/or waist circumference (WC), in children/adolescents and adults (Ribeiro et al. 2020). The study from Radke et al. considers that the currently available evidence was inadequate to assess associations between obesity and phthalate exposure. Claudia Ribeiro et al. (2019) pointed out that the inconsistencies found between studies did not allow to reach a definitive conclusion. Nevertheless, most of the results included in those reviews did not reach statistical significance, a positive association between phthalates and adiposity measures was found, especially in adults (Ribeiro et al. 2019). Also, Mohsen Golestanzadeh et al. (2019) showed that most studies confirmed a positive correlation between exposure to phthalates and obesity (Golestanzadeh, Riahi, and Kelishadi 2019).

Swedish Prospective Investigation of the Vasculature in Uppsala Seniors (PIVUS) study and the National Health and Nutrition Examination Survey (NHANES) are the two main data sources that have explored the relationship between BMI and other adiposity measures and phthalates. Lind et al., using the PIVUS study (elderly population), found significant relationships between serum MiBP metabolite and adiposity measures (BMI, WC, and total fat mass) in women aged 70 years or older but not in men (Huo, Lyons, and Magliano 2016, Lind et al. 2012). Using NHANES data, Hatch et al. reported associations of urinary phthalates with BMI and waist circumference which differed by age and sex (Hatch et al. 2008, Zarean and Poursafa 2019). Women were found to have higher levels of all metabolites in urine, but the strongest direct association with BMI was seen among 20- to 59-year-old males for MBzP, MEHHP and MEOHP. For women, BMI was positively associated with MEP but inversely associated with MEHP and MBzP. Regarding MBP, also in the NHANES study, a negative association for older females was found, but the opposite was shown in young males (Hatch et al. 2008). Stalhut et al. showed a relationship between MEP, MBzP and waist circumference in men but not in women (Zarean and Poursafa 2019, Stahlhut et al. 2007). Several other studies have presented significant relationships between urinary phthalates metabolites and BMI in adults (Hatch et al. 2008, Stahlhut et al. 2007, Stojanoska et al. 2017, Buser, Murray, and Scinicariello 2014, Lind, Zethelius, and Lind 2012, Dong et al. 2017, James-Todd et al. 2016, Yaghjyan et al. 2015, Dirtu et al. 2013, Starling et al. 2015, Milosevic et al. 2017, Olsen, Lind, and Lind 2012, Svensson et al. 2011, Peck et al. 2010), but not all of these analyses were adjusted for key covariates such as creatinine (Huo, Lyons, and Magliano 2016, Goodman, Lakind, and Mattison 2014). Other methodological factors make the relationship difficult to understand and compare results, namely a possible age- and gender-dependent association, and some of the studies did not evaluate these interactions, possibly leading to conflicting results (Huo, Lyons, and Magliano 2016, Ribeiro et al. 2019).

In children, the evidence is also conflicting. MEP, the DEP metabolite, was found to be positively associated with BMI among Chinese school-aged children (Wang et al. 2012) and among overweight girls (6–8-year-old) 1 year later in New York City (Huo, Lyons, and Magliano 2016, Zarean and Poursafa 2019, Teitelbaum et al. 2012). Also, for MEP, the NHANES study showed a positive trend of increasing BMI with increasing MEP in 12 to 19-year-olds, but not in other age groups (Hatch et al. 2008). Among Danish 4 to 9-year-old children, the relationship between phthalates and BMI was significant but in the opposite direction (Regnier and Sargis 2014).

Association between Phthalates Exposure and Other Metabolic Alterations

A growing number of *in vitro*, *in vivo*, and epidemiological studies documented not only the link of phthalates exposure with obesity but also with diabetes, and metabolic syndrome and its compounds, which are among the most relevant underlying factors for the development of non-communicable diseases (Stojanoska et al. 2017, Zarean and Poursafa 2019). A positive association has already been shown between phthalates and the development of hypertension and atherosclerosis in adults (Lind and Lind 2011, Lu et al. 2018, Mariana and Cairrao 2020). The available data showed DEHP, DEP and DBP as the phthalates that have the greatest impact on the development of metabolic disorders (Stojanoska et al. 2017).

Recently, two systematic reviews regarding metabolic outcomes and phthalates exposure were published (Golestanzadeh, Riahi, and Kelishadi 2019, Radke et al. 2019). The results from Radke et al. were based on seven studies in adults, including six cross-sectional, three studies in adolescents and four studies in children (Radke et al. 2019). Their results support that phthalate exposure at levels seen in human populations may have metabolic effects, namely the diabetes risk, despite none of the associations in this review reached the level of "robust" evidence (Radke et al. 2019). The single prospective study in adult women (Sun et al. 2014) in this systematic review (Radke et al. 2019) that examined incident diabetes as an outcome, reported strong associations for multiple phthalates (butyl phthalates and total phthalate metabolites) among middle-aged U.S. female nurses (Sun et al. 2014). Additionally, several studies reported associations with insulin resistance (Lind, Zethelius, and Lind 2012, Stahlhut et al. 2007, James-Todd et al. 2012, Huang et al. 2014). When coherence across these outcomes was analyzed, DEHP, DBP, and DIBP had moderate evidence of an association, and DINP, BBP, and DEP had slight evidence of an association (Radke et al. 2019). The data from the NHANES (2001–2008) suggested that urinary PAEs metabolites, such as mono-n-butyl phthalate (MnBP), monobenzyl phthalate (MBzP), mono-isobutyl phthalate (MiBP) and three DEHP metabolites, including mono(2-ethylhexyl) phthalate (MEHP), mono(2-ethyl-5-hydroxy-hexyl) phthalate (MEHHP), and mono (2-ethyl- 5-oxohexyl) phthalate (MEOHP), were positively associated with diabetes among women (James-Todd et al. 2012, Duan et al. 2017). Some studies suggested this association was racial/ethnic-dependent. In a study of phthalates and phthalate-associated insulin resistance, an association was observed in Mexican Americans and African- Americans but not in non-Hispanic whites (Trasande et al. 2013). In another study, phthalates were associated with worse glucose control and more severe insulin resistance in African-Americans and Mexican Americans compared with non-Hispanic whites (Huang et al. 2014). An additional study examining the link between phthalates and Gestational Diabetes Mellitus (GDM) suggested a potentially higher phthalate-associated risk among Asians (Shaffer et al. 2019). According to data from the European Union, it is estimated that five EDCs alone add €18–29 billion annually to obesity- and diabetes-associated healthcare costs (Legler et al. 2015, Sargis and Simmons 2019). So, it is urgent to implement political actions to reduce EDC exposure. Urinary DEHP concentrations were associated with increased insulin resistance in a cross-sectional study of adolescents (Trasande et al. 2013). However, in this study, it is not clear whether insulin-resistant children consume food with higher phthalate content, or insulin-resistant children excrete more DEHP.

The association between phthalate metabolites and cardiometabolic risk factors in children and adolescents such as obesity, hypertension, hyperglycemia, and dyslipidemia was analysed in a meta-analysis by Golestanzadeh et al. (2019) (Golestanzadeh, Riahi, and Kelishadi 2019). A positive association was found with some cardiometabolic risk factors, such as BMI, BMI z-score, and blood pressure both systolic as well as diastolic blood pressure (Katsikantami et al. 2016, Golestanzadeh, Riahi, and Kelishadi 2019), but there are still few data on other specific cardiovascular effects of phthalates (Mariana and Cairrao 2020). However, no consistent information was found between different phthalates and WC, HDL, and TG, as well as birth weight (Golestanzadeh, Riahi, and Kelishadi 2019). Also, Golestanzadeh et al. (2019) concluded that the currently available evidence is still insufficient to evaluate the correlation between phthalate exposure and cardiometabolic risk factors in children and adolescents (Golestanzadeh, Riahi, and Kelishadi 2019).

Conclusion

Scientific, governmental, and public concern exist over the potential adverse human health risks related to ubiquitous exposures to plastic additives, such as phthalates, among the general population. Some legislative actions have been implemented in the European Union regarding the concentration of these compounds, namely in children's products. This has instigated the industry to search for alternative chemicals. Thus, manufacturers have begun to remove HMW phthalates from their products, replacing them with phthalate analogs.

Despite its potential to promote adipogenesis, the association between phthalates and adiposity measures among humans remains unclear since epidemiological studies show inconsistencies that could be explained by methodological limitations. In general, most of the available epidemiological data about phthalates comes from cross-sectional studies making the conclusions prone to bias and reverse causality.

Additionally, studies covering foetal and perinatal life are scarce although these are critical periods of development when environmental factors can permanently change the structure and function of the body, a phenomenon known as programming. So, longitudinal studies covering pregnancy and the early life years are needed to provide a comprehensive understanding of the interaction between genetic and environmental effects on obesity and metabolic-related outcomes.

References

Bateman, M. E., A. L. Strong, J. A. McLachlan, M. E. Burow, and B. A. Bunnell. 2016. "The effects of endocrine disruptors on adipogenesis and osteogenesis in mesenchymal stem cells: a review." *Front Endocrinol (Lausanne)* 7:171. doi: 10.3389/fendo.2016.00171.

Blount, B. C., M. J. Silva, S. P. Caudill, L. L. Needham, J. L. Pirkle, E. J. Sampson, G. W. Lucier, R. J. Jackson, and J. W. Brock. 2000. "Levels of seven urinary phthalate metabolites in a human reference population." *Environ Health Perspect* 108 (10):979-82. doi: 10.1289/ehp.00108979.

Boberg, Julie, Kit Granby, Terje Svingen, and Anne Marie Vinggaard. 2018. "Plastics." In *Encyclopedia of Reproduction (Second Edition)*, edited by Michael K. Skinner, 619-623. Oxford: Academic Press.

Bornehag, C. G., and E. Nanberg. 2010. "Phthalate exposure and asthma in children." *Int J Androl* 33 (2):333-45. doi: 10.1111/j.1365-2605.2009.01023.x.

Bouma, K., and D. J. Schakel. 2002. "Migration of phthalates from PVC toys into saliva simulant by dynamic extraction." *Food Addit Contam* 19 (6):602-10. doi: 10.1080/02652030210125137.

Buser, M. C., H. E. Murray, and F. Scinicariello. 2014. "Age and sex differences in childhood and adulthood obesity association with phthalates: analyses of NHANES 2007-2010." *Int J Hyg Environ Health* 217 (6):687-94. doi: 10.1016/j.ijheh.2014.02.005.

Cao, Y. F., Z. Du, Z. T. Zhu, H. Z. Sun, Z. W. Fu, K. Yang, Y. Z. Liu, C. M. Hu, P. P. Dong, F. J. Gonzalez, and Z. Z. Fang. 2017. "Inhibitory effects of fifteen phthalate esters in human cDNA-expressed UDP-glucuronosyltransferase supersomes." *Chemosphere* 185:983-990. doi: 10.1016/j.chemosphere.2017.07.105.

Casals-Casas, C., J. N. Feige, and B. Desvergne. 2008. "Interference of pollutants with PPARs: endocrine disruption meets metabolism." *Int J Obes (Lond)* 32 Suppl 6:S53-61. doi: 10.1038/ijo.2008.207.

Chiang, H. C., Y. T. Kuo, C. C. Shen, Y. H. Lin, S. L. Wang, and T. C. Tsou. 2016. "Mono (2-ethylhexyl)phthalate accumulation disturbs energy metabolism of fat cells." *Arch Toxicol* 90 (3):589-601. doi: 10.1007/s00204-014-1446-9.

Corton, J. C., and P. J. Lapinskas. 2005. "Peroxisome proliferator-activated receptors: mediators of phthalate ester-induced effects in the male reproductive tract?" *Toxicol Sci* 83 (1):4-17. doi: 10.1093/toxsci/kfi011.

Desvergne, B., J. N. Feige, and C. Casals-Casas. 2009. "PPAR-mediated activity of phthalates: A link to the obesity epidemic?" *Mol Cell Endocrinol* 304 (1-2):43-8. doi: 10.1016/j.mce.2009.02.017.

Dirtu, A. C., T. Geens, E. Dirinck, G. Malarvannan, H. Neels, L. Van Gaal, P. G. Jorens, and A. Covaci. 2013. "Phthalate metabolites in obese individuals undergoing weight loss: Urinary levels and estimation of the phthalates daily intake." *Environ Int* 59:344-53. doi: 10.1016/j.envint.2013.06.023.

Dong, R., T. Zhou, J. Chen, M. Zhang, H. Zhang, M. Wu, S. Li, L. Zhang, and B. Chen. 2017. "Gender- and age-specific relationships between phthalate exposures and obesity in Shanghai adults." *Arch Environ Contam Toxicol* 73 (3):431-441. doi: 10.1007/s00244-017-0441-6.

Duan, Y., L. Wang, L. Han, B. Wang, H. Sun, L. Chen, L. Zhu, and Y. Luo. 2017. "Exposure to phthalates in patients with diabetes and its association with oxidative stress, adiponectin, and inflammatory cytokines." *Environ Int* 109:53-63. doi: 10.1016/j.envint.2017.09.002.

Elobeid, M. A., and D. B. Allison. 2008. "Putative environmental-endocrine disruptors and obesity: a review." *Curr Opin Endocrinol Diabetes Obes* 15 (5):403-8. doi: 10.1097/MED.0b013e32830ce95c.

Engel, A., T. Buhrke, F. Imber, S. Jessel, A. Seidel, W. Volkel, and A. Lampen. 2017. "Agonistic and antagonistic effects of phthalates and their urinary metabolites on the steroid hormone receptors ERalpha, ERbeta, and AR." *Toxicol Lett* 277:54-63. doi: 10.1016/j.toxlet.2017.05.028.

Feige, J. N., L. Gelman, D. Rossi, V. Zoete, R. Metivier, C. Tudor, S. I. Anghel, A. Grosdidier, C. Lathion, Y. Engelborghs, O. Michielin, W. Wahli, and B. Desvergne. 2007. "The endocrine disruptor monoethyl-hexyl-phthalate is a selective peroxisome proliferator-activated receptor gamma modulator that promotes adipogenesis." *J Biol Chem* 282 (26):19152-66. doi: 10.1074/jbc.M702724200.

Foster, P. M., E. Mylchreest, K. W. Gaido, and M. Sar. 2001. "Effects of phthalate esters on the developing reproductive tract of male rats." *Hum Reprod Update* 7 (3):231-5. doi: 10.1093/humupd/7.3.231.

Frederiksen, H., N. E. Skakkebaek, and A. M. Andersson. 2007. "Metabolism of phthalates in humans." *Mol Nutr Food Res* 51 (7):899-911. doi: 10.1002/mnfr.200600243.

Giuliani, A., M. Zuccarini, A. Cichelli, H. Khan, and M. Reale. 2020. "critical review on the presence of phthalates in food and evidence of their biological impact." *Int J Environ Res Public Health* 17 (16). doi: 10.3390/ijerph17165655.

Golestanzadeh, M., R. Riahi, and R. Kelishadi. 2019. "Association of exposure to phthalates with cardiometabolic risk factors in children and adolescents: a systematic review and meta-analysis." *Environ Sci Pollut Res Int* 26 (35):35670-35686. doi: 10.1007/s11356-019-06589-7.

Goodman, M., J. S. Lakind, and D. R. Mattison. 2014. "Do phthalates act as obesogens in humans? A systematic review of the epidemiological literature." *Crit Rev Toxicol* 44 (2):151-75. doi: 10.3109/10408444.2013.860076.

Gruss, S. M., K. Nhim, E. Gregg, M. Bell, E. Luman, and A. Albright. 2019. "public health approaches to type 2 diabetes prevention: the US National Diabetes Prevention Program and beyond." *Curr Diab Rep* 19 (9):78. doi: 10.1007/s11892-019-1200-z.

Hao, C., X. Cheng, H. Xia, and X. Ma. 2012. "The endocrine disruptor mono-(2-ethylhexyl) phthalate promotes adipocyte differentiation and induces obesity in mice." *Biosci Rep* 32 (6):619-29. doi: 10.1042/BSR20120042.

Hatch, E. E., J. W. Nelson, M. M. Qureshi, J. Weinberg, L. L. Moore, M. Singer, and T. F. Webster. 2008. "Association of urinary phthalate metabolite concentrations with body mass index and waist circumference: a cross-sectional study of NHANES data, 1999-2002." *Environ Health* 7:27. doi: 10.1186/1476-069X-7-27.

Heindel, J. J., and B. Blumberg. 2019. "Environmental Obesogens: Mechanisms and Controversies." *Annu Rev Pharmacol Toxicol* 59:89-106. doi: 10.1146/annurev-pharmtox-010818-021304.

Heindel, J. J., R. Newbold, and T. T. Schug. 2015. "Endocrine disruptors and obesity." *Nat Rev Endocrinol* 11 (11):653-61. doi: 10.1038/nrendo.2015.163.

Hruby, A., and F. B. Hu. 2015. "The epidemiology of obesity: a big picture." *Pharmacoeconomics* 33 (7):673-89. doi: 10.1007/s40273-014-0243-x.

Huang, T., A. R. Saxena, E. Isganaitis, and T. James-Todd. 2014. "Gender and racial/ethnic differences in the associations of urinary phthalate metabolites with markers of diabetes risk: National Health and Nutrition Examination Survey 2001-2008." *Environ Health* 13 (1):6. doi: 10.1186/1476-069X-13-6.

Huo, L., J. Lyons, and D. J. Magliano. 2016. "Infectious and environmental influences on the obesity epidemic." *Curr Obes Rep* 5 (3):375-82. doi: 10.1007/s13679-016-0224-9.

Jackson, E., R. Shoemaker, N. Larian, and L. Cassis. 2017. "adipose tissue as a site of toxin accumulation." *Compr Physiol* 7 (4):1085-1135. doi: 10.1002/cphy.c160038.

James-Todd, T. M., T. Huang, E. W. Seely, and A. R. Saxena. 2016. "The association between phthalates and metabolic syndrome: the National Health and Nutrition Examination Survey 2001-2010." *Environ Health* 15:52. doi: 10.1186/s12940-016-0136-x.

James-Todd, T., R. Stahlhut, J. D. Meeker, S. G. Powell, R. Hauser, T. Huang, and J. Rich-Edwards. 2012. "Urinary phthalate metabolite concentrations and diabetes among women in the National Health and Nutrition Examination Survey (NHANES) 2001-2008." *Environ Health Perspect* 120 (9):1307-13. doi: 10.1289/ehp.1104717.

Kahn, L. G., C. Philippat, S. F. Nakayama, R. Slama, and L. Trasande. 2020. "Endocrine-disrupting chemicals: implications for human health." *Lancet Diabetes Endocrinol* 8 (8):703-718. doi: 10.1016/S2213-8587(20)30129-7.

Katsikantami, I., M. N. Tzatzarakis, V. Karzi, A. Stavroulaki, P. Xezonaki, E. Vakonaki, A. K. Alegakis, S. Sifakis, A. K. Rizos, and A. M. Tsatsakis. 2020. "Biomonitoring of bisphenols A and S and phthalate metabolites in hair from pregnant women in Crete." *Sci Total Environ* 712:135651. doi: 10.1016/j.scitotenv.2019.135651.

Katsikantami, I., S. Sifakis, M. N. Tzatzarakis, E. Vakonaki, O. I. Kalantzi, A. M. Tsatsakis, and A. K. Rizos. 2016. "A global assessment of phthalates burden and related links to health effects." *Environ Int* 97:212-236. doi: 10.1016/j.envint.2016.09.013.

Kavlock, R., K. Boekelheide, R. Chapin, M. Cunningham, E. Faustman, P. Foster, M. Golub, R. Henderson, I. Hinberg, R. Little, J. Seed, K. Shea, S. Tabacova, R. Tyl, P. Williams, and T. Zacharewski. 2002. "NTP Center for the Evaluation of Risks to Human Reproduction: phthalates expert panel report on the reproductive and developmental toxicity of di(2-ethylhexyl) phthalate." *Reprod Toxicol* 16 (5):529-653. doi: 10.1016/s0890-6238(02)00032-1.

Kim, S. H., and M. J. Park. 2014. "Phthalate exposure and childhood obesity." *Ann Pediatr Endocrinol Metab* 19 (2):69-75. doi: 10.6065/apem.2014.19.2.69.

Koniecki, D., R. Wang, R. P. Moody, and J. Zhu. 2011. "Phthalates in cosmetic and personal care products: concentrations and possible dermal exposure." *Environ Res* 111 (3):329-36. doi: 10.1016/j.envres.2011.01.013.

La Merrill, M. A., L. N. Vandenberg, M. T. Smith, W. Goodson, P. Browne, H. B. Patisaul, K. Z. Guyton, A. Kortenkamp, V. J. Cogliano, T. J. Woodruff, L. Rieswijk, H. Sone, K. S. Korach, A. C. Gore, L. Zeise, and R. T. Zoeller. 2020. "Consensus on the key characteristics of endocrine-disrupting chemicals as a basis for hazard identification." *Nat Rev Endocrinol* 16 (1):45-57. doi: 10.1038/s41574-019-0273-8.

Larsen, S. T., and G. D. Nielsen. 2008. "Structure-activity relationship of immuno-stimulatory effects of phthalates." *BMC Immunol* 9:61. doi: 10.1186/1471-2172-9-61.

Lauretta, R., A. Sansone, M. Sansone, F. Romanelli, and M. Appetecchia. 2019. "Endocrine disrupting chemicals: effects on endocrine glands." *Front Endocrinol (Lausanne)* 10:178. doi: 10.3389/fendo.2019.00178.

Lefterova, M. I., A. K. Haakonsson, M. A. Lazar, and S. Mandrup. 2014. "PPARgamma and the global map of adipogenesis and beyond." *Trends Endocrinol Metab* 25 (6):293-302. doi: 10.1016/j.tem.2014.04.001.

Legler, J., T. Fletcher, E. Govarts, M. Porta, B. Blumberg, J. J. Heindel, and L. Trasande. 2015. "Obesity, diabetes, and associated costs of exposure to endocrine-disrupting chemicals in the European Union." *J Clin Endocrinol Metab* 100 (4):1278-88. doi: 10.1210/jc.2014-4326.

Lind, P. M., B. Zethelius, and L. Lind. 2012. "Circulating levels of phthalate metabolites are associated with prevalent diabetes in the elderly." *Diabetes Care* 35 (7):1519-24. doi: 10.2337/dc11-2396.

Lind, P. M., and L. Lind. 2011. "Circulating levels of bisphenol A and phthalates are related to carotid atherosclerosis in the elderly." *Atherosclerosis* 218 (1):207-13. doi: 10.1016/j.atherosclerosis.2011.05.001.

Lind, P. M., V. Roos, M. Ronn, L. Johansson, H. Ahlstrom, J. Kullberg, and L. Lind. 2012. "Serum concentrations of phthalate metabolites are related to abdominal fat distribution two years later in elderly women." *Environ Health* 11:21. doi: 10.1186/1476-069X-11-21.

Lu, X., X. Xu, Y. Lin, Y. Zhang, and X. Huo. 2018. "Phthalate exposure as a risk factor for hypertension." *Environ Sci Pollut Res Int* 25 (21):20550-20561. doi: 10.1007/s11356-018-2367-6.

Lyche, Jan L. 2011. "Chapter 48 - Phthalates." In *Reproductive and Developmental Toxicology*, edited by Ramesh C. Gupta, 637-655. San Diego: Academic Press.

Maloney, E. K., and D. J. Waxman. 1999. "Trans-activation of PPARalpha and PPARgamma by structurally diverse environmental chemicals." *Toxicol Appl Pharmacol* 161 (2):209-18. doi: 10.1006/taap.1999.8809.

Maresca, M. M., L. A. Hoepner, A. Hassoun, S. E. Oberfield, S. J. Mooney, A. M. Calafat, J. Ramirez, G. Freyer, F. P. Perera, R. M. Whyatt, and A. G. Rundle. 2016. "Prenatal exposure to phthalates and childhood body size in an urban cohort." *Environ Health Perspect* 124 (4):514-20. doi: 10.1289/ehp.1408750.

Mariana, M., and E. Cairrao. 2020. "Phthalates implications in the cardiovascular system." *J Cardiovasc Dev Dis* 7 (3). doi: 10.3390/jcdd7030026.

Milosevic, N., N. Milic, D. Zivanovic Bosic, I. Bajkin, I. Percic, L. Abenavoli, and M. Medic Stojanoska. 2017. "Potential influence of the phthalates on normal liver function and cardiometabolic risk in males." *Environ Monit Assess* 190 (1):17. doi: 10.1007/s10661-017-6398-0.

Muscogiuri, G., L. Barrea, D. Laudisio, S. Savastano, and A. Colao. 2017. "Obesogenic endocrine disruptors and obesity: myths and truths." *Arch Toxicol* 91 (11):3469-3475. doi: 10.1007/s00204-017-2071-1.

Olsen, L., L. Lind, and P. M. Lind. 2012. "Associations between circulating levels of bisphenol A and phthalate metabolites and coronary risk in the elderly." *Ecotoxicol Environ Saf* 80:179-83. doi: 10.1016/j.ecoenv.2012.02.023.

Parlett, L. E., A. M. Calafat, and S. H. Swan. 2013. "Women's exposure to phthalates in relation to use of personal care products." *J Expo Sci Environ Epidemiol* 23 (2):197-206. doi: 10.1038/jes.2012.105.

Peck, J. D., A. M. Sweeney, E. Symanski, J. Gardiner, M. J. Silva, A. M. Calafat, and S. L. Schantz. 2010. "Intra- and inter-individual variability of urinary phthalate metabolite concentrations in Hmong women of reproductive age." *J Expo Sci Environ Epidemiol* 20 (1):90-100. doi: 10.1038/jes.2009.4.

Pereira-Fernandes, A., C. Vanparys, L. Vergauwen, D. Knapen, P. G. Jorens, and R. Blust. 2014. "Toxicogenomics in the 3T3-L1 cell line, a new approach for screening of obesogenic compounds." *Toxicol Sci* 140 (2):352-63. doi: 10.1093/toxsci/kfu092.

Pereira-Fernandes, A., H. Demaegdt, K. Vandermeiren, T. L. Hectors, P. G. Jorens, R. Blust, and C. Vanparys. 2013. "Evaluation of a screening system for obesogenic compounds: screening of endocrine disrupting compounds and evaluation of the PPAR dependency of the effect." *PLoS One* 8 (10):e77481. doi: 10.1371/journal.pone.0077481.

Radke, E. G., A. Galizia, K. A. Thayer, and G. S. Cooper. 2019. "Phthalate exposure and metabolic effects: a systematic review of the human epidemiological evidence." *Environ Int* 132:104768. doi: 10.1016/j.envint.2019.04.040.

Regnier, S. M., and R. M. Sargis. 2014. "Adipocytes under assault: environmental disruption of adipose physiology." *Biochim Biophys Acta* 1842 (3):520-33. doi: 10.1016/j.bbadis.2013.05.028.

Ribeiro, C. M., B. T. S. Beserra, N. G. Silva, C. L. Lima, P. R. S. Rocha, M. S. Coelho, F. A. R. Neves, and A. A. Amato. 2020. "Exposure to endocrine-disrupting chemicals and anthropometric measures of obesity: a systematic review and meta-analysis." *BMJ Open* 10 (6):e033509. doi: 10.1136/bmjopen-2019-033509.

Ribeiro, C., V. Mendes, B. Peleteiro, I. Delgado, J. Araujo, M. Aggerbeck, I. Annesi-Maesano, D. Sarigiannis, and E. Ramos. 2019. "Association between the exposure to phthalates and adiposity: A meta-analysis in children and adults." *Environ Res* 179 (Pt A):108780. doi: 10.1016/j.envres.2019.108780.

Sargis, R. M., and R. A. Simmons. 2019. "Environmental neglect: endocrine disruptors as underappreciated but potentially modifiable diabetes risk factors." *Diabetologia* 62 (10):1811-1822. doi: 10.1007/s00125-019-4940-z.

Sathyanarayana, S., C. J. Karr, P. Lozano, E. Brown, A. M. Calafat, F. Liu, and S. H. Swan. 2008. "Baby care products: possible sources of infant phthalate exposure." *Pediatrics* 121 (2):e260-8. doi: 10.1542/peds.2006-3766.

Shaffer, R. M., K. K. Ferguson, L. Sheppard, T. James-Todd, S. Butts, S. Chandrasekaran, S. H. Swan, E. S. Barrett, R. Nguyen, N. Bush, T. F. McElrath, S. Sathyanarayana, and Tides Study team. 2019. "Maternal urinary phthalate metabolites in relation to gestational diabetes and glucose intolerance during pregnancy." *Environ Int* 123:588-596. doi: 10.1016/j.envint.2018.12.021.

Sonkar, R., C. A. Powell, and M. Choudhury. 2016. "Benzyl butyl phthalate induces epigenetic stress to enhance adipogenesis in mesenchymal stem cells." *Mol Cell Endocrinol* 431:109-22. doi: 10.1016/j.mce.2016.04.025.

Stahlhut, R. W., E. van Wijngaarden, T. D. Dye, S. Cook, and S. H. Swan. 2007. "Concentrations of urinary phthalate metabolites are associated with increased waist circumference and insulin resistance in adult U.S. males." *Environ Health Perspect* 115 (6):876-82. doi: 10.1289/ehp.9882.

Starling, A. P., L. S. Engel, A. M. Calafat, S. Koutros, J. M. Satagopan, G. Yang, C. E. Matthews, Q. Cai, J. P. Buckley, B. T. Ji, H. Cai, W. H. Chow, W. Zheng, Y. T. Gao, N. Rothman, Y. B. Xiang, and X. O. Shu. 2015. "Predictors and long-term reproducibility of urinary phthalate metabolites in middle-aged men and women living in urban Shanghai." *Environ Int* 84:94-106. doi: 10.1016/j.envint.2015.07.003.

Stojanoska, M. M., N. Milosevic, N. Milic, and L. Abenavoli. 2017. "The influence of phthalates and bisphenol A on the obesity development and glucose metabolism disorders." *Endocrine* 55 (3):666-681. doi: 10.1007/s12020-016-1158-4.

Sun, Q., M. C. Cornelis, M. K. Townsend, D. K. Tobias, A. H. Eliassen, A. A. Franke, R. Hauser, and F. B. Hu. 2014. "Association of urinary concentrations of bisphenol A and phthalate metabolites with risk of type 2 diabetes: a prospective investigation in the Nurses' Health Study (NHS) and NHSII cohorts." *Environ Health Perspect* 122 (6):616-23. doi: 10.1289/ehp.1307201.

Svensson, K., R. U. Hernandez-Ramirez, A. Burguete-Garcia, M. E. Cebrian, A. M. Calafat, L. L. Needham, L. Claudio, and L. Lopez-Carrillo. 2011. "Phthalate exposure associated with self-reported diabetes among Mexican women." *Environ Res* 111 (6):792-6. doi: 10.1016/j.envres.2011.05.015.

Teitelbaum, S. L., N. Mervish, E. L. Moshier, N. Vangeepuram, M. P. Galvez, A. M. Calafat, M. J. Silva, B. L. Brenner, and M. S. Wolff. 2012. "Associations between phthalate metabolite urinary concentrations and body size measures in New York City children." *Environ Res* 112:186-93. doi: 10.1016/j.envres.2011.12.006.

Trasande, L., A. J. Spanier, S. Sathyanarayana, T. M. Attina, and J. Blustein. 2013. "Urinary phthalates and increased insulin resistance in adolescents." *Pediatrics* 132 (3):e646-55. doi: 10.1542/peds.2012-4022.

Wang, H. X., Y. Zhou, C. X. Tang, J. G. Wu, Y. Chen, and Q. W. Jiang. 2012. "Association between bisphenol A exposure and body mass index in Chinese school children: a cross-sectional study." *Environ Health* 11:79. doi: 10.1186/1476-069X-11-79.

Wang, Y., H. Zhu, and K. Kannan. 2019. "A Review of biomonitoring of phthalate exposures." *Toxics* 7 (2). doi: 10.3390/toxics7020021.

Yaghjyan, L., S. Sites, Y. Ruan, and S. H. Chang. 2015. "Associations of urinary phthalates with body mass index, waist circumference and serum lipids among females: National Health and Nutrition Examination Survey 1999-2004." *Int J Obes (Lond)* 39 (6):994-1000. doi: 10.1038/ijo.2015.8.

Yin, L., K. S. Yu, K. Lu, and X. Yu. 2016. "Benzyl butyl phthalate promotes adipogenesis in 3T3-L1 preadipocytes: A High Content Cellomics and metabolomic analysis." *Toxicol In Vitro* 32:297-309. doi: 10.1016/j.tiv.2016.01.010.

Zarean, M., and P. Poursafa. 2019. "The role of environmental disruptor chemicals in the development of non communicable disease." *Adv Exp Med Biol* 1121:21-31. doi: 10.1007/978-3-030-10616-4_3.

Chapter 4

Genotoxic and Mutagenic Effects of Phthalates

Emel Atlı*

Department of Mathematics and Science Education,
Nevsehir Haci Bektas Veli University, Nevsehir, Turkey

Abstract

Phthalates are widely used in industry to make the hard and brittle structure of plastics made of polyvinyl chloride (PVC) soft and flexible. In addition, since it can be used in many different areas such as solvent, lubricating oil, cleaner, it is inevitable for living things to be exposed to phthalates. It has been determined that phthalates have different biological effects on living things due to their large production volumes and widespread use. Although these compounds, which are environmental chemicals, stand out with their endocrine-disrupting properties, it has been determined that they also have genotoxic effects. In this study, the genotoxic and mutagenic effects of phthalates will be summarized.

Keywords: phthalates, genotoxic effects, mutagenic effects

Introduction

Phthalates are a family of industrial chemicals used for various purposes, such as plasticizers that add flexibility and durability to polyvinyl chloride (pvc)

---

* Corresponding Author's Email: emelatli@nevsehir.edu.tr.

In: Phthalates: Environmental and Health Effects
Editors: Müfide Aydoğan Ahbab and Nurhayat Barlas
ISBN: 978-1-68507-970-3

products (Lyche et al. 2009). They are produced by the addition of an excess of branched or normal alcohols to phthalic anhydride in the presence of a catalyst (Peijnenburg, 2008). The most used phthalates are di(2-ethylhexyl)-phthalate (DEHP), diisononyl phthalate (DINP), dimethyl phthalate (DMP), diethyl phthalate (DEP), diisodecyl phthalate (DIDP), benzyl butyl phthalate (BBP), and dibutyl phthalate (DBP) (Erkekoglu and Kocer-Gumusel 2014). The molecular formulas of different phthalates are given in Figure 1 (Paluselli et al. 2018). These compounds, which are used in many products such as personal care products, toys, paints, adhesives, lubricants, furnishings, food packaging nutritional supplements, medical devices (cardiac catheters, endotracheal tubes, some implanted devices, etc.) and building materials, personal care products, electronics, medical devices, have become an inevitable part of modern life (Hannon and Flaws 2015, Liu et al. 2022). Because phthalates are non-covalently bound to plastics, these substances often leach into the atmosphere, soil, and environmental resources such as sediments and natural water bodies (Bergé 2013), and thus organisms are widely exposed to phthalates. Additionally, human exposure is widespread as a result of the ubiquitous use of phthalates in personal care and consumer products. Exposure through ingestion, inhalation, and skin contact is considered important routes of exposure for the general population (Meeker et al. 2009).

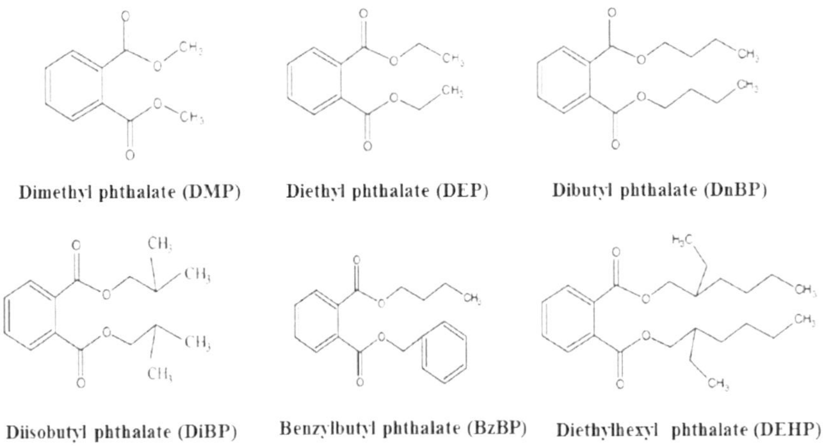

Figure 1. The molecular formulas of different phthalates (Paluselli et al. 2018).

As with many environmental chemicals, phthalates can cause cytogenetic damage in animals and humans. Recent studies have shown that these compounds also have genotoxic and mutagenic effects. Many *in vivo* and *in vitro* test systems such as Ames test, chromosome aberration test, unscheduled DNA synthesis (UDS) test, micronucleus assay, hypoxanthine guanine phosphoribosyl transferase (HGPRT) mutation assay, Comet assay have been used to determine the genotoxic and mutagenic activities of phthalates (Philips et al. 1982, Philips et al. 1986 Kleinsasser et al. 2000, Kleinsasser et al. 2004, Ahbab et al. 2014, Erkekoglu and Kocer-Gumusel 2014, Chang et al. 2017, Karabulut and Barlas, 2018, Balabanic et al. 2021). Before taking a look at these studies, it is useful to get information about these techniques.

Genotoxicity and Mutagenicıty Tests

The Ames test is a method in which mutant strains of *Salmonella typhimurium* containing various mutations in different regions of the histidine operon are used. This test is based on the principle that strains of *S. typhymurium* that lost their histidine synthesizing ability, which was created by artificial mutation, after being treated with the test compound in the presence or absence of mammalian liver post mitochondrial supernatant (S9) containing cytochrome P-450 enzymes, undergo a second mutation and grow in a histidine-free environment. The mutagenicity is determined by counting the self-mutating colonies that allow them to grow in a histidine-free medium (Figure 2). TA-1531, TA100, TA102, or TA104 strains are used to determine point mutations, and TA-1537, TA-1538, TA97a, or TA98 strains are used for frameshift mutations (Mortelmans and Zeiger 2000, Sekeroglu and Sekeroglu 2011, Erkekoglu and Kocer-Gumusel 2014).

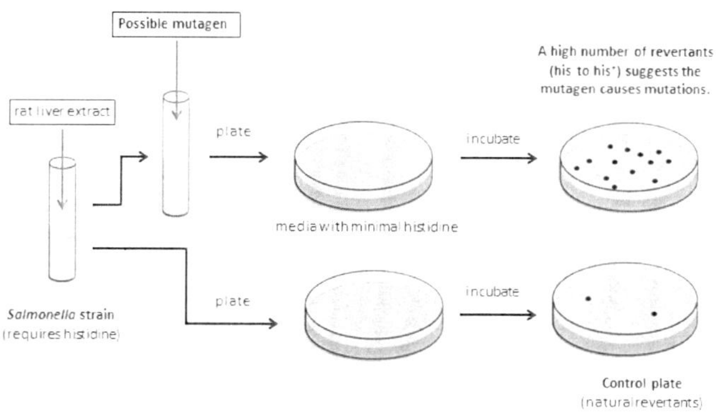

Figure 2. Ames test procedure.

The *in vitro* mammalian cell chromosome aberration test is a method used to induce structural chromosomal abnormalities, such as breaks and exchanges. It can be performed in primary human peripheral blood lymphocytes (HPBL) or established cell lines, such as Chinese hamster ovary (CHO) cells. First, mammalian somatic cells are cultured *in vitro*. Later, the cells are exposed to a test substance, harvested, and stained. Metaphase cells are analyzed microscopically for the presence of chromosome aberrations (OECD 1997, Clare 2012) (Figure 3).

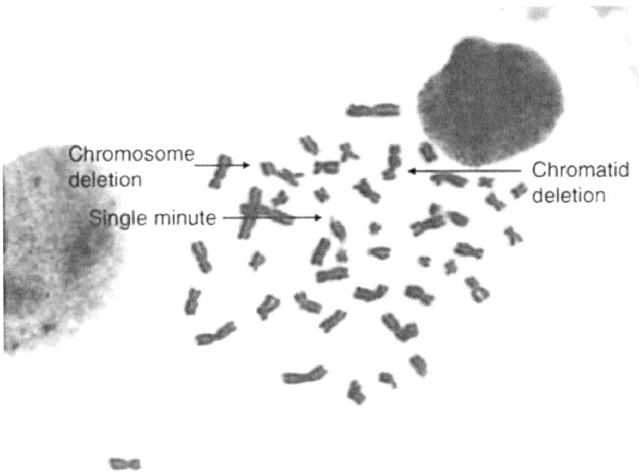

Figure 3. Structural aberrations (Clare 2012).

The *in vivo* unprogrammed DNA synthesis (UDS) test with mammalian liver cells is another method used in genotoxicity studies. The purpose of this method is to identify substances that induce DNA repair after removal of a DNA sequence containing a site of damage in the liver induced by chemical or physical agents. The test is generally based on the incorporation of tritium-labeled thymidine (3H-TdR) into the DNA of liver cells with a low cell frequency in the S-phase of the cell cycle. 3H-TdR uptake is usually determined by autoradiography (OECD 1997).

Micronucleus assays are one of the most frequently used methods in genotoxicity studies because they can be applied *in vitro* and *in vivo* on all cell types. Micronuclei are structures that usually result from deficiencies in genes that control the cell cycle, defects in the mitotic spindle, kinetochore, or other parts of the mitotic apparatus, and chromosomal damage. These structures that emerge during the mitotic division of the cell are formations that are not included in the main nucleus and originate from all chromosomes or acentric chromosome fragments. The increase in the number of micronuclei is evaluated as an indirect indicator of chromosomal irregularities in cells caused by various agents and genomic instability in somatic cells (Fenech 2000, Sekeroglu and Sekeroglu 2011) (Figure 4).

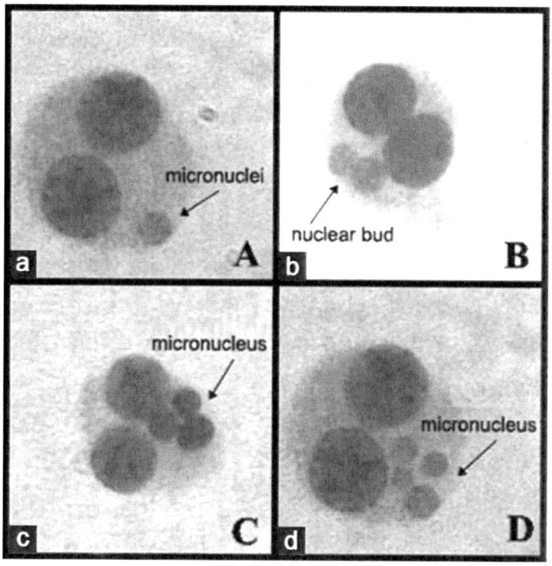

Figure 4. Microscopic view of binucleated cells with 1 MN (a), 2 MNs (b), 3 MNs (c), and 4 MNs (d) (arrows) at × 1000. MN: Micronucleus (Syafudin et al. 2018).

The hypoxanthine (guanine) phosphoribosyl transferase (HPRT) assay is an *in vitro* technique and measures the ability of a test chemical to cause mutations at the hprt locus in mammalian cells. The hprt gene is located on the X chromosome and codes for the HPRT enzyme (Stearns 2007). This assay is based on the detection of mutations that destroy the functionality of the HPRT gene (and/or protein) by positive selection using a toxic analog, and the observation of HPRT mutants as viable colonies (Erkekoglu and Kocer-Gumusel 2014).

The Comet assay (single-cell gel electrophoresis) is a method for measuring DNA strand breaks caused by genotoxic chemicals in eukaryotic cells. Cells embedded in agarose on the microscope slide are lysed with detergent and high salt to form nucleoids containing supercoiled DNA loops attached to the nuclear matrix. While undamaged DNAs do not form comets (tails) in the preparations examined with a fluorescent microscope, since the fragments in damaged DNA molecules have different molecular weights and different electrical charges, they migrate outward from the nucleus by moving at different speeds in the electrical field and form a comet appearance (Figure 5). The comet's density relative to the head reflects the number of DNA breaks (Collins 2004, Sekeroglu and Sekeroglu 2011, Karabulut and Barlas 2018).

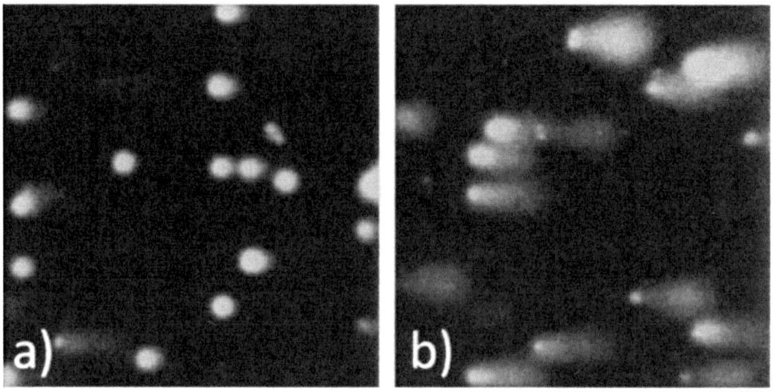

Figure 5. Representative microscopic appearances of the Comet assay. Control cell (a) and DNA- damaged cell (b) (Suzuki et al. 2015).

Genotoxicity and Mutagenicity of Phthalates

The genotoxic and mutagenic effects of phthalates were examined using different tests. In a study investigating the genotoxic effects of phthalates, it was determined that DEHP induced single chromatid aberrations and sister chromatid exchange (SCE) in human lymphocytes. In addition, DEHP induced lymphatic mitotic inhibition and an increase in human lymphocyte doubling time after 4 hours of exposure (Turner et al. 1974). In another study with human lymphocyte cells, DEHP caused chromosome breaks, increase or decrease in chromosome gaps, and decrease in mitotic rate. DEHP treatments also induced polyploidy and aneuploidy in human fetal lung cells (Stenchever et al. 1976).

Seed (1982) evaluated the mutagenic activities of several phthalate esters in an 8-azaguanine resistance assay in *Salmonella typhimurium*. As a result of this study, DMP, DEP, DBP, and DEHP's metabolite 2-ethylhexanol (EH) were found to be mutagenic, while it was determined that phthalate esters such as DEHP, di-n-octyl phthalate (DNOP), diallyl phthalate (DAP), diisobutyl phthalate (DIBP) and DIDP were not mutagenic. In another study, Tomita et al. (1982) examined the mutagenic activities of DEHP and mono-2-ethylhexyl phthalate (MEHP) in bacteria and mammalian cells. MEHP but not DEHP exerted a dose-dependent DNA damaging effect to *Bacillus subtilis* in Rec-assay. DEHP and MEHP showed mutagenic activities to *Salmonella typhimurium* TA-100, with and without S-9 mix, respectively. MEHP caused the mutation in *Escherichia coli* WP2B/r and sister chromatid exchanges (SCE) in Chinese hamster V79 cells. Induction of SCE was thought to be a sensitive reflection of DNA repair-related toxicities. It also induced 8AG/6TG-resistant gene mutations and chromosomal aberrations in the V79 cells. Transplacental administration of DEHP or MEHP to the Syrian golden hamster embryos was carried out by administering DEHP or MEHP to gravid animals on day 11 of gestation, followed by the cultivation of embryonic cells for 15-20 days. Both DEHP and MEHP induced 8AG/6TG-resistant mutation, chromosomal aberrations, and morphological transformation in the embryonic cells of the Syrian golden hamster.

In a study by Philips et al. (1982), DEHP and its major metabolites MEHP, EH, and phthalic acid (PA) were tested for clastogenic activity in cultured CHO cells. Only MEHP was found to cause chromosome damage. In addition, MEHP was found to be ineffective in SCE and HPRT assay in CHO cells. In another study by Philips et al. (1986), MEHP was applied to cells of two culture lines derived from CHO cells and rat liver cells (RL4). Chromosomal aberrations were observed in the cells of both culture lines. In CHO cells, the capability of MEHP to cause chromosome breakage was unaffected by the presence of an exogenous metabolic activation system (S-9 mix) which activates many mutagens. In another study investigating the genotoxic effects of phthalates, DEHP was found to induce SCE in human lymphocytes co-cultured with rat liver cells for 3-6 h (Lindahl-Kiessling et al. 1989).

In a study by Song et al. (2005) to determine the genotoxicities of DEHP and its metabolites, EHA (2-ethylhexanoic acid) and DEP were analyzed using chromosome aberration (CA), sister chromatid exchange (SCE), micronucleus (MN), and single-cell gel electrophoresis. No increase in CA frequency was observed by DEHP and its two metabolites. While DEHP increased the frequency of SCE and MN, EHA only increased the frequency of SCE. DEP increased the frequency of SCE, but the increase was not statistically significant. DEHP and DEP also caused DNA damage. In another study, both chromatid and chromosomal type chromosomal aberrations (break and exchange) were detected in the lymphocytes of B6C3F1 mice after DBP exposures (5000 ppm DBP containing diet for 6 h/day for 16, 32, and 52 weeks) and these aberrations showed marked increases while the week of exposure increased. In the supravital micronucleus test, it was determined that the micronuclear reticulocyte counts increased compared to the control, but this increase was not dependent on time (Kim et al. 2002).

In a study by Huang et al. (2012) to determine the reproductive hazards and genomic alterations of DEHP, it was determined that the testicles of Big Blue® transgenic mice exposed with DEHP for 4 weeks had an approximately 3-fold increase in the frequency of genomic DNA mutations compared to controls. In another study investigating the effects of MEHP on human hepatocellular liver carcinoma HepG2 cells demonstrated MEHP-induced oxidative DNA damage in exposure groups. It was stated that DNA damage occurred because MEHP caused oxidative stress. It is known that oxidative stress is caused by the imbalance between the production of reactive oxygen species (ROS) and cellular antioxidant defense mechanisms, and oxygen-derived free radicals cause DNA damage. (Yang et al. 2012). Recently, Sicińska et al. (2021) investigated the genotoxic potential of some phthalates (DBP, BBP, mono-n-butylphthalate (MBP), mono-benzylphthalate (MBzP)). Phthalates exposures were found to induce DNA single and double strand breaks and more strongly oxidized purines than pyrimidines in human peripheral blood mononuclear cells (PBMCs). It was stated that DNA damage of PBMCs exposed to the tested phthalates and their metabolites may be due to increased ROS production and accumulation.

In recent years, the Comet assay has been frequently used to test the genotoxicity of phthalates. In a study by Anderson et al. (1999), DEHP and MEHP were tested for their potential for genotoxicity in human leukocytes using the Comet test. Both of these chemicals were found to cause an increase in DNA damage. As a result, it was determined that both DEHP and MEHP were genotoxic. Kleinsasser et al. (2000) investigated the genotoxic effects of DBP and diisobutyl phthalate (DIBP) using the Comet assay. Tissue biopsy samples taken during oropharyngeal and lower nasal turbinate surgery were used to prepare mucosal cell cultures. It has been determined that DBP and DIBP are genotoxic and cause significant DNA damage in mucosal cells in all patient groups. A subsequent study by Kleinsasser et al. (2004) used the Comet assay to detect single-stranded breaks and alkali-labile regions of DNA after incubation of human nasal mucosa cells and peripheral lymphocytes with MEHP, the major hydrolysis product of DEHP. MEHP showed a dose-dependent increase of DNA migration in both human mucosal cells and lymphocytes. This effect demonstrated the genotoxic potential of MEHP.

Duty et al. (2003) provided semen samples from 168 subjects to determine whether environmental phthalate levels were associated with altered DNA integrity in human sperm. Semen samples were analyzed for five phthalate metabolites (monoethyl phthalate (MEP), monobenzyl phthalate (MBzP), mono n-butyl phthalate (MBP), MEHP, monomethyl phthalate (MMP) and sperm DNA damage. It was used with the Comet assay to determine DNA damage. As a result, it was determined that only MEP caused DNA damage and other phthalates were ineffective.

In a study on HeLa cells, DEHP was tested for genotoxicity potential using the Comet assay. DEHP was genotoxic above the 90µM dose, as evidenced by significant increases in tail moment. In contrast, DNA strand breaks were not observed at lower concentrations (Park and Choi 2007). In another study by Choi et al. (2010), the genotoxic effects of DEHP on human hepatocyte cells (HepG2) were investigated using the Comet assay. HepG2 cells were exposed to various concentrations of DEHP (0, 2.5, 5, 10, 25, 50, 100 and 250 µM) for 24 or 48 hours. It was determined that DEHP was genotoxic and caused DNA damage. In studies by Erkekoglu et al. (2010a, 2010b), it was reported that DEHP and its main metabolite MEHP caused increases in the Comet assay parameters (tail intensity, tail moment) in LnCAP (human prostatic cell line) and MA-10 Leydig cells (mouse Leydig cells). As a result of these studies, both DEHP and MEHP were determined to be genotoxic in LnCAP and MA-10 cells. In these studies, oxidative stress caused by phthalate applications was shown as the cause of genotoxicity, similar to previous studies. It was emphasized that oxidative stress may have caused DNA damage.

Ahbab et al. (2014) investigated the possible genotoxicity of di-n-hexyl phthalate (DHP) and dicyclohexyl phthalate (DCHP) in male rat pups using the Comet test. Researchers administered DCHP and DHP via gavage to pregnant rats at doses of 0 (control), 20, 100, and 500 µmg/kg/day from gestation day 6 (GD6) to GD19. Male rats were allowed to grow up to different ages after birth. Blood lymphocytes and testis samples from adult male rats were analyzed by the Comet assay. The results showed that tail length, tail density, olive tail moment (OTM), and percentage of DNA present in the tail increased in a dose-dependent manner after DHP was applied. DHP significantly induced genotoxicity at doses of 100 and 500 µmg/kg/day compared to the control; however, it was determined that DCHP did not cause genotoxicity. In a study by Karabulut and Barlas (2018) genotoxic effects of DEHP was tested in blood and sperm samples in male rats using the Comet assay method. For this purpose, the rats exposed to doses of 100, 200 and 400 mg/kg/day DEHP for 28 days. The study revealed that increases in the DNA damage level in both blood lymphocytes and sperm. They were concluded that the tail intensity showed a significant increase in the 100 mg/kg/day, 200 mg/kg/day and 400 mg/kg/day dose groups compared to the control group in blood samples.

Wang et al. (2015) found that exposure of the human embryonic kidney cell line 293 (HEK-293) to DEHP resulted in a significant dose-dependent increase in DNA strand breaks in the Comet assay. The results of this study demonstrated that DEHP exerts DNA damage effects in HEK-293 cells, possibly via the oxidative stress pathway, and that lysosome and mitochondria may be vital targets in DEHP-induced toxicity. Later, it was investigated the genotoxicity and mutagenicity of MEHP using mammalian CHO cells by Chang et al. (2017). It was determined that MEHP exposure increased the production of reactive oxygen species (ROS), which caused genotoxicity. The Comet assay was used to detect ROS-induced DNA damage and it was observed that single strand breaks occurred in cells as a result. It was also detected mutations that were dominated by G:C to A:T and A:T to G:C transitions in the guaninehyoxanthine phosphoribosyltransferase (*gpt*) gene in AS52 cells.

In a recent study, Balabanic et al. (2021) evaluated genotoxic activities of endocrine disrupting compounds, including DMP, DEP, DBP, BBP, DEHP. None of the tested phthalates was genotoxic in *Salmonella typhimurium* (SOS/*umu*C assay). However, phthalate exposures resulted in a statistically significant increase of DNA damage in the Comet assay with human hepatocellular carcinoma (HepG2) cells. The results of this study showed that genotoxicity testing with bacterial models is insufficient and may give misleading results regarding the genotoxic potential of EDCs, including phthalates. The researchers stated that eukaryotic cell lines, especially hepatocellular carcinoma cells of human origin and metabolically active, are a very useful model for the assessment of DNA damage caused by pure chemicals as well as complex mixtures with known and unknown chemicals.

There has been an increase in the presence of phthalates in freshwater and marine ecosystems due to the increased consumption of consumer products such as plasticizers and the inappropriate release of polluted water and wastewater. For this reason, the effects of phthalates on aquatic organisms have also become one of the researched subjects. The effects of DEP on the genetic toxicity of carp were investigated by Zhang and Wang (2014). As a result, it was determined that the percentage of micronucleated erythrocytes and nuclear anomalies increased significantly in DEP treatment groups compared to the control groups. In a study by Benli et al. (2016), it was tested whether 10 mg/L DBP caused genotoxicity in Nile tilapia (*Oreochromis niloticus*) erythrocytes. The results showed that the mean MN frequencies in the DBP treatment group were significantly different from the control and solvent control groups and that DBP had a genotoxic effect. In a similar study, the genotoxicity of DBP was examined in juvenile Nile tilapia (*Oreochromis niloticus*) by the Comet assay. The results showed that there was a significant increase in DNA damage (Khalil et al. 2016). Later, Molino et al. (2019) investigated the genotoxic and mutagenic effects of DEHP in the European sea bass (*Dicentrarchus labrax*) embryonic cell line (DLEC) using the Comet and Cytokinesis-block micronucleus (CBMN) assays. In conclusion, DEHP was determined to cause DNA damage and micronucleus induction. In another study, Boran and Terzi (2019) determined the potential toxic effects of DEHP to larval (72h post fertilization) zebrafish (*Danio rerio*) by analyzing changes in expression levels of stress-related genes (p53, rad51, and xrcc5) by the quantitative real-time polymerase chain reaction (PCR). Some significant differences in the induction of stress-related genes were observed in larvae exposed to DEHP compared to control. Also, there was a concentration-related increase in DNA damage in cells from larvae exposed (96 h) to DEHP. Recently, Jiang et al. (2022) examined the toxic effects of DBP exposure for 7, 14, 21 and 28 days on zebrafish (*Danio rerio*) brain. As a result, it was determined that DBP increased oxidative stress and DNA damage in zebrafish brain and disrupted the expression of antioxidant (*Cu/Zn-sod, gpx*) and apoptosis-related (*caspase-3, p53*) genes of the zebrafish. The results of these studies have shown that exposure to phthalates has potential risks for the healthy development of aquatic organisms and ecosystems, and may cause genotoxic effects in these organisms.

The genotoxic effects of phthalates were also investigated using plants. In a study investigating the genotoxic effects of DEHP, the root tip of *Vicia faba* was exposed to different concentrations (0.01, 0.1, 1, 10 mg•mL $^{-1}$) of DEHP and it was determined that DEHP increased the micronucleus ratio. The types of chromosomal aberrations found were chromatid gaps, chromatid breaks, acentric fragments, and dicentrics (Gao et al. 2009). In a study by Kumari et al. (2021) that used the *Allium cepa* test to investigate the cytotoxicity and genotoxicity of BBP and DBP, it was observed that phthalates significantly reduced the mitotic index (MI) after 24 and 48 hours of exposure. A significant increase in the percent of chromosomal abnormalities was also induced by the phthalates. Additionally, Pietrini et al. (2022) examined the genotoxic effects of DMP on duckweed plants (*Lemna minor* L. and *Spirodela polyrhiza* (L.) Schleid.). The Comet assay in 24 h-treated plants revealed genotoxic damage induced by DMP. These studies with plants showed the negative effects of soil and water pollution caused by phthalates on flora and underlined the need to limit the widespread use of these chemicals.

In some of the studies investigating the genotoxic and mutagenic effects of phthalates, no significant changes were observed. Agarval et al. (1985) tested the mutagenic potential of DMP, DEP, DBP, DEHP, and metabolites of DEHP (MEHP, EH, and PA) in cultures of *Salmonella typhimurium* using the Ames test procedure for base-pair substitution or frameshift-type mutations. As a result, it was determined that these compounds were not mutagenic. Later, the mutagenicity of plasticizers DEHP and MEHP was investigated in vitro using *Salmonella typhimurium* TA102, a strain susceptible to mutations that occur as a cause of oxidative DNA damage. In addition, DNA amplification in Chinese hamster cells transformed with SV40 and DNA damage in rat and hamster hepatocytes were investigated. The two compounds were not genotoxic in any of the test systems (Schmezer et al. 1988).

Elliott and Elcombe (1987) applied DEHP to rat hepatocytes and tested the genotoxic effects of this chemical. As a result, it was determined that DEHP did not cause DNA damage. In another study, DEHP did not induce sister chromatid exchange (SCE) or DNA damage in CHO cells and did not increase the numbers of peripheral blood micronuclei (Douglas et al. 1986). In a study investigating the genotoxic effects of phthalates, DEHP and its two major metabolites, MEHP and EH, were evaluated for their ability to induce chromosomal damage in male Fischer 344 rats after oral administration. All test chemicals (5.0, 1.7 and 0.5 ml/kg/day for DEHP; 0.14, 0.05 and 0.01 ml/kg/day for MEHP; and 0.21, 0.07 and 0.02 ml/kg/day for EH) and control (corn oil) were administered by gavage for five consecutive days. 50 metaphase bone marrow cells of each animal were examined. As a result, no significant increase in chromatid and chromosome breaks or structural rearrangements was noted for DEHP, MEHP, and EH (Putman et al. 1983).

The ability of DEHP to induce DNA damage or repair was examined by Butterworth et al. (1984) *in vivo* and *in vitro* in rat hepatocytes and *in vitro* in human hepatocytes. UDS was measured by incorporation of [^{3}H]thymidine into primary hepatocyte cultures immediately isolated from exposed animals with 12.000 ppm DEHP or hepatocyte cultures incubated directly with 0.1, 1.0 and 10.0 mM DEHP. DNA damage was also measured by alkaline elution of cellular DNA from the same cultures. No chemically induced DNA damage or repair was observed in rat or human hepatocytes *in vivo* or *in vitro* under any of the conditions used.

Müller-Tegethoff et al. (1995) investigated the genotoxic effects of 21 different chemicals and it was determined that DEHP did not induce micronuclei formation in rat hepatocytes. The genotoxic and mutagenic effects of DEHP and its two major metabolites (MEHP and EH) were investigated using both the *Salmonella*/mammalian microsome mutagenicity (Ames) test and the L5178Y TK+/— mouse lymphoma cell mutagenicity assay. DEHP, MEHP, and EH did not exhibit any significant mutagenic activity in strains TA-98, TA-100, TA-1535, TA-1537, and TA-1538 in the Ames test and L5178Y TK+/ — mouse lymphoma cell mutagenicity assay (Kirby et al. 1983). In a study by Zeiger et al. (1985), DEHP was tested for mutagenicity in *Salmonella typhimurium* strains TA98, TA100, TA1535, and TA1537 without metabolic activation and in the presence of rat and hamster liver S-9 metabolic activation systems. No mutagenic activity was observed. In another study, four metabolites of DEHP (MEHP, mono-(2-ethyl-5-hydroxyhexyl)phthalate, mono-(2-ethyl-5-oxohexyl)phthalate, and mono-(5-carboxy-2-ethylpentyl) phthalate) and 3 structurally related derivatives of di(2-ethylhexyl)adipate (DEHA) (mono-(2-ethylhexyl)adipate, mono-(2-ethyl-5-hydroxyhexyl)adipate, and mono-(2-ethyl-5-oxohexyl)-adipate) were tested for mutagenicity in the Ames test using *Salmonella typhimurium* strains TA97, TA98, TA100, and TA102. Concentrations of these compounds up to 1000 μg/plate were negative with all tester strains in the presence or absence of metabolic activation (Dirven et al. 1991).

In a study by Astill et al. (1986) with rat hepatocytes, the effects of DEHP were investigated using different test systems (Ames test, mouse lymphoma activation assay, micronucleus test, UDS, and cell transformation tests) and it was determined that this chemical did not have a genotoxic effect. Similarly, Lee et al. (2019) examined the genotoxic effects of DEHP by Ames test with histidine-requiring *Salmonella typhimurium* (TA98, TA100, TA1535, and TA1537) and tryptophan-requiring *Escherichia coli* (WP2uvrA(pKM101)) strains, chromosomal aberration test with Chinese hamster lung (CHL/IU) cells and micronucleus test with bone marrow cells of CD-1 mice. No genotoxic effect of DEHP was found in any of the test systems used.

In a study by Mckee et al. (2000) to investigate the mutagenic effects of phthalates, DINP was evaluated in the Ames test, in vitro cytogenetics, and mouse micronucleus assays, and DIDP in a mouse micronucleus test. All tests performed gave negative results. As a result, it was determined that none of the tested phthalates were mutagenic. In another study, the genotoxicities of PA and terephthalic acid (TPA) were examined using Ames, chromosomal aberration, and micronucleus tests. In the Ames test, both test chemicals did not produce any mutagenic response on *Salmonella typhimurium* strains TA98, TA100, TA102, TA1535, or TA1537 in the absence or presence of the

S9 mixture. The CA test also showed that PA and TPA did not exert a significant cytogenetic effect on CHO cells. In the mouse micronucleus test, no significant changes in the formation of micronucleated polychromatic erythrocytes were observed in ICR male mice administered these chemicals at all doses (0, 20, 100, 500, 2500, or 12,500 μM/kg). The results of this study using *in vitro* and *in vivo* mutagenic test systems showed that PA and TPA produced no such mutagenic effect (Lee and Lee 2007).

In a study by Okai and Higashi-Okai (2000) to determine the genotoxicity of DEHP, the umu C gene expression system was used in *Salmonella typhimurium* (TA 1535/pSK 1002), which reflects the SOS response to genotoxin-induced DNA damage. DEHP itself had no significant effect on umu C gene expression in test bacteria at 0.5 to 4 mM. However, higher concentrations of DEHP (2 and 4 mM) resulted in weak induction of umu C gene expression in the presence of rat liver S-9 mixture. As a result, it was determined that DEHP had very low or no genotoxicity.

The mutagenic and genotoxic effects of phthalates were also investigated with *Drosophila melanogaster*, which is a frequently used model organism in genetic studies. In comprehensive studies involving 45 different chemicals by Yoon et al. (1985), and 22 different chemicals by Zimmering et al. (1989), the mutagenicity of DEHP was investigated in *D. melanogaster* using the sex linked recessive lethal test. As a result, it was determined that DEHP was not mutagenic. Later, in a study by Kawai (1998), the genotoxic and mutagenic effects of DEHP were examined in *D. melanogaster* using different test systems. In the somatic mutation and recombination test (SMART), no mutagenic effect of DEHP was found. Additionally, somatic DNA damage and DNA double strand breaks were not detected in the DNA repair test. In a study by Fahim et al. (2018), it was investigated the genotoxic effects of DBP and di-octyl phthalate (DOP) at 30μg/ml concentration using the SMART, and these chemicals were determined to be mutagenic.

Conclusıon

There is public concern about phthalates because of their widespread use, including in products for children, and their potential effects on human health. Therefore, the biological effects of phthalates have been examined in many studies. In this context, the genotoxic and mutagenic effects of phthalates were also investigated. In some studies, genotoxic and mutagenic effects were determined, while in others, no effect was observed. However, the results of studies conducted in recent years prove the genotoxic effects of these chemicals. In many European Union countries, the UK and Canada, the use of some phthalates such as BBP, DBP, DEHP, DIDP, DINP, and DNOP in toys, childcare products, and cosmetics are banned and restricted. Considering their harmful biological effects, the use of these chemicals should be banned or restricted all over the world, and less harmful or harmless alternatives should be used.

References

Agarwal, D. K., W. H. Lawrence, L. J. Nunez, and J. Autian. 1985. "Mutagenicity evaluation of phthalic acid esters and metabolites in *Salmonella typhimurium* cultures." *Journal of Toxicology and Environmental Health* 16, no. 1: 61-69.

Ahbab, M. A., Ü. Ündeğer, N. Barlas, and N. Başaran. 2014. "In utero exposure to dicyclohexyl and di-n-hexyl phthalate possess genotoxic effects on testicular cells of male rats after birth in the comet and TUNEL assays." *Human and Experimental Toxicology* 33, no. 3 (March):230–239.

Anderson, D., T. W. Yu, and F. Hincal. 1999. "Effect of some phthalate esters in human cells in the Comet assay." *Teratogenesis, Carcinogenesis, and Mutagenesis* 19, no. 4 (July): 275–280.

Astill, B., E. Barber, A. Lington, E Moran, A. Mulholland, E. Robinson, and B. Scheider. 1986. "Chemical industry voluntary test program for phthalate esters: health effects studies." *Environmental Health Perspectives* 65, (March): 329–336.

Balabanič, D., M. Filipič, A. K. Klemenčič, and B. Žegura. 2021. "Genotoxic activity of endocrine disrupting compounds commonly present in paper mill effluents." *Science of The Total Environment* 794, (November) : 148489.

Benli, A. C., B. Erkmen, and F. Erkoc. 2016. "Genotoxicity of sub-lethal di-n-butyl phthalate (DBP) in Nile tilapia (*Oreochromis niloticus*)." *Archives of Industrial Hygiene and Toxicology* 67, no. 1 (March):25-30.

Bergé, A., M. Cladière, J. Gasperi, A. Coursimault, B. Tassin, and R. Moilleron. 2013. "Meta-analysis of environmental contamination by phthalates." *Environmental Science and Pollution Research International* 20, no. 11 (August): 8057–8076.

Boran, H., and S. Terzi. 2019. "Bis(2-ethylhexyl) phthalate induces DNA strand breaks and gene expression alterations in larval zebrafish *Danio rerio*." *Toxicology and Industrial Health* 35, no. 8 (August): 520-529.

Butterworth, B. E., E. Bermudez, T. Smith-Oliver, L. Earle, R. Cattley, J. Martin, J. A. Popp, S. Strom, R. Jirtle, and G. Michalopoulos. 1984. "Lack of genotoxic activity of di(2-ethylhexyl)phthalate (DEHP) in rat and human hepatocytes." *Carcinogenesis* 5, no. 10 (October): 1329–1335.

Chang, Y. J., C. Y. Tseng, P. Y. Lin, Y. C. Chuang, and M. W. Chao. 2017. "Acute exposure to DEHP metabolite, MEHP cause genotoxicity, mutagenesis and carcinogenicity in mammalian Chinese hamster ovary cells." *Carcinogenesis* 38, no. 3 (March): 336–345.

Choi, S, S. Y. Park, J. Jeong, E. Cho, S. Phark, M. Lee, D. Kwak, J. Y. Lim, W. W. Jung, and D. Sul. 2010. "Identification of toxicological biomarkers of di(2-ethylhexyl) phthalate in proteins secreted by HepG2 cells using proteomic analysis." *Proteomics* 10, no. 9 (May):1831–1846.

Clare, G. 2012. "The in vitro mammalian chromosome aberration test." In *Methods in Molecular Biology*, edited by J. Parry and E.Parry, 69–91. New York : Springer. https://doi.org/10.1007/978-1-61779-421-6_5.

Collins, A. R. 2004. "The comet assay for DNA damage and repair: principles, applications, and limitations." *Molecular Biotechnology* 26, no. 3 (March): 249–261.

Dirven, H. A. A. M., J. L. G. Theuws, F. J. Jongeneelen, and R. P. Bos. 1991. "Non-mutagenicity of 4 metabolites of di(2-ethylhexyl)phthalate (DEHP) and 3 structurally related derivatives of di(2-ethylhexyl)adipate (DEHA) in the *Salmonella* mutagenicity assay." *Mutation Research/Genetic Toxicology* 260, no. 1 (May): 121-130.

Douglas, G. R., A. P. Hugenholtz, and D. H. Blakey. 1986. "Genetic toxicology of phthalate esters: mutagenic and other genotoxic effects." *Environmental Health Perspectives* 65, no. 1 (March):255–262.

Duty, S. M., N. P. Singh, M. J. Silva, D. B. Barr, J. W. Brock, L. Ryan, R. F. Herrick, D. C. Christiani, and R. Hauseret. 2003. "The relationship between environmental exposures to phthalates and DNA damage in human sperm using the neutral Comet assay." *Environmental Health Perspectives* 111, no. 9 (July): 1164–1169.

Elliott, B. M., and C. R. Elcombe. 1987. "Lack of DNA damage or lipid peroxidation measured *in vivo* in the rat liver following treatment with peroxisomal proliferators." *Carcinogenesis* 8, no. 9 (September):1213–1218.

Erkekoglu P, W. Rachidi, V. De Rosa, B. Giray, A. Favier, and F. Hincal. 2010a. "Protective effect of selenium supplementation on the genotoxicity of di(2-ethylhexyl) phthalate and mono(2-ethylhexyl) phthalate treatment in LNCaP cells." *Free Radical Biology and Medicine* 49, no. 4 (August): 559–566.

Erkekoglu, P. and B. Kocer-Gumusel. 2014. "Genotoxicity of phthalates." *Toxicology Mechanisms and Methods* 24, no. 9 (September) : 616-626.

Erkekoglu, P., W. Rachidi, O. G. Yuzugullu, B. Giray, A. Favier, M. Ozturk, F. Hincal. 2010b. "Evaluation of cytotoxicity and oxidative DNA damaging effects of di(2-ethylhexyl)-phthalate (DEHP) and mono(2-ethylhexyl)-phthalate (MEHP) on MA-10 Leydig cells and protection by selenium." *Toxicology and Applied Pharmacology* 248, no. 1 (October): 52-62.

Fahim, H., N. Alsonosy, M. Khallaf, Y. Abdeldaim, and H. Elsheshetawy. 2018. "Genetic effect of migratory compounds from bottled natural drinking water stored under direct sunlight." *Arab Universities Journal of Agricultural Sciences* 26, no. 2C (May) :1907-1916.

Fenech, M. 2000. "The in vitro micronucleus technique. " *Mutation Research* 455, no. 1-2 (November): 81–95.

Gao, N., Q. Chang, Y. Zheng and S. Ding. 2009. "Effects of di-(2-ethylhexyl) phthalate on root tips of *Vicia faba* seedlings." Paper presented at *3rd International Conference on*

Bioinformatics and Biomedical Engineering, Beijing, China, June 11-13, 2009. https://doi.org/10.1109/ICBBE.2009.5162735.

Hannon, P. R., and J. A. Flaws. 2015. "The effects of phthalates on the ovary." *Frontiers in Endocrinology* 6, no. 8 (February): 1-9.

Huang, X. F., Y. Li, Y. H. Gu, M. Liu, Y. Xu, Y. Yuan, F. Sun, H. Q. Zhang, and H. J. Shi. 2012. "The Effects of di-(2-ethylhexyl)-phthalate exposure on fertilization and embryonic development in vitro and testicular genomic mutation *in vivo*." *PLoS ONE* 7, no. 11 (November): e50465.

Jiang, N., P. Song, X. Li, L. Zhu, J. Wang, X. Yin, and J. Wang. 2022. "Dibutyl phthalate induced oxidative stress and genotoxicity on adult zebrafish (*Danio rerio*) brain." *Journal of Hazardous Materials* 424, (February): 127749.

Karabulut, G., and N. Barlas. 2018. "A dose–response study following in vivo exposure to di(2-ethylhexyl)-phthalate (DEHP): Genotoxic, histologic, immunohistochemical, morphometric and hormonal effects on reproductive systems in pre-pubertal male rats." *Toxicology Research* 7, no. 5 (September): 859-873.

Kawai, K. 1998. "Enhancement of the DNA damaging activity of N-nitrosodimethylamine by di-(2-ethylhexyl) phthalate in somatic cells *in vivo* of *Drosophila melanogaster*." *Biological and Pharmaceutical Bulletin* 21, no. 6 (June): 579-582.

Khalil, S. R., Y. Abd Elhakim, and A. E. El-Murr. 2016. "Sublethal concentrations of di-n-butyl phthalate promote biochemical changes and DNA damage in juvenile Nile tilapia (*Oreochromis niloticus*)." *The Japanese Journal of Veterinary Research* 64, no. 1 (February): 67-80.

Kim, M. Y., Y. C. Kim, and M. H. Cho. 2002. "Combined treatment with 4-(N-methyl-N-nitrosamino)-1-(3-pyridyl)-1-butanone and dibutyl phthalate enhances ozone-induced genotoxicity in B6C3F1 mice." *Mutagenesis* 17, no. 4 (July): 331–336.

Kirby, P. E., R. F.Pizzarello, T. E Lawlor, S. R. Haworth, and J. R. Hodgson. 1983. "Evaluation of di-(2-ethylhexyl) phthalate and its major metabolites in the Ames test and L5178Y mouse lymphoma mutagenicity assay." *Environmental Mutagenesis* 5: 657-663.

Kleinsasser, N. H., E. R. Kastenbauer, H. Weissacher, R. K. Muenzenrieder, and U. A. Harréus. 2000. "Phthalates demonstrate genotoxicity on human mucosa of the upper aerodigestive tract." *Environmental and Molecular Mutagenesis* 35, no. 1 (February): 9–12.

Kleinsasser, N. H., U. A. Harréus, E. R. Kastenbauer, B. C. Wallner, A. W. Sassen, R. Staudenmaier, and A. W. Rettenmeier. 2004. "Mono(2-ethylhexyl)phthalate exhibits genotoxic effects in human lymphocytes and mucosal cells of the upper aerodigestive tract in the comet assay." *Toxicology Letters* 148, no. 1-2 (March): 83-90.

Kumari, A., S. Arora, and R. Kaur. 2021. "Comparative cytotoxic and genotoxic potential of benzyl-butyl phthalate and di-n-butyl phthalate using *Allium cepa* assay." *Energy, Ecology and Environment* 6, no. 3 (September): 244–257.

Lee, J. W., S. J. Lee, M. C. Gye, and E. Y. Moon. 2019. "Genotoxicity and glucose tolerance induction by acetyltriethylcitrate, substitute plasticizer compared to di(2-ethylhexyl)phthalate." *Scientific Reports* 9, (August): 12237.

Lee, K. H., and B. M. Lee. 2007. "Study of mutagenicities of phthalic acid and terephthalic acid using *in vitro* and *in vivo* genotoxicity tests." *Journal of Toxicology and Environmental Health A* 70, (July):1329–1335.

Lindahl-Kiessling, K., I. Karlberg, and A. M. Olofsson. 1989. "Induction of sister-chromatid exchanges by direct and indirect mutagens in human lymphocytes, co-cultured with intact rat liver cells. Effect of enzyme induction and preservation of the liver cells by freezing in liquid nitrogen. " *Mutation Research* 211, no. 1 (March):77–87.

Liu, M., L. Zhao, L. L. Liu, W.T. Guo, H. H. Yang, S. Chen, J. Yu, M. Li, Q. Fang, X. F. Lai, L. L. Yang, R. Zhu, and X. M. Zhang. 2022. "Urinary phthalate metabolites mixture, serum cytokines and renal function in children: a panel study." *Journal of Hazardous Materials* 422, no : 2 (January): 126963.

Lyche, J. L., A. C. Gutleb, A. Bergman, G. S. Eriksen, A. J. Murk, E. Ropstad, M. Saunders, and J. U. Skaare. 2009. "Reproductive and developmental toxicity of phthalates." *Journal of Toxicology and Environmental Health, Part B* 12, no. 4 (August): 225-249.

McKee, R. H., R. T. Przygoda, M. A. Chirdon, G. Engelhardt, and M. Stanley. 2000. "Di(isononyl) phthalate (DINP) and di(isodecyl) phthalate (DIDP) are not mutagenic." *Journal of Applied Toxicology* 20, no. 6 (November): 491–497.

Meeker, J. D., S. Sathyanarayana, and S. H. Swan. 2009. "Phthalates and other additives in plastics: human exposure and associated health outcomes." *Philosophical Transactions of the Royal Society of London. Series B, Biological Sciences* 364, no. 1526 (July): 2097–2113.

Molino, C., S. Filippi, G. A. Stoppiello, R. Meschini, and D. Angeletti. 2019. "In vitro evaluation of cytotoxic and genotoxic effects of Di(2-ethylhexyl)-phthalate (DEHP) on European sea bass (*Dicentrarchus labrax*) embryonic cell line." *Toxicology in Vitro* 56, no. 3 (April): 118-125.

Mortelmans, K., and E. Zeiger. 2000. "The Ames Salmonella/microsome mutagenicity assay." *Mutation Research* 455, no. 1-2 (November): 29–60.

Müller-Tegethoff, K., P. Kasper, and L. Müller. 1995. "Evaluation studies on the in vitro rat hepatocyte micronucleus assay." *Mutation Research* 335, no. 3 (December): 293–307.

OECD. 1997. "Test No. 473: In vitro Mammalian Chromosome Aberration Test." In *OECD Guidelines for the Testing of Chemicals*, Paris: OECD Publishing. https://doi.org/10.1787/9789264071261-en.

OECD. 1997. "Test No. 486: Unscheduled DNA Synthesis (UDS) Test with Mammalian Liver Cells *in vivo*." In *OECD Guidelines for the Testing of Chemicals*, Paris: OECD Publishing. https://doi.org/10.1787/9789264071520-en.

Okai, Y., and K. Higashi-Okai. 2000. "Enhancing effect of a plastic plasticizer, di-2-ethylhexyl phthalate on umu C gene expression in *Salmonella typhimurium* (TA 1535/pSK 1002)." *Journal of University of Occupational and Environmental Health* 22, no. 4 (December): 305-315.

Park, S. Y., and J. Choi. 2007. "Cytotoxicity, genotoxicity and ecotoxicity assay using human cell and environmental species for the screening of the risk from pollutant exposure." *Environment International* 33, no. 6 (August): 817–822.

Peijnenburg, W. J. G. M. 2008. "Phthalates." In *Encyclopedia of Ecology,* edited by S. E. Jørgensen and B. D. Fath, 2733-2738. Amsterdam: Academic Press. https://doi.org/10.1016/B978-008045405-4.00419-5.

Phillips, B. J., D Anderson, S. D. Gangolli. 1986. "Studies on the genetic effects of phthalic acid esters on cells in culture." *Environmental Health Perspectives* 65, no. 1 (March):263–266.

Phillips, B. J., T. E. James, and S. D. Gangolli. 1982. "Genotoxicity studies of di(2-ethylhexyl)phthalate and its metabolites in CHO cells." *Mutation Research* 102, no. 3 (October):297–304.

Pietrini, F., V. Iannilli, L. Passatore, S. Carloni, G. Sciacca, M. Cerasa, and M. Zacchini. 2022. "Ecotoxicological and genotoxic effects of dimethyl phthalate (DMP) on *Lemna minor* L. and *Spirodela polyrhiza* (L.) Schleid. plants under a short-term laboratory assay." *Science of The Total Environment* 806, no. 4 (February): 150972.

Putman, D. L., W.A. Moore, L.M. Schechtman, and J. R. Hodgson. 1983. "Cytogenetic evaluation of di-(2-ethylhexyl) phthalate and its major metabolites in fischer 344 rats." *Environmental and Molecular Mutagenesis* 5: 227-231.

Schmezer, P., B. L. Pool, R. G. Klein, D. Komitowski, and D. Schmähl. 1988. "Various short-term assays and two long-term studies with the plasticizer di(2-ethyl-hexyl)phthalate in the Syrian golden hamster." *Carcinogenesis* 9, no. 1 (January): 37-43.

Seed, J. L. 1982. "Mutagenic activity of phthalate esters in bacterial liquid suspension assays." *Environmental Health Perspectives* 45, (November): 111-114.

Sekeroglu, Z. A., and V. Sekeroglu. 2011. "Genetik toksisite testleri." *TUBAV Bilim Dergisi* 4, no. 3 (September): 221-229.

Sicińska, P., K. Mokra, K. Wozniak, J. Michałowicz, and B. Bukowska. 2021. "Genotoxic risk assessment and mechanism of DNA damage induced by phthalates and their metabolites in human peripheral blood mononuclear cells." *Scientific Reports* 11, no. 1 (January): 1658-1670.

Song, J. Y., Y. H. Cho, Y. J. Kim, and H. W. Chung. 2005. "Genotoxicity of di-2-ethylhexyl phthalate, 2-ethylhexanoic acid and di-2-ethyl phthalate in human lymphocytes *in vitro*." *Environmental Mutagens and Carcinogens* 25, no. 3 (September): 110-117.

Stearns, D. M. 2007. "Evaluation of chromium (III) genotoxicity with cell culture and in vitro assays." In *The Nutritional Biochemistry of Chromium (III),* edited by J. B. Vincent, 209-224. Elsevier. https://doi.org/10.1016/B978-044453071-4/50011-4.

Stenchever, M. A., M. A. Allen, L. Jerominski, and R.V. Petersen. 1976. "Effects of bis(2-ethylhexyl) phthalate on chromosomes of human leukocytes and human fetal lung cells." *Journal of Pharmaceutical Sciences* 65, no. 11 (November):1648–1651.

Suzuki, Y., N. Ohta, Y. Takahashi, S. Shibata, S. Kakehata, and Y. Okamoto. 2015. "Pharmacodynamics of anti-inflammatory drugs–intranasal corticosteroid and DNA damage." In *Recent Advances in Rhinosinusitis and Nasal Polyposis,* edited by H. Kawauchi, D. Passali, R. Mladina, A. Lopatin and D. Zabolotnyi, 117-126. Amsterdam: Kugler Publications.

Syaifudin, M., V. P. Defiyandra, S. Nurhayati, S. Purnami, and E. Pudjadi. 2018. "Micronucleus assay-based evaluation of radiosensitivity of lymphocytes among inhabitants living in high background radiation area of Mamuju, West Sulawesi, Indonesia." *Genome Integrity* 9, no. 2 (May): 1-5.

Tomita, I., Y. Nakamura, N. Aoki, and N. Inui. 1982. "Mutagenic/carcinogenic potential of DEHP and MEHP." *Environmental Health Perspectives* 45, (November): 119-125.

Turner, J. H., J. C. Petricciani, M. L. Crouch, and S. Wenger. 1974. "An evaluation of the effects of diethylhexyl phthalate (DEHP) on mitotically capable cells in blood packs. " *Transfusion* 14, no. 6 (December): 560–566.

Wang, X., L. Jiang, L. Ge, M. Chen, G. Yang, F. Ji, L. Zhong, Y. Guan, and X. Liu. 2015. "Oxidative DNA damage induced by di-(2-ethylhexyl) phthalate in HEK-293 cell line." *Environmental Toxicology and Pharmacology* 39, no. 3 (May):1099-1106.

Wikipedia. 2022. *Ames Test*. https://en.wikipedia.org/wiki/Ames_test.

Yang, G., X. Zhou, J. Wang, W. Zhang, H. Zheng, W. Lu, J. Yuan. 2012. "MEHP-induced oxidative DNA damage and apoptosis in HepG2 cells correlates with p53-mediated mitochondria-dependent signaling pathway." *Food and Chemical Toxicology* 50, no. 7 (July): 2424-2431.

Yoon, J. S., J. M. Mason, R. Valencia, R. C. Woodruff, and S. Zimmering. 1985. "Chemical mutagenesis testing in *Drosophila*. IV. Results of 45 coded compounds tested for the national toxicology program." *Environmental Mutagenesis* 7, no. 3 (January): 349-367.

Zeiger, E., S. Haworth, K. Mortelmans, and W. Speck. 1985. "Mutagenicity testing of di(2-ethylhexyl)phthalate and related chemicals in *Salmonella*." *Environmental Mutagenesis* 7, no. 2: 213–232.

Zhang, G., and Y. Wang. 2014. "Genotoxic effects of diethyl phthalate on the non-specific immune function of carp." *Toxin Reviews* 33, no. 4 (March): 139-145.

Zimmering, S., J. M. Mason, and R. Valencia. 1989. "Chemical mutagenesis testing in *Drosophila*. VII. Results of 22 coded compounds tested in larval feeding experiments." *Environmental and Molecular Mutagenesis* 14, no. 4 (January): 245-251.

Chapter 5

Are Phthalates Diabetogenic Chemicals?

Fulya Dal Yöntem[1]
and Müfide Aydoğan Ahbab[2,*]
[1]Koç University, Faculty of Medicine,
Department of Biophysics, Istanbul, Turkey
[2]University of Health Sciences Turkey,
Hamidiye Vocational School of Health Services,
Istanbul, Turkey

Abstract

Diabetes mellitus is a chronic metabolic disorder caused by interaction of genetics and environmental factors resulted high blood glucose levels. The global prevalence of diabetes is ascending, and the evidence suggests a positive relationship between diabetes and human exposure to phthalates. Phthalates are a group of plasticizers used for plastic material production. The epidemiological and experimental studies indicate that phthalate metabolites are associated with oxidative stress, loss of beta cells, impaired insulin secretion, disrupted insulin signaling pathway and altered glucose metabolism. Indeed, some phthalate metabolites were found to be associated with reduced insulin sensitivity, increased insulin resistance and inflammatory cytokines. There is limited research indicating that maternal phthalate exposure might be a risk factor for glucose intolerance and gestational diabetes. Moreover, prenatal and/or lactational exposure to phthalate metabolites might cause high blood glucose levels with reduced insulin levels, reduction in pancreatic beta cell mass and epigenetic changes in genes related to beta cell development in offspring. Thus, phthalates can be a potential risk factor

---

* Corresponding Author's Email: mufideaydogan.ahbab@sbu.edu.tr

In: Phthalates: Environmental and Health Effects
Editors: Müfide Aydoğan Ahbab and Nurhayat Barlas
ISBN: 978-1-68507-970-3

to promote diabetes mellitus. Further prospective and experimental studies are needed to confirm this potential mode of action implicating phthalates in the rising rates of diabetes.

Keywords: phthalates, diabetes mellitus, glucose homeostasis, insulin resistance, endocrine disrupting chemicals

Introductıon

In the last 50 years, as the technology and modern production techniques developed, various chemicals have been widely produced and released to the environment to be used in multiple products, especially in increasing agricultural production. These chemicals, which are banned in most countries because they cause serious adverse effects on human and natural life, include mainly herbicides, fungicides, insecticides, plasticizers, polychlorinated biphenyls and alkylphenolic compounds. Recent studies have shown that these chemicals, which are still in use and commonly found in the environment, cause significant reproductive problems in humans and animals, attracting considerable attention among the scientific world and the public. Numerous studies showed that there has been a decline in human semen quality over the last 50-70 years (Carlsen et al. 1992, Toppari et al. 1996). The fact that similar reproductive problems are observed in many wildlife species suggests that these problems arise due to the increased use of chemicals released into the environment because of industrial production (Toppari et al. 1996).

Humans and wildlife are exposed to various chemical agents and many of them are ubiquitous and short-lived chemicals in the environment. Increased scientific evidence shows that some of the environmental chemicals, which are natural or human made, disrupt the endocrine system of human or wildlife by interfering with hormonal homeostasis (Chang et al. 2021). These chemicals are called as endocrine disrupting chemicals/agents (EDCs) and/or endocrine disruptors which cause adverse health effects even at very low concentrations. EDCs can mimic or block hormone action in various ways, either by directly activating or inactivating hormone receptors or by disrupting the synthesis of hormones (Giulivo et al. 2016).

EDCs are quite diverse, including chlorinated pesticides, polychlorinated biphenyls and dioxins, compounds associated with plastics production like bisphenol A (BPA) and phthalates. Of all known chemicals, almost 1000 chemicals are thought to be potential endocrine disruptors (Street et al. 2018).

EDCs are classified as persistent chemicals, such as PCBs, and non-persistent chemicals, such as BPA and phthalates (Song et al. 2016). Among EDCs, it is now well-known that phthalates have the capacity to act as endocrine disruptors (Monneret 2017, Fénichel and Chevalier 2017). In addition to teratogenic, mutagenic, and carcinogenic effects of phthalates on cells and animals, exposure to several phthalates and their metabolites have been shown to interfere with the endocrine system and cause reproductive toxicity in *in vivo* studies (Mylchreest et al. 2002, Foster 2005, Foster 2006, Saillenfait et al. 2008, Saillenfait et al. 2013, Shi et al. 2019). Recently, it has been suggested that phthalates, which have various adverse effects on the reproductive system, may also have an effect on metabolic homeostasis suggesting that exposure to phthalates could be a risk of diabetes (Svensson et al. 2011). In this chapter, the relationship between phthalates and diabetes risk will be discussed.

Phthalates

Phthalates are diesters of phthalic acids used widely as plasticizers and additives in the manufacture of plastic materials (Net et al. 2015). They are used in industries as solvents, plasticizers, and additives in polyvinyl chloride (PVC) plastics or personal care and consumer products used in food packaging materials. Besides they can be found in medical devices, tubes, and bags. Phthalates make the rigid plastic materials flexible (Latini 2005). They release from the plastic overtime because of their non-covalent nature and disperse easily throughout the ecosystem (Latini 2005, Nam et al. 2020).

Phthalates can be classified by their molecular weight and carbon chain length of subgroups (Wu et al. 2017) (Table 1). Low-molecular weight (LMW) phthalates have 1-6 carbon atom chain length and are usually used in the production of personal care and cosmetic products such as nail polish and fragrances. DMP, DEP, DBP and BBP are well-known LMW phthalates. High-molecular weight (HMW) phthalates have 7 and more carbon atom chain length in their subgroups. HMW phthalates are especially used in the industry to produce rigid polymers to make them more flexible and elastic such as PVC. The most widely used HMW phthalates are DEHP, DINP and DIDP (Wang et al. 2019).

Phthalates exist ubiquitous in different environmental compartments of water, aquatic sediments, biota, soil and air. It has been revealed by many studies that phthalates can be found in indoors, human urine, consumer foods, human milk and amniotic fluid (Dargnat et al. 2009, Sánchez-Avila et al. 2009, Mok et al. 2022, Cao et al. 2021, Bräuner et al. 2022). Since phthalates do not covalently bound to the plastic material or polymer, they leach, migrate or vapor to the surrounding environment (Benjamin et al. 2017). Humans are exposed to phthalates through various routes such as ingestion, inhalation, dermal absorption, parenteral administration, and medication. The route of exposure varies by structure of phthalate and the usage area (Wang et al. 2019). The main route of exposure to certain phthalates is oral intake with food or drink (Serrano et al. 2014). In addition, the inhalation and dermal exposures to phthalates are also noteworthy routes to intake these chemicals into the human body (Lyche 2011).

Most of phthalates are lipophilic chemicals. Once absorbed to the body, they are generally metabolized to their metabolites (Table 1). They are transformed chemically in the human body by two phase reactions before excreted by urine, feces, or other body fluids. At the first phase, phthalate diesters are hydrolyzed to their monoesters catalyzed by lipases and esterases, so they become hydrophilic chemicals (Frederiksen et al. 2007). The monoester phthalates can be further metabolized by various oxidation and hydroxylation steps. In the second phase, monoester phthalate metabolites can be conjugated with glucuronide or sulphate. After conjugation, they can be excreted easily from the body (Chang et al. 2021).

It has been revealed by *in vitro, in vivo* and epidemiologic studies that certain phthalates have endocrine disrupting effects and cause abnormalities in the development of the male reproductive system leading to the inhibition of testosterone production (Gray Jr et al. 2000, Parks et al. 2000, Desdoits-Lethimonier et al. 2012, Enangue Njembele and Tremblay 2021). Due to the risks to human health (endocrine-disrupting and reproductive effects of phthalates), especially to children, certain phthalates have been listed in Substance of Very High Concern (SVHC) on The European Commission's REACH (Regulation concerning the Registration, Evaluation, Authorisation and Restriction of Chemicals) (Eureach_Annex_Xvii 2007, ECHA 2018). In Europe, DEHP was the first phthalate diester to be restricted in toys and other childcare products that could come in direct contact with children's mouths in 1999 (Eureach_Annex_Xvii 2007). Subsequently, DBP, BBP, DINP, DIDP, DOP and DIBP, especially DEHP, are limited by REACH to a maximum content of 0.1% by weight in all consumer products offered to the EU market (ECHA 2018). In addition, the Consumer Product Safety Commission (CPSC) has banned the use of certain phthalates greater than 0.1% by weight in children's toys and childcare products in the United States (CPSC 2017).

Table 1. Some parent phthalates and their metabolites with abbreviations

	Parent Chemical		Metabolites	
LMW Phthalates	Di-methyl phthalate	DMP	Mono-methyl phthalate	MMP
	Di-ethyl phthalate	DEP	Mono-ethyl phthalate	MEP
	Di-allyl phthalate	DAP	Mono-allyl phthalate	MAP
	Benzylbutyl phthalate	BZBP	Monobenzyl phthalate Mono-n-butyl phthalate	MBZP MBP
	Di-isobutyl phthalate	DIBP	Mono-isobutyl phthalate	MIBP
	Di-n-butyl phthalate	DBP	Mono-n-butyl phthalate	MBP
	Di-n-hexyl phthalate	DHP	Mono-hexyl phthalate	MHP
	Di-cyclohexyl phthalate	DCHP	Mono-cyclo-hexyl phthalate	MCHP
	Di-n-pentyl-phthalate	DPP	Mono-n-pentyl phthalate	MPP
HMW Phthalates	Di(2-ethylhexyl) phthalate	DEHP	Mono(2-ethylhexyl) phthalate Mono(2-ethyl-5-carboxypentyl) phthalate Mono(2-ethyl-5-hydroxyhexyl) phthalate Mono(2-ethyl-5-oxohexyl) phthalate Mono-(2-carboxymethylhexyl) phthalate	MEHP MECPP MEHHP MEOHP MCMHP
	Di-octyl phthalate	DOP	Mono-n-octyl phthalate Mono-3-carboxypropyl phthalate	MOP MCPP
	Di-isononyl phthalate	DINP	Mono-isononyl phthalate Mono-(hydroxyisononyl) phthalate Mono-(carboxyisooctyl) phthalate Mono-(oxoisononyl) phthalate Mono-(4-methyl-7-hydroxyoctyl) phthalate Mono-(4-methyl-7-oxooctyl) phthalate Mono-(4-methyl-7-carboxyheptyl) phthalate	MINP MHINP MCIOP MOINP MMHOP MMOOP MMCHP
HMW Phthalates	Di-iso-decylphthalate	DIDP	Mono-isodecyl phthalate Mono-(hydroxyisodecyl) phthalate Mono-(oxoisodecyl) phthalate Mono-(carboxyisononyl) phthalate Mono-(2-propyl-6-carboxyhexyl) phthalate	MIDP MHIDP MOIDP MCINP MPCHP
	Di-(2-propylheptyl) phthalate	DPHP	Mono-(2-propyl-6-hydroxyheptyl) phthalate Mono-(2-propyl-6-oxoheptyl) phthalate Mono-(2-propyl-6-carboxyhexyl) phthalate	MPHHP MPOHP MPCHP

Kato et al. 2005, Silva et al. 2007, Joensen et al. 2014, Piecha et al. 2016.

DEHP is the most commonly used phthalate derivative in consumer products and the concentration of DEHP in plastics may reach up to 40% by weight (Halden 2010). DEHP is rapidly metabolized into various substances once it enters to human body and the toxic effects of DEHP is related to the main metabolite of DEHP, mono-ethylhexyl phthalate (MEHP) (Shea and American Academy of Pediatrics Committee on Environmental 2003). MEHP was found in 80.6% of 10.031 subject in the study investigating phthalate traces in human urine samples between 1999 and 2006 (Ferguson et al. 2011).

Phthalates and phthalate metabolites can bind to molecular targets in the cell and disrupt hormonal homeostasis in the body, leading to various disorders in fetuses, infants, children, and adults. Studies have shown that phthalates and their monoesters are associated with reproductive system disorders, cardiovascular diseases, neurological disorders, respiratory system diseases, as well as metabolic diseases such as thyroid diseases, diabetes, obesity and metabolic syndrome (Chang et al. 2021, Jones 2010). Certain phthalates and phthalate metabolites have been shown to be reproductive and developmental toxicants in *in vivo* studies (Ema and Miyawaki 2002, Gray Jr et al. 2000, Parks et al. 2000, Saillenfait et al. 2008, Saillenfait et al. 2013). Phthalates act mainly as anti-androgens (Latini et al. 2006, Mahood et al. 2005). Some of the toxic effects of phthalates result from the interactions with peroxisome proliferator-activated receptors (PPARs) (Ventrice et al. 2013). Phthalates have been shown to interact with three different receptor isoforms of PPAR (PPARα, PPARβ, PPARγ) (Casals-Casas et al. 2008). In the presence of an agonist, PPARs form heterodimers with the retinoid X receptor (RXR), and PPAR/RXR heterodimers bind to peroxisome proliferator response elements (PPRE) located in the promoter region of PPAR-regulated genes (Qi et al. 2000). PPARα is expressed mainly in liver tissue, but also in heart and skeletal muscle, brown adipose tissue, kidney and intestine, and plays a key role in fatty acid oxidation. PPARγ, described as 'thrifty gene', has crucial function in energy storage and adipocyte differentiation (Evans et al. 2004, Casals-Casas et al. 2008). A prolonged activation of PPARγ by agonists, such as pharmaceutical treatments used for type 2 diabetes mellitus (T2DM), can trigger fat storage, resulting in weight gain as a side effect (Auwerx 1999, Svensson et al. 2011). PPARβ is detected in all tissues with a wide variety of roles, from cell differentiation and survival to both systemic and tissue-specific fatty acid metabolism. Three PPAR isoforms together control different aspects of fatty acid metabolism, energy balance, insulin sensitivity, and glucose homeostasis, through difference in tissue distribution and activation of specific target genes (Evans et al. 2004).

Diabetes and Phthalates

Diabetes is classified mainly as Type 1 Diabetes Mellitus (T1DM), T2DM, the specific types of diabetes and gestational diabetes mellitus (GDM) (ADA 2020). In both T1DM and T2DM, various genetic and environmental factors can result in the progressive loss of beta cell mass and/or function that cause hyperglycemia (ADA 2020). T1DM occurs because of islet autoimmune antibody production against pancreatic beta cells leading to insulin deficiency. T2DM is characterized by insulin resistance concomitant with the progressive loss of adequate beta cell insulin secretion (ADA 2014). The prevalent feature of all types of diabetes is dysfunction or destruction of pancreatic beta cells that caused by genetic abnormalities, epigenetic changes, insulin resistance, autoimmunity, concurrent illnesses, inflammation, and environmental factors (WHO 2019).

Diabetes encloses many disorders characterized by hyperglycaemia (WHO 2019). Measurement of fasting blood glucose (FBG), oral glucose tolerance test (OGTT), plasma glycosylated hemoglobin (HbA1c) levels, and a random blood glucose in the presence of signs and symptoms of diabetes should be tested for diagnosis of diabetes (WHO 2019). Disturbances in insulin production and function are key pathways in the etiology of diabetes. Insulin resistance refers to the combined inability of peripheral tissues to facilitate glucose uptake and suppress glucose output of the liver in response to increasing amounts of insulin (Khan and Pessin 2002).

In recent years, several scientific papers start to reveal the possible harmful health effects of EDCs that are strongly linked to chronic diseases of the endocrine system. In the 1990s, various EDCs were associated with glucose and insulin metabolism and the pathogenesis of T2DM (Alonso-Magdalena et al. 2011, Song et al. 2016). Any chemical that has the potential to damage pancreatic beta cells and alter their hormonal function can lead the onset and development of diabetes (Deng et al. 2018). Studies are accumulating showing that phthalate exposure may be a risk factor for diabetes. There are various *in vitro* (Table 2), *in vivo* (Table 3), and epidemiologic studies (Table 4) suggesting the relationship between phthalate exposure and diabetes (Shi et al. 2020, Li et al. 2021, James-Todd et al. 2012, Stahlhut et al. 2007, Svensson et al. 2011, Lin et al. 2011b, Rajesh and Balasubramanian 2014a, 2015, Mangala Priya et al. 2014). DEHP and/or MEHP has been found to cause hepatic, reproductive and developmental toxicities *in vivo*. A study conducted with rats indicated that low levels of DEHP developed symptoms of diabetes including higher blood sugar and lower insulin levels. When DEHP administration was removed all the symptoms were back to normal levels (Gayathri et al. 2004).

Table 2. Summary of *in vitro* studies assessing the association between phthalate exposure, oxidative stress and apoptosis

Author (year)	Cell Type	Exposure time	Phthalate	Concentrations	Outcome
Mondal and Mukherjee (2020)	L6 myo-tubes	24 hours	DEHP	50 and 100 µM	Increase in the lipid peroxidation, OH*, H_2O_2, and NO levels in DEHP-treated L6 myotubes
Shi L et al. (2019)	INS-1	24 hours	MEHP	25 µM	Increase of ROS and MDA, and decrease of SOD and GSH levels in a dose dependent manner. Apoptosis was induced through mitochondrial membrane potential depolarization and cytochrome c release following activation of caspase 9 and 3
Li L et al. (2021)	INS-1	24 hours	DEHP and DBP	30 µM	DEHP alone, DBP alone and DEHP + DBP combination increased apoptosis rates and ROS levels. Apoptosis was induced through PI3K/Akt/Bcl-2 pathway
Ding et al. (2019)	Insulin resistant BRL cells	24 hours	DEHP	50 µM	DEHP elevated apoptosis in a dose dependent manner at insulin resistant BRL cells compared to non-resistant control BRL cells
Sun et al. (2015)	INS-1	24 hours	DEHP	625 µM	DEHP increased ROS generation and decreased Nrf2 amount both in nucleus and cytosol. Apoptosis was induced with DEHP treatment
She et al. (2017)	INS-1	1 hour	DEHP	400 µM	DEHP increased intracellular ROS levels, decreased mitochondrial membrane potential and significantly induced lysosomal membrane permeability

In the cross-sectional study with 2330 participants having self-reported diabetes and cardiovascular disease designed by Dong et al. (2017), the urinary levels of MEOHP, MEHHP and MECPP were found to be positively associated with DM. In another study carried out by the Korean National Environmental Health Survey (KoNEHS) between 2015–2017 (Cycle 3), the researchers determined that the higher the urinary phthalate metabolites, the higher the prevalence of diabetes (Nam et al. 2020). In an exploratory cross-sectional study, Svensson et al. (2011) found that participants with self-reported diabetes had significantly higher total DEHP metabolite concentrations and lower levels of MBZP compared to participants without diabetes. MBP, MEHHP, MEOHP and MECPP concentrations were found to be significantly increased in patients with T2DM compared to non-diabetic subjects in Prague (Piecha et al. 2016).

Glucose Homeostasis and Phthalates

Glucose homeostasis is essential for life and long-term health for both humans and animals. Liver, skeletal muscle, and adipose tissue for glucose uptake in the body are key to maintaining effective glucose homeostasis in many chronic diseases (Hiriart et al. 2014, Yang 2014). The transition from early metabolic abnormalities that occur before diabetes (impaired fasting glucose and impaired glucose tolerance) to diabetes may take many years, but most of these people with pre-diabetes eventually develop diabetes (Nathan et al. 2007). In numerous animal studies, the link between exposure to phthalates and changes in glucose homeostasis and/or DM was observed. DEHP, the most abundant phthalate, exposure to animals can induce high plasma glucose concentration (Martinelli et al. 2006, Rajesh et al. 2013).

Impaired glucose tolerance is defined by an elevated 2-h plasma glucose concentration after OGTT that demonstrates abnormal glucose homeostasis. DEHP and DBP exposure to animals exhibited impaired glucose tolerance in adipose and muscle tissues (Zhang et al. 2017, Deng et al. 2018). DEHP induced glucose tolerance caused by abnormal glucose intermediate metabolite contents in liver and skeletal muscle *in vivo* (Martinelli et al. 2006).

Table 3. Summary of *in vivo* studies assessing the association between phthalate exposure and glucose homeostasis

Author (Year)	Species	Exposure Time	Phthalate	Dose/Route	Outcome
Mondal and Mukherjee (2020)	Male Swiss albino mice	from 8 weeks of age during 3 months	DEP	1 and 10 mg/kg bw/day dietary	Decreased GLUT2 and GLUT4 protein concentration in isolated hepatic and adipocyte cells of mice exposed to DEP
Boberg et al. (2008)	Wistar rats	gestational (GD 7-21)	DIBP	600 mg/kg bw/day oral gavage	Reduced fetal plasma insulin levels in offspring at GD 19 or 21 after DIBP exposure along with rosiglitazone
Zhang et al. (2020)	Male and female C57BL/6J mice	from 8 weeks of age during 16 weeks	BBP	4 µg/kg bw/day, 169 µg/kg bw/day, 3 mg/kg bw/day, 50 mg/kg bw/day dietary	Increased body weight, liver and adipose tissue weight, FBG, glucose intolerance and insulin intolerance in male mice exposed to 3 mg/kg body weight/day BBP on a high-fat diet compared to high fed diet alone. No similar effects in female mice
Venturelli et al. (2019)	Wistar rats	Gestational and lactational (GD 13-PND 21)	DEHP, DBP	7, 70, 700 mg/kg bw/day for DEHP 5, 50, 500 mg/kg bw/day for DBP oral gavage	Increased FBG at adulthood after highest dose DEHP and DBP
Martinelli et al. (2006)	Male Wistar rats	21 Days	DEHP	2% DEHP dietary	High blood glucose, deficiency in muscle glucose and lactate transport, a reduction of the flux through muscle hexokinase and hepatic glucokinase, and a reduction in glycogen synthesis
Lin et al. (2011a)	Wistar rats	Gestational and lactational (GD 0- PND 21)	DEHP	1.25 and 6.25 mg/kg bw/day oral gavage	High blood sugar, low serum insulin, impaired glucose tolerance and insulin secretion in female offspring at adulthood Increased serum insulin levels in male offspring at adulthood

Author (Year)	Species	Exposure Time	Phthalate	Dose/Route	Outcome
Rajesh et al. (2013)	Male Wistar rats	30 days at adulthood	DEHP	10, 100 mg/kg bw/day gastric intubation	Elevated H_2O_2, hydroxyl radical levels and lipid peroxidation in adipose tissue of DEHP exposed group Disruption of IR, IRS-1, pIRS-1 protein levels, decreased plasma membrane GLUT4 level leading to decreased glucose uptake and oxidation Elevated FBG after DEHP exposure
Mangala Priya et al. (2014)	Wistar rats	Lactational	DEHP	1, 10, 100 mg/kg bw/day oral gavage	Reduced the oxidation of glucose and impaired insulin signaling in cardiac muscle of F1 female albino rats at 58th day
Rajesh and Balasubramanian (2014b)	Wistar rats	Gestational (GD 9-21)	DEHP	1, 10 and 100 mg/kg bw/day oral gavage	Elevated FBG, impaired serum insulin, glucose tolerance and insulin tolerance, and glucose uptake and oxidation in the muscle at PD 60
Rajesh and Balasubramanian (2014b) *(cont.)*	Wistar rats	Gestational (GD 9-21)	DEHP	1, 10 and 100 mg/kg bw/day oral gavage	Diminished plasma membrane INSR protein and its phosphorylated form Increased serine phosphorylated IRS1 and GLUT4
Venturelli et al. (2015)	Wistar rats	Lactational (PD 1-21) or pubertal (PD 22-52)	DEHP	7.5 and 75 mg/kg bw/day oral gavage	Increased FBG, decreased insulin sensitivity and lower insulin secretion in isolated pancreatic islets of adult rats after lactational DEHP exposure Hyperglycemia at adulthood after prebubertal DEHP exposure
Rajesh and Balasubramanian (2015)	Wistar rats	Gestational (GD 9-21)	DEHP	1, 10 and 100 mg/kg bw/day oral gavage	Disruption in insulin and glucose tolerance, insulin secretion stimulated by glucose, elevated blood glucose, and decreased pancreatic insulin content in DEHP exposed offspring at PND60. The expression of genes related to the development and function of pancreatic beta cells decreased Overall level of DNA methylation increased

Table 3. (Continued)

Author (Year)	Species	Exposure Time	Phthalate	Dose/Route	Outcome
Zhou et al. (2015)	Female Apoe−/− mice	From 6 weeks of age for 11 weeks	DEHP	100 mg/kg bw/day via drinking water	Insulin tolerance testing on non-fasting mice with little effect of DEHP on insulin sensitivity 3 weeks after treatment, but higher glucose concentration after DEHP exposure
Wang et al. (2016)	Male Balb/c mice	55 days at adulthood	DEHP	10, 50 or 250 mg/kg/day oral gavage	Lowers serum insulin levels in animals exposed to DEHP
Zhang et al. (2017)	SD rats	15 weeks at adulthood	DEHP	0.05, 5 and 500 mg/kg bw/day oral gavage	Decreased insulin secretion level after DEHP exposure in response to OGTT at 3 weeks. Slower decreasing FBG after DEHP exposure during the OGTT at 5 weeks. Blood glucose levels of DEHP exposed groups rose much higher and fell off much slower during OGTT in all DEHP
Zhang et al. (2017) *(cont.)*	SD rats	15 weeks at adulthood	DEHP	0.05, 5 and 500 mg/kg bw/day oral gavage	exposed rats at 15 weeks. Decreased glucose tolerance and insulin tolerance along with expression of insulin receptor and GLUT4 proteins in liver tissues
Deng et al. (2018)	Male Balb/c mice	From 5-6 weeks of age during 7 weeks	DBP	0.5, 5, 50 mg/kg bw/day oral gavage	Decreased insulin secretion and glucose intolerance but no effect on insulin resistance in high levels DBP exposed rats. Exacerbated glucose intolerance, insulin tolerance and insulin resistance by disrupting PI3K expression and AKT phosphorylation and decreasing the level of GLUT-2 in the pancreas after DBP along with STZ exposure and a high fat diet

Author (Year)	Species	Exposure Time	Phthalate	Dose/Route	Outcome
Zhang et al. (2018)	SD rats	Gestational and lactational	DEHP	600 mg/kg bw/day intragastrically	Increased insulin levels with no change in indexes for pancreas islet function at 14 weeks aged males
Rajagopal et al. (2019a)	Wistar rats	Gestational and lactational (GD 9- PND 21)	DEHP	10 and 100 mg/kg/day oral gavage	Decreased glucose uptake and oxidation, decreased insulin receptor and GLUT2 mRNA levels, and decreased GLUT2 protein levels in the cytosol of male offsping at adulthood
Rajagopal et al. (2019b)	Wistar rats	Gestational and lactational (GD 9- PND 21)	DEHP	10 and 100 mg/kg/day oral gavage	Hyperglycemia and hyperinsulinemia with impaired glucose and insulin tolerance after maternal DEHP exposure to male offspings at adulthood Decreased expressions of IRS1, Akt and their phosphorylated forms and reduced glycogen synthase activity and glycogen concentration
Parsanathan et al. (2019)	Wistar rats	Lactational	DEHP	1, 10, and 100 mg/kg bw/day oral gavage	Lower body weight, decreased 14C-2-deoxyglucose uptake in heart muscle of DEHP-exposed pups Increased FBG in the high-dose DEHP group Decrease in protein levels of InsRβ, IRS, pIRS1, pAkt and GLUT4 and increase in pGLUT4
Ding et al. (2021)	ICR mice	Pubertal 3 weeks exposure	DEHP	0.18, 1.8, 18 and 180 mg/kg bw/day	Exposure to DEHP aggravated metabolic disturbances in female pubertal T2DM mice. Increased insulin and C-peptide levels in DEHP-treated female pubertal T2DM mice

Table 4. Summary of epidemiologic studies assessing the association between phthalate exposure and glucose homeostasis

Author (Year), Country	Study Design	Age	Sample Size	Matrix/Phthalate metabolite Analyzed	Outcome
Stahlhut et al. (2007) USA	Cross-sectional	> 18	1451 (Male)	Urinary/MBP, MEP, MEHP, MBZP, MEHHP, MEOHP	MBP, MBZP, MEP associated with HOMA in males
James-Todd et al. (2012) USA	Cross-sectional	20-79	2350 Female	Urinary/MEP, MBP, MIBP, MBZP, MCPP, MEHP, MEHHP, MEOHP	Higher urine levels of MBP, MIBP, MBZP, MCPP and ΣDEHP metabolites associated with increased odds of diabetes compared with women with the lowest levels of these phthalates after adjusting for certain confounders. Women in the highest quartile for MBZP and MIBP had almost twice the odds of diabetes compared with women in the lowest quartile Among women without self-reported diabetes, MIBP positively associated with FBG, and MIBP and ΣDEHP metabolites positively associated with HOMA-IR
Kim et al. (2013) Korea	Follow-up, cross-sectional	≥60	560 (146 Male, 414 Female)	Urinary/MEHHP, MEOHP, MBP	No relation between MBP and HOMA-IR. MEHHP and MEOHP significantly associated with HOMA-IR in the elderly population, especially with a history of DM and females
Trasande et al. (2013) USA	Cross-sectional	12-19	5829 (424 Male, 342 Female)	Urinary/MEP, MBP, MIBP, MBP, MBZP, MCPP, MEHP, MECPP, MEHHP, MEOHP	DEHP metabolites significantly associated with HOMA-IR in adolescents subjects

Author (Year), Country	Study Design	Age	Sample Size	Matrix/Phthalate metabolite Analyzed	Outcome
Huang et al. (2014) USA	Cross-sectional	12-<80	3083 (1620 Male, 1463 Female)	Urinary/MEP, MBP, MIBP, MBZP, MCPP, MEHP, MEHHP, MEOHP	MIBP, MCPP, MEHP, MEHHP, MEOHP positively associated with FBG, HOMA-IR and insulin with no difference in gender. MBZP linked only with insulin and HOMA-IR
Dirinck et al. (2015) Belgium	Cross-sectional	41±12.5	123 (38 Male, 85 Female)	Urinary/MMP, MCPP, MEP, MECPP, MEHHP, MIBP, MEOHP, MBP, MBZP, MEHP	Exposure to phthalates associated with increased insulin resistance, decreased insulin sensitivity, and possibly impaired beta cell function in overweight and obese subjects. MEP levels were predictive for increasing HOMA-IR indices, levels of MCPP were predictive for decreased Belfiore indices
Chen et al. (2017) Taiwan	Follow-up, cross-sectional	12-30	786	Urinary/MMP, MEP, MnBP, MBzP, MEHP, MEHHP, MEOHP	Urinary MEHP-related insulin resistance and lower male testosterone levels in young adults, but not adolescents. Impaired glucose homeostasis by urinary MEHP metabolites only in young adults. HMW phthalates more closely associated with insulin resistance than LMW phthalates in young Taiwanese subjects
Dales et al. (2018) Canada	Cross-sectional	12-79	4437	Urinary/MBP, MIBP, MBZP, MCPP, MEHHP, MEHP, MEOHP, MEP, MMP, MINP, MOP	2119 of 4437 participants to have FBG and at least one phthalate metabolite above detection limits. MBzP, MCPP, MEHP, MEHHP, MIBP, and DEHP metabolites positively associated with increased HbA1C. Positive association with DEHP metabolites and increased FBG, insulin, HOMA-IR and HOMA-β.

Table 4. (Continued)

Author (Year), Country	Study Design	Age	Sample Size	Matrix/Phthalate metabolite Analyzed	Outcome
Li et al. (2019b) USA	Cross-sectional	37.44 ± 21.51	1605 (817 Male, 788 Female)	Urinary/MEHP, MEOHP, MEHHP, MECPP, MBZP, MBP, MIBP, MEP, MCPP	DEHP metabolite concentrations between the 25th percentile and the 75th percentile associated with higher log HOMA-IR. Lower HOMA-IR associated with urinary MEP. No relation between other phthalate metabolites to HOMA-IR.Weakened DEHP metabolite concentrations and HOMA-IR association at higher serum β-carotene concentrations
Svensson et al. (2011) USA	Case-control study	(60.5±8.5, 52.4±12.8)	221 (Female)	Urinary/MEP, MBP, MIBP, MBzP, MEHP, MEHHP, MEOHP, MECPP, MCPP	Significantly higher total DEHP metabolite concentrations, but lower levels of MBZP in participants with diabetes compared to without diabetes. After adjusting for key confounders, considerable significant positive associations with diabetes status with MEHHP and MEOHP over tertiles.
Olsén et al. (2012) USA	Cross-sectional	70	1016	Serum/MEHP, MEP, MIBP, MMP	Relation with MIBP to FBG
Lind et al. (2012) Sweden	Cross-sectional	70	1016	Serum/MEHP, MEP, MIBP, MMP	High levels of MMP, MIBP and MEP, but not MEHP, associated with an increased prevalence of diabetes after adjusting for certain confounders. MIBP mainly related to poor insulin secretion determined by proinsulin-to-insulin ratio. MEP and MMP mainly related to IR determined by HOMA-IR.

Author (Year), Country	Study Design	Age	Sample Size	Matrix/Phthalate metabolite Analyzed	Outcome
Piecha et al. (2016) Czech Republic	Pilot study	52.7 (23.4)	168	Urinary/MMP, MEP, MBP, MIBP, MBZP, MCHP, MEHP, MEHHP, MEOHP MECPP, MCMHP, MCPP, MOP, MINP, MHINP, MOINP, MCIOP, MMHOP, MMOOP, MMCHP, MIDP, MHIDP, MOIDP, MCINP, MPHHP, MPOHP, MPCHP	MBP, MEHHP, MEOHP and MECPP concentrations significantly increased in patients with T2DM compared to non-diabetic subjects
James-Todd et al. (2016a) USA	Cross-sectional	20-80	2719	Urinary/MEP, MBP, MIBP, MBZP, MCPP	MBzP and ΣDEHP metabolites associated with hyperglycemia as a result of changes in glucose dysregulation
Saengkaew et al. (2017) Thailand	Cross-sectional, case-control	7-18	155	Urinary/MMP, MBP	Higher MBP Concentration in participants with abnormal FBG than in those with normal FBG. Positively correlated MBP levels in normal weight group with HbA1c, negatively correlated with MBP levels in the overweight/obesity group
Dong et al. (2017) China	Cross-sectional	53(41,64)	2330 (1108 Male, 1222 Female)	Urinary/MMP, MEP, MnBP, MiBP, MBzP, MEHP, MEOHP, MEHHP, MECPP, MCMHP	The urinary levels of MEOHP, MEHHP and MECPP positively associated with DM. MEHHP, MEOHP, MECPP, MCMHP and the sums of the oxidative metabolites of DEHP significantly related to diabetes in males, but not in females

Table 4. (Continued)

Author (Year), Country	Study Design	Age	Sample Size	Matrix/Phthalate metabolite Analyzed	Outcome
Castro-Correia et al. (2018) Portugal	Cross-sectional, follow up	0.9-11.3	38	Urinary/MIBP, MBP	Higher MIBP concentrations associated with a tendency to new-onset diabetes
Li et al. (2019a) Saudi Arabia	Case-control study	28–68	101 (52 T2DM and 47 controls)	Urinary/MMP, MEP, MBP, MIBP, MIPP, MPEP, MEHP, MECPP, MEHHP, MEOHP, MCMHP, MCPP, MCHP, MBZP, MHP, MOP, MINP, MIDP	12 phthalate metabolites positively related with higher urinary concentrations of oxidative stress biomarkers
Duan et al. (2019) China	Case-control study	58 ± 10 and 51 ± 10	500 (250 with T2DM and 250 controls)	Urinary/MMP, MBP, MIBP, MEHP, MEP, MBZP, MCPP, MEHHP, MEOHP, MECPP, MCMHP	Significant positive associations between urinary concentrations of MEOHP, MEHP, MCPP, MIBP, MMP and sum of DEHP metabolites with T2DM. MEHHP positively related to HbA1c levels in controls. The associations of exposure to phthalates with T2DM, FBG, and HbA1c may differ between gender, BMI, or age
Nam et al. (2020) Korea	Cross-sectional	≥19	3781 (1648 Male and 2133 Female)	Urinary/DEHP, MEHHP, MEOHP, MECCP, MnBP, MBzP, MCOP, MCNP, MCPP	Higher the urinary phthalate metabolites, higher the prevalence of diabetes
Milošević et al. (2020) Serbia	Cross-sectional	18-50	305	Urinary/MEP, MEHP, MMP, MPP, MBP, MAP, MCHP, MBZP, MOP	Urinary MEP concentration positively correlated with the HOMA-IR in T2DM subgroup, while urinary MEHP levels associated with glucose serum levels in T2DM subgroup

Author (Year), Country	Study Design	Age	Sample Size	Matrix/Phthalate metabolite Analyzed	Outcome
Duan et al. (2021) China	Cross-sectional	56 ± 7	120 (60 control and 60 T2DM)	Urinary/MMP, MEP, MBP, MIBP, MEHP, MBZP, MCPP, MEHHP, MEOHP, MECPP, MCMHP	Phthalate exposure may contribute to T2DM risk through disturbing galactose metabolism, amino acid metabolism, and pyrimidine metabolism
Lee et al. (2021) Korea	Cross-sectional	≥19	3782	Urinary/MEHHP, MEOHP, MECCP, MnBP, MBzP, MCOP, MCNP, MCPP	Overall decrease in ORs for phthalate metabolites, following specific gravity adjustment, for diabetes

Glucose is the main energy source for many tissues of the body. Glucose transporters (GLUTs), which are facilitating glucose transporters, are involved in the metabolism of glucose and other hexoses, including absorption, distribution, and excretion/recovery. Although GLUT2 is more abundant in pancreatic beta cells and hepatocytes, it is also found in the intestine, kidney and central nervous system. While GLUT2 facilitates the uptake of glucose for the cell depending on the blood glucose level in hepatocytes, it triggers glucose-stimulated insulin secretion in pancreatic beta cells (Chadt and Al-Hasani 2020). In the basal state, GLUT4 is localized in the tubulovesicular system inside the cell. In the presence of insulin, GLUT4 translocates to the plasma membrane in adipose, skeletal and cardiac muscle cells. Translocation of GLUT4 to the plasma membrane is one of the rate-limiting steps in which insulin stimulates glucose uptake in muscle and fat (Khan and Pessin 2002). Dietary exposure of DEP (1 and 10 mg/kg body weight/day) to adult male Swiss albino mice for 3 months induced GLUT2 and GLUT4 protein concentration in isolated hepatic and adipocyte cells of mice suggested insufficient cellular glucose uptake (Mondal and Mukherjee 2020). In another study, decreased plasma membrane GLUT4 levels by DEHP led to decreased glucose uptake and oxidation in adipose tissue, and in consequence elevated FBG (Rajesh et al. 2013). Exposure to DBP along with streptozotocin (STZ), a toxin that specifically destroys islet β cells, and a high fat diet exacerbated glucose intolerance and decreased the level of GLUT2 in the pancreas (Deng et al. 2018).

The relationship between human phthalate exposure and glucose homeostasis is a critical issue that has recently been studied by researchers (Stahlhut et al. 2007, James-Todd et al. 2012, Nam et al. 2020, Dong et al. 2017, Castro-Correia et al. 2018). In cross-sectional epidemiologic studies, DEHP metabolites were found to be related with elevated FBG with no difference in gender (Huang et al. 2014, Dales et al. 2018, James-Todd et al. 2016a). Although MIBP, a LMW phthalate metabolite, was also determined to be associated with FBG of women with self-reported diabetes (James-Todd et al. 2012), the association between FBG and MIBP was observed in cross-sectional studies with no gender difference (Huang et al. 2014, Olsén et al. 2012). MBZP and MBP are other phthalate metabolites that have also been found to be related with FBG (James-Todd et al. 2016a, Saengkaew et al. 2017).

Maternal exposure to DEHP resulted in hyperglycemia, impaired glucose tolerance, decreased glucose uptake and oxidation, decreased insulin receptor and GLUT2 mRNA levels, and decreased GLUT2 protein levels in the cytosol of liver cells, without any changes in the membrane (Rajagopal et al. 2019a, b). The authors concluded that exposure to DEHP alters the regulation of GLUT2 transcription and triggers epigenetic modification in the insulin receptor and GLUT2 gene promoters that is substantial in the development of the metabolic abnormality in adult F1 male offspring (Rajagopal et al. 2019a, b).

It is well known that exposure to chemicals is associated with chronic diseases during critical periods of development (Lin et al. 2011a). Developmental exposure to DEHP during GD 9-21 resulted elevated FBG and glucose tolerance after OGTT at adulthood in the F1 offspring (Rajesh and Balasubramanian 2014b). In utero and lactational (from GD13 to PD 21) exposure to DEHP (7, 70, and 700 mg/kg bw/day) and DBP (5, 50, and 500 mg/kg bw/day) resulted increased FBG in male and female offspring exposed to the highest doses of DEHP and DBP at adulthood (Venturelli et al. 2019). In another study by Venturelli et al. (2015), lactational or pubertal exposure to DEHP (7.5 and 75 mg/kg bw/day) caused increased FBG. In cardiac muscle, lactational exposure to DEHP at dose of 1, 10, and 100 mg/kg bw/day decreased 14C-2-deoxyglucose uptake in heart muscle of all DEHP-exposed pups, when FBG increased in the high-dose group with decreased GLUT4 protein level and increased pGLUT4 protein level (Parsanathan et al. 2019). The authors concluded that lactational DEHP exposure caused F1 male offspring to cardiac glucometabolic disorders at PND22 (Parsanathan et al. 2019). Additionally, in a previous study, glucose uptake was significantly reduced by disrupted insulin signaling because of impaired GLUT4 translocation in cardiac muscle cells of F1 female albino rats lactationally exposed to DEHP (Mangala Priya et al. 2014). The authors reported that chronic activation of PPARα by DEHP may partly lead to reduced glucose uptake inside the cell. In a study by Hines et al. (2009), urinary DEHP metabolites were found to be positively associated with serum glucose levels in lactating women.

HbA1c is an important indicator of long-term glycemic control, with its ability to provide information about cumulative glycemic history of an individual for the previous two to three months, which is the estimated half-life of red blood cells (Sherwani et al. 2016). MBZP, MCPP, MEHP, MEHHP and MIBP were found to be associated with an increased HbA1c levels, except for MEP (Dales et al. 2018). A cross-sectional case-control study (Saengkaew et al. 2017) in Thailand was conducted with normal weight and overweight/obesity stratified participants (155 children), aged 7-18 years, to evaluate the association between urinary phthalate metabolites (MMP and

MBP) and metabolic abnormalities. The concentration of MBP in participants with abnormal FBG was significantly higher than in those with normal FBG. HbA1c in normal weight group was positively correlated with MBP levels, whereas negatively correlated with MBP levels in the overweight/obesity group. In a case-control study on Chinese people (250 with T2DM and 250 controls), Duan et al. (2019) stated that urinary concentrations of MEHHP were positively related to HbA1c levels in controls. The authors reported that the significant positive associations between urinary phthalate metabolite concentrations (MEOHP and sum of DEHP metabolites) and HbA1c levels were more presumedly to be found in the lower body mass index (BMI) subgroup (< 25 kg/m^2). In other studies (Dirinck et al. 2015, James-Todd et al. 2012), the association between phthalate metabolites and HbA1c levels was not observed.

Total and saturated fat intake was associated with a higher risk of T2DM, but these associations were not independent of BMI (van Dam et al. 2002). There are *in vivo* studies to understand the effects of phthalate exposure on the development of diabetes with high fat diet. Male mice exposed to 3 mg/kg bw/day BBP on a high-fat diet had significant increases in body weight, liver and adipose tissue weights, FBG and glucose intolerance compared to high fat diet only. Pregnant Sprague-Dawley rats were exposed to DEHP (300 mg/kg/day) orally on gestational day 6 to postnatal day (PND) 21 (Strakovsky et al. 2015). At adulthood, male and female offspring were exposed to a high fat dietary challenge. Males exposed to DEHP maternally and fed with high-fat diet had increased energy intake and body weight, leading to glucose intolerance.

Metabolic syndrome is associated with elevated blood pressure, impaired glucose tolerance or insulin resistance, atherogenic dyslipidemia and increase susceptibility of developing T2DM (Cook 2007, Grundy et al. 2004). Apolipoprotein E-deficient (Apoe-/-) mice were characterized by a number of age-related diseases such as rapidly developing atherosclerosis and Alzheimer (Shen et al. 2018). Loss of insulin signaling in endothelial cells accelerates atherosclerosis in Apoe-/- mice (Rask-Madsen et al. 2010). These mice develop significant hyperglycemia and T2DM when fed with a Western diet (Su et al. 2006). Female Apoe−/− mice fed with a Western diet and exposed to DEHP or not (100 mg/kg) had significantly elevated FBG levels and tended to have increased glucose intolerance compared to control mice after two weeks of exposure (Zhou et al. 2015). 3 weeks after treatment, insulin tolerance testing on non-fasting mice was found to have little effect of DEHP on insulin sensitivity, although it resulted in a higher glucose concentration in mice after DEHP exposure. The authors concluded that exposure to DEHP caused a brief interference of glucose homeostasis but has little impact on the development of T2DM and atherosclerosis in Apoe−/− mice (Zhou et al. 2015).

Insulin Secretion and Signaling Pathway

Insulin is released due to the increase in blood glucose and plays a very important role in controlling glucose homeostasis. Pancreatic beta cells secrete insulin in response to an increase in blood glucose after every meal. In recent years, the incidence of T1DM has increased in many European countries (IDF 2021). T1DM may occur because of the damage to insulin-secreting pancreatic beta cells as a result of an autoimmune process resulting in insulin deficiency. T1DM can develop in genetically predisposed individuals and can be triggered by various environmental factors. There is increasing evidence that exposure to EDCs during critical periods of development can program gene expression, causing permanent changes and unexpected effects on metabolism (Fénichel and Chevalier 2017). Evidence for some associations between T1DM and environmental chemicals and air pollutants such as PFAS, PCBs, arsenic, BPA, phthalates, pesticides, ozone and nitric oxides has been reported in epidemiologic and laboratory studies (Howard 2019, 2018, Shapiro et al. 2015). Castro-Correia et al. (2018) investigated the relationship between urine concentrations of phthalate metabolites of prepubertal children with new-onset diabetes, prepubertal children diagnosed of T1DM, and healthy control children. It was found that though the concentrations of DBP and DIBP metabolites were statistically similar in all children, the authors concluded that there was a clear trend for higher levels of DIBP metabolites in the children with new-onset diabetes.

Insulin is the only hormone that is able to lower body glucose among the hormones released in the body (Rorsman and Braun 2013). Any disturbance in insulin secretion leads to the development of diabetes. DEHP metabolites, MBZP and MIBP were associated with elevation of fasting insulin levels with reduction in glucose controls and beta cell function (Dales et al. 2018, Huang et al. 2014). Basal proinsulin (a precursor molecule of insulin) levels were increased in T2DM compared to control, the increase in proinsulin level was thought to be an indicator of onset of T2DM (Mykkänen et al. 1995). Proinsulin/insulin ratio might represent beta cell function and early sign of failing pancreas (Kim et al. 2000). The study by Lind et al. (2012) determined a significant relation with MEHP and MIBP exposure with a high proinsulin-to-insulin ratio in elderly. In an *in vivo* study, dietary DEHP (5, 50 and 500 mg/kg bw/day) exposure to rats for 4 weeks resulted with an increased insulin level at high dose DEHP exposure (Jia et al. 2016).

Disruption of insulin signaling throughout the body leads to insulin resistance and eventually to T2DM (Khan and Pessin 2002). Homeostatic Model Assessment for Insulin Resistance (HOMA-IR) is an index to estimate insulin sensitivity derived from FPG and insulin concentrations (Bergman et al. 2020). Dales et al. (2018) suggested that phthalate exposure may possibly impair the control of blood glucose and thus cause prediabetes predisposition. In epidemiologic studies, phthalate metabolites were associated with insulin resistance (Li et al. 2019, Trasande et al. 2013). Stahlhut et al. (2007) showed that, several common phthalate metabolites (MBP, MBZP, MEP) were positively correlated with abdominal obesity and insulin resistance in adult US men in a large national cross-sectional sample. Trasande et al. (2013) reported that DEHP was significantly associated with HOMA-IR in a cross-sectional study carried out with 766 fasting adolescents aged between 12-19 in the 2003-2008 NHANES. Kim et al. (2013) found that the molar sum of DEHP metabolites (MEHHP and MEOHP) significantly associated with HOMA-IR, and the association was evident among participants with a history of DM and among females. There was no relation observed between MBP and HOMA-IR. In another study, Dirinck et al. (2015) evaluated the relationship between urinary levels of several phthalate metabolites and glucose metabolism, assessed by a standard 75 g OGTT, both in overweight and obese subjects. The authors reported that exposure to phthalates is associated with increased insulin resistance, decreased insulin sensitivity, and possibly impaired beta cell function in this population (Dirinck et al. 2015). In this study, MEP levels were predictive for increasing HOMA-IR indices, levels of MCPP were predictive for decreased Belfiore indices (OGTT based estimates of insulin resistance), and several phthalate metabolites were predictive for decreased insulin sensitivity, as assessed by the Matsuda index (estimates insulin sensitivity) even after correction for BMI in the regression model. The authors suggested that these findings pointed out a possible insulin resistance induced by diabetogenic effects of phthalate metabolites as well as their obesogenic effects. High levels of DBP were shown to decrease the insulin secretion but had no effect on insulin resistance (Deng et al. 2018). The researchers concluded that DBP aggravated T2DM by disrupting the insulin signaling pathway and impairing insulin secretion. In an *in vivo* study, BBP increased the risk of T2DM in male mice, not female, by increasing insulin intolerance (Zhang et al. 2020).

The study by James-Todd et al. (2012) compared the association between urinary phthalate metabolite concentrations and prevalence of self-reported diabetes in 2350 adult women aged 20-79 who participated in a NHANES cross-sectional study between 2001 and 2008. The results of the study showed that MIBP and sum of DEHP metabolites were positively associated with HOMA-IR suggesting phthalates might affect T2DM risk either through glucose dysregulation or insulin resistance. Lind et al. (2012) determined that MEP and MMP were mainly related to insulin resistance determined by HOMA-IR in elderly. Besides, MBZP, MBP, MIBP, MCPP, and DEHP metabolites (MEHP, MEHHP, MEOHP) were found to be positively associated with HOMA-IR with no difference in gender (Huang et al. 2014).

In a cross-sectional study by Dales et al. (2018), HOMA-IR and HOMA-β were determined to have positive associations with DEHP metabolites that indicated β-cell disfunction and insulin resistance, thereby may predispose to pre-diabetes. MEP was also found to be positively correlated to HOMA-IR in T2DM subgroup in a study by Milošević et al. (2020).

Zhang et al. (2017) conducted a study to understand the possible mechanism of the DEHP exposure to male Sprague Dawleyrats and revealed significant liver damage, glucose tolerance, and insulin tolerance, along with decreased expression of insulin receptor and GLUT4 proteins in liver tissue. In the adipose tissue, decreased insulin receptor, IRS-1, pIRS-1 protein levels were observed after DEHP exposure at adulthood (Rajesh et al. 2013). Dietary exposure of DEP to adult male Swiss albino mice for 3 months induced insulin resistance onset even at low levels (Mondal and Mukherjee 2020). IRS-1, one of the major substrate for insulin receptor kinase, is included in insulin signaling (Khan and Pessin 2002). DEHP reduced the expression of the IRS-1 and phosphorylated Akt protein, which may be due to increased ROS production, and therefore led to defective translocation of GLUT4 to the membrane (Mangala Priya et al. 2014). Srinivasan et al. (2011) investigated the effect of DEHP (10 and 100 mg/kg body weight) on insulin signaling and glucose oxidation in skeletal muscle of adult male albino rats via gastric intubation for 30 days. It was found that DEHP exposure caused to elevate the H_2O_2, hydroxyl radical levels and lipid peroxidation which disrupt the membrane integrity and insulin receptor. The authors reported their results as DEHP disrupted insulin signaling, glucose uptake and oxidation through decreased translocation of the plasma membrane GLUT4, which may be partially responsible for the high FBG levels. They concluded that DEHP affected glucose oxidation in skeletal muscle and mediated through enhanced lipid peroxidation, impaired insulin signaling and GLUT4 translocation in plasma membrane. A study by Mangala Priya et al. (2014) reported that lactational DEHP exposure to F1 female albino rats reduced the oxidation of glucose and impaired insulin signaling in cardiac muscle suggesting a possible role of DEHP in the development of T2DM.

There is growing appreciation that exposure to exogenous EDCs during gestational and lactational periods is particularly susceptible to the effects that can lead to lifelong consequences (Gore et al. 2015). It is suspected that phthalates among these chemicals may have the same effect. Therefore, *in vivo* studies have investigated whether phthalates cause metabolic disorders during critical developmental periods. DEHP-exposed offspring exhibited impaired serum insulin, and insulin tolerance at PD 60 (Rajesh and Balasubramanian 2014b). Plasma membrane INSR and pINSR protein levels, glucose uptake and oxidation reduced in the muscle and the IRS-1 protein levels in 10 and 100 mg/kg bw/day DEHP exposed males and all doses of DEHP exposed females were decreased. Serine phosphorylation of IRS1 and GLUT4 levels were increased in DEHP-exposed groups. In a follow-up study by the same researchers (Rajesh and Balasubramanian 2015), disruption of insulin and glucose tolerance, insulin secretion stimulated by glucose, elevated blood glucose, and decreased pancreatic insulin content were observed in DEHP exposed offspring. In DEHP-exposed groups, the expressions of genes related to the development and function of pancreatic beta cells decreased in the islets, when the overall level of DNA methylation increased. In a study with DIBP, the rats exposed to DIBP (600 mg/kg bw/day) and rosiglitazone from GD 7–21 had reduced fetal plasma insulin levels in offspring at GD 19 or 21 (Boberg et al. 2008).

Insulin resistance leads to the hyperinsulinemia typically seen in the early stages of T2DM and metabolic syndrome (Heindel et al. 2017). Hyper-insulinemia with impaired insulin tolerance were observed after maternal DEHP exposure (Rajagopal et al. 2019b). Besides, the levels of insulin signaling molecules (IRS1, Akt and their phosphorylated forms) as well as glycogen synthase activity and glycogen concentration were decreased significantly. The authors concluded that maternal DEHP exposure may disrupt insulin signaling and alter glucoregulatory events leading to the development of T2DM in F1 male offspring (Rajagopal et al. 2019b). Based on the results from these studies, DEHP exposure during gestational and lactational periods may affect insulin secretion in rats and cause disruption in insulin signaling.

Gestational and lactational exposure to DEHP resulted in abnormal beta cell structure, decreased beta cell mass and pancreatic insulin content, as well as changes in the expression of genes related to pancreatic development and beta cell function in the weaned offspring (Lin et al. 2011a). At adulthood, high blood sugar, low serum insulin, impaired glucose tolerance and insulin secretion were seen in female offspring developmentally exposed to DEHP. In male offspring exposed to DEHP, serum insulin was elevated during fasting. The results of the study suggested that developmental exposure to DEHP led to beta cell dysfunction and whole body glucometabolic abnormalities in the rat.

It has been determined that children and young people are more easily exposed to phthalates than adults due to their lifestyles and eating habits that include nourishment with fast food and plastic packaged foods, besides using personal care products (Ding et al. 2019). A study in Brussels, Belgium revealed1.7 times higher levels of DEHP metabolites in urine collected from children (6–11 years) than the levels from mothers because of the food consumption and daily activities at home (Fang et al., 2019; Koppen et al., 2019). Besides, high dose in utero and lactational DEHP (700 mg/kg bw/day) exposure (from GD13 to PD 21) decreased rate of glucose degradation following insulin administration and decreased insulin secretion in the GSIS test. Lactational exposure (PND 1-21) to DEHP (7.5 and 75 mg/kg bw/day) led to male offspring revealed changes in the glycemic homeostasis in adulthood, characterized by the increased FBG, decreased insulin sensitivity and low insulin secretion in isolated pancreatic islets (Venturelli et al. 2015). The protein levels of insulin signaling molecules such as insulin receptor subunit β (InsRβ) and insulin receptor substrate 1 (IRS1) decreased in DEHP-exposed offspring after lactational exposure (Parsanathan et al. 2019).

Ding et al. (2021) investigated the sex differences, metabolic toxicity, and the underlying mechanisms of the effect of DEHP on pubertal T2DM mice. The researchers found that exposure to DEHP aggravated metabolic disturbances in female pubertal T2DM mice, and these mice were more sensitive to effects of DEHP exposure than pubertal control mice. The authors also reported that DEHP exposure could further inhibit glucose utilization and metabolism in female pubertal T2DM mice. On the other hand, the authors observed increased insulin and C-peptide levels in DEHP-treated female pubertal T2DM mice, indicating compensation for impaired insulin sensitivity by DEHP. HbA1c increased after high dose DEHP (180 mg/kg/day) exposure at normal pubertal mice. DEHP increased phosphorylated Jun-N-terminal kinase (p-JNK) and disrupted insulin sensitivity in the liver, which were major causes of DEHP-aggravated metabolic disturbance in pubertal T2DM mice. The authors suggested that overactivation of JNK by DEHP and inflammation disturbed the hepatic cellular regeneration in the T2DM mice, which eventually induced further severe oxidative damage and apoptosis (Ding et al. 2021).

Accumulated evidence suggests a link between reduced testosterone plasma levels, T2DM, and insulin resistance (Zhong et al. 2021, Bianchi and Locatelli 2018). Total testosterone is inversely related to insulin concentration and insulin resistance in men (Jones 2010). Chen et al. (2017) evaluated glucose homeostasis and testicular function in relation to seven urinary phthalate metabolites among adolescents (aged 12-20) and young adults (aged 20-30) in total 786 subjects in Taiwan from 2006 to 2008. A decrease in male testosterone and an increase in creatinine adjusted urinary MEHP levels were observed throughout four quartiles of HOMA-IR. The authors reported that urinary MEHP-related insulin resistance and decreased male testosterone levels in young adults, but not adolescents, may occur because of MEHP-related HOMA-IR and testicular dysfunction varied with age. They concluded that impaired metabolic homeostasis of glucose by urinary MEHP metabolites were observed only in young adults. Their findings, which showed increased insulin resistance exclusively with HMW phthalates, also suggested that HMW phthalates are more closely associated with insulin resistance than LMW phthalates in young Taiwanese subjects (Chen et al. (2017).

In order to reveal the role of metabolism in the relation between phthalate metabolites, bisphenols and T2DM (Duan et al. 2021), fasting blood and spot urine samples of 60 T2DM cases and 60 control volunteers were evaluated for non-targeted metabolomics analysis and phthalate metabolite and bisphenol determinations. The findings of the study indicated that phthalate exposure may contribute to T2DM risk through disturbing galactose, amino acid, and pyrimidine metabolism.

Bodin et al. (2015) investigated the effects of oral exposure to Bisphenol A, a mixture of phthalates (DEHP, DBP, BBP and DIBP) or a combination of BPA and the phthalate mixture through drinking water from conception and throughout life to examine possible development of T1DM in non-obese diabetic mice. They concluded that exposure to BPA, but not to phthalates or mixed exposure to BPA and phthalates, accelerated diabetes development. Likewise, OGTT was carried out to 8 weeks old male offspring exposed to maternal and lactational DEHP (600 mg/kg bw/day) and resulted increased insulin levels with no change in indexes for pancreas islet function at male offspring aged 14 weeks (Zhang et al. 2018). C57BL/6J male mice were exposed to 2 mg/kg bw/day DEHP for 15 weeks to understand the effect of DEHP on insulin signaling regulatory pathway in skeletal muscle (Wei et al. 2020). FBG increased in DEHP exposed mice, whereas no change in fasting blood insulin levels were found. When systemic insulin sensitivity and quantitative insulin sensitivity check index after DEHP exposure decreased, HOMA-IR was found to be higher compared to control. The expression and phosphorylation of INSR and insulin receptor substrate-1 decreased in the muscle of DEHP exposed group.

Epidemiologic studies showed that phthalate exposure is related with obesity, and the obesity increases the risk of T2DM. There are *in vivo* studies to understand the effects of phthalate exposure on the development of diabetes with high fat diet. To determine the diabetes-like effects of DEHP, Wang et al. (2016) conducted a study with male Balb/c mice grouped as follows: vehicle control; 10, 50 or 250 mg/kg bw/day DEHP with normal diet; diabetes model (STZ and high fat diet); 10, 50 or 250 mg/kg bw/day DEHP and diabetes model. DEHP did not directly induce diabetes but lowers serum insulin levels in animals exposed to DEHP alone. It has been suggested that dose-related damage to the pancreas of DEHP plus STZ-exposed mice occurred that caused by the oxidative mechanism. In another study, BBP at various doses (4 μg/kg bw/day, 169 μg/kg bw/day, 3 mg/kg bw/day, 50 mg/kg bw/day) mixed with chow diet or high fat diets was exposed to C57BL/6 male and female mice for 16 weeks to examine the detrimental and sex-specific metabolic disorders (Zhang et al. 2020). Male mice exposed to 3 mg/kg bw/day BBP on a high-fat diet had significant increases in body weight, liver and adipose tissue weights, and showed significant increases in FBG, glucose intolerance and insulin intolerance compared to high fed diet alone. These effects were not observed in female mice. With these results of the studies, DEHP, DBP and BBP may increase the risk of T2DM in rats by decreasing the serum insulin levels and worsen high fat- and STZ-induced diabetes conditions.

Oxidative Stress, Apoptosis, Beta Cell Loss and Phthalates

Oxidative stress is defined as increasement of reactive oxygen species (ROS) and reactive nitrogen species (RNS) or imbalance between antioxidative defense mechanisms and oxidants. Potential oxidative stress generating sources are production of ROS through mitochondrial oxidative phosphorylation, exposure to ionizing radiation, metabolism of exogenous compounds and pathological processes such as diabetes, atherosclerosis and cancer. Oxidative damage of ROS can be categorized as free oxygen radicals and non-radical ROS. Free oxygen radicals are any chemicals that has an ability to be found unbound and has one or more unpaired electrons (Thannickal and Fanburg 2000). When free radicals react with non-radical ROS, a new radical is formed and this can end up with chain reaction of free radical formulation (Thannickal and Fanburg 2000). Molecular oxygen is needed for life to exist however it accepts electrons easily and therefore free radicals, including ROS, can widely increase. These short-lived free radicals can carry their damaging effects above their limited diffusion periods. Excessive ROS generation induces oxidative stress, cell function loss and as a result apoptosis and necrosis (Halliwell et al. 2000). Once ROS is produced, it reacts with oxidative damage susceptible parts of the cell (lipids on the cell membrane, nucleotides at DNA, sulfhydryl groups at proteins and cross-linking parts of ribonucleoproteins) and causes alterations at cellular structure and functions.

Presence of DEHP, MBP and DBP were positively correlated with the oxidative stress markers such as serum gamma glutamyl transferase (GGT) and C-reactive protein (CRP) (Ferguson et al. 2011). An *in vitro* study revealed that when L6 myotubes were exposed to various concentrations of DEHP, insulin receptor and GLUT4 gene expression, insulin receptor protein concentration, glucose uptake and oxidation, and enzymatic and non-enzymatic antioxidants significantly reduced in a dose dependent manner. At the same study, glutamine fructose-6-phosphate amidotransferase, nitric oxide (NO), lipid peroxidation, and ROS levels also elevated in a dose dependent manner (Rajesh and Balasubramanian 2014a). Moreover, clinical studies showed the connection between phthalates and oxidative damage at diabetes patients. A total of 329 patient clinical study investigated levels of 11 phthalate metabolites including MBP, MIBP, MBZP, MCPP, MEHP, MEHHP, MEOHP, MMP, MEP, MECPP, and MCMHP in urine samples. The levels of lipid peroxidation were assessed at the same study by using malondialdehyde (MDA) which is induced after excessive ROS production. All the 11 phthalates investigated were found to positively associate with increased oxidative stress leves in T2DM patients (Duan et al. 2017).

Mitochondria is the major source of the ROS production in the cell. Through the oxidative phosphorylation process, electrons transfer from one complex to another (NADH: ubiquinone oxidoreductase (complex I), succinate dehydrogenase (complex II), coenzyme Q: cytochrome c reductase (complex III), cytochrome C oxidase (complex IV)) within the mitochondrial inner membrane generating a proton gradient which drives ATP synthase (complex V) resulting with ATP production. ROS are formed by the electron leakage from complex I, II and III with one electron reduction of oxygen to superoxide ($O_2^{\bullet-}$) (Goncalves et al. 2015, Chouchani et al. 2014). At normal and healthy cells, ROS levels are controlled by antioxidants such as superoxide dismutase (SOD), glutathione peroxidase (GPX) and catalase. However, at diabetes, intracellular hyperglycemia, which is known as major complication of diabetes, increases mitochondrial membrane potential to a threshold that blocks electron transfer from complex III and reverses electron transport (RET) which increases superoxide formation (Korshunov et al. 1997). This triggers a maladaptive response by overproducing superoxide anions and affects several metabolic and signaling pathways which are involved in diabetic complications.

ROS, such as superoxide and H_2O_2, can be converted into H_2O and O_2 by antioxidant enzymes (SOD, GPX and CAT) and phthalates has the ability to decrease the capacity of these antioxidants (Abdollahi et al. 2014). DEHP, for instance, can decrease SOD and therefore lead the accumulation of MDA in islet beta cells (INS-1) (She et al. 2017). MEHP, which is 20 times more toxic than DEHP in rats, also reduces SOD and glutathione (GSH) levels of INS-1 cells in a dose dependent manner (Shi et al. 2020).

Damaged cells within a multi-cellular organism are removed from the body mainly with a process called apoptosis (also known as programmed cell death). Apoptosis is mediated by intrinsic (mitochondrial) and extrinsic (receptor mediated) pathways. Intrinsic pathway can be activated by oxidative stress and various extra and intra cellular stresses. Regulation of intrinsic pathway depends on the balance between pro- and anti- apoptotic members of the Bcl-2 protein family and susceptibility of the cells to apoptosis is determined by Bcl-2 (anti-apoptotic protein)/Bax (pro- apoptotic protein) ratio. When this ratio is decreased, mitochondrial outer membrane disruption increases which leads to release of cytochrome c into the cytoplasm. Released cytochrome c activates a caspase cascade ending with caspase 3 triggering apoptosis. *In vivo* and *in vitro* studies revealed that in both T1DM and T2DM, beta cell death occurs by apoptosis. In T1DM, destruction of beta cells was mediated by macrophages and T cells which release chemokines and cytokines to the microenvironment of the islets and then deliver pro-apoptotic signals (Cnop et al. 2005, Thomaidou et al. 2018). In T2DM, reduced beta cell mass was linked to increased beta cell apoptosis (Butler et al. 2003, Yoon et al. 2003).

Phthalate exposure has been linked to pancreatic beta cell apoptosis by several groups. Two of the mainly exposed phthalates, DEHP and DBP and their combination, increased ROS levels and induced apoptosis at INS-1 cells (rat insulinoma cells) by inhibiting the PI3K/Akt/Bcl-2 signaling pathway (Li et al. 2021). DEHP and DBP combination exposure increased susceptibility of INS-1 cells to apoptosis compared to DEHP and DBP alone groups. Caspase 8 protein expression level was also increased with DEHP and DBP alone or combination exposure suggesting that extrinsic pathway acts on inducing apoptosis at INS-1 cells (Li et al. 2021). In another study with the same cell line (INS-1), exposure to MEHP, main metabolite of DEHP, also induced apoptosis through mitochondrial membrane potential depolarization and cytochrome c release following activation of caspase 9 and 3 (Shi et al. 2020).

In silico studies revealed the link between 44 DEHP and DBP mutual genes linked to T2DM where apoptosis and oxidative stress were the main mechanisms of work (Baralic et al. 2021). Data mining results from the same study showed that DEHP and DBP interacted with genes which encode both pro-apoptotic (BAX) and anti-apoptotic members of the Bcl2 family (BCL2). When DBP decreased the expression of mRNA expression of BAX, DEHP both increased and decreased its expression suggesting the response is dose- and exposure time- dependent. Besides, both DEHP and DBP were found to interact with CASP3 and CASP8 (Baralic et al. 2021). Although there are several reports demonstrating the role of oxidative stress and apoptosis at phthalate toxicity, a clear relationship and the main cause is still under question since beta cell apoptosis is difficult to detect *in vivo*.

Phthalates, Inflammation and Diabetes

Besides oxidative stress and apoptosis, it was reported that inflammatory cytokines play important roles in the pathogenesis of diabetes (S et al. 2014, Ghoshal and Bhattacharyya 2015, Liu et al. 2016, Tong et al. 2017). Pathogen invasion, tissue injury or irritants can cause an important physiological response called inflammation. High glucose concentrations and oxidative stress can mediate the release of the inflammatory mediators such as cytokines. In T1DM, destruction of beta cells was mediated by macrophages and T cells which release chemokines and cytokines such as interferon gamma (IFN-γ), TNF- α and IL-1 beta to the microenvironment of the islets. When these inflammatory molecules act together, they upregulate the inducible nitric oxide synthase (iNOS) with subsequent production of nitric oxide (NO) however it was shown that NO is not implicated in the pancreatic beta cell damage (Thomas et al. 2002, Arif et al. 2011). In T2DM, islet inflammation is also seen at several experimental models and beta cell damage is caused mainly by inflammasome/IL-1 beta signaling pathway (Sauter et al. 2008). It was suggested by Maedler et al. (2003) that hyperglycemia induces IL-1 beta production via free fatty acid stimulation (pro apoptotic receptor) at pancreatic beta cells. These free fatty acids also cause production and secretion of IL-1 beta and IL-1-dependent pro-inflammatory cytokines in pancreatic islets. IL-1 beta production is regulated by auto stimulation at pancreatic beta cells and this process increases NO production which leads to decreased ATP production in mitochondria causing beta cell dysfunction along with reduced insulin secretion (Boni-Schnetzler et al. 2009).

In vivo and *in vitro* studies report that exposure to phthalate metabolites increases the production of pro-inflammatory cytokines (Zhou et al. 2019, Bolling et al. 2020, Nishioka et al. 2012). Duan et al. (2017) stated that urinary phthalate metabolite concentrations were positively associated with urinary MDA levels (oxidative stress biomarker) in a study conducted with diabetic patients aged from 29 to 93. It has been revealed that decreased levels of adiponectin (a secretory protein produced by adipose tissue) in serum is associated with chronic inflammation of metabolic disorders including T2DM (Choi et al. 2020). In the same study, Duan et al. (2017) revealed that MMP concentrations in the urine had inverse association with serum adiponectin levels however other phthalate metabolites (MECPP, MCMHP, MEHHP, MEOHP, MBZP, MCPP, MBP, MIBP, and sum of phthalate metabolites) were positively related. TNF-α is a 26 kDa cell surface transmembrane protein and its actions were mediated by two distinct membrane receptors called TNFR-1 and TNFR-2 (Idriss and Naismith 2000). TNF-α is found in white adipose tissue and in human fat, and positively correlated with obesity or hyperinsulinemia (Hotamisligil et al. 1995, Kern et al. 1995). *In vivo* studies also revealed that TNF-α levels were positively correlated with MMP concentrations whereas MECPP, MEHHP, MEOHP, MBZP, MBP, and MIBP were negatively associated (Duan et al. 2017).

Inflammation biomarkers such as CRP, alkaline phosphatase (ALP), absolute neutrophil count (ANC) and ferritin were reported to be positively associated with urinary phthalate metabolites (MBZP, MIBP, MEHHP, MEOHP, MBP, MCPP, MECPP, and MEHP) in a study carried out between 1999 to 2006 in U.S. population (NHANES 1999-2006) (Ferguson et al. 2011, 2012). It was also revealed that TNF-α, IL-6, IL-8, or IL-1β levels were elevated at human umbilical vein endothelial cells, macrophages, corneal endothelial cells, bronchial epithelial cells, endometrial cells, and epithelial cells exposed to increased levels of DEHP and DBP (Nishioka et al. 2012, Jepsen et al. 2004, Kruger et al. 2012). However, our knowledge about the relationship between inflammation biomarkers and phthalate concentrations at diabetes are still limited.

Phthalate Exposure and Epigenetics of Diabetes

Epigenetics is defined as alterations at gene expressions in a cell that are not caused by DNA sequence changes (Waterland 2006). Epigenetic mechanisms which alter the gene expression are DNA methylation, histone modifications and RNA based mechanisms (non-coding RNAs). It has been revealed that epigenetics influence gene expression profiles of most organs and cell types and can act on human health and diseases (Schwartz and Collins 2007, Perera and Herbstman 2011). Role of epigenetic factors in the pathogenesis of T2DM were partly revealed by data mining studies however due to the limitations of getting target tissue from diabetes patients, only several number of studies has examined the epigenetic changes (Wren and Garner 2005). Alterations of DNA methylation, histone modifications and long non-coding RNAs (lncRNA) were observed at autopsy samples of human islets from subjects with T2DM (Moran et al. 2012, Stitzel et al. 2010, Volkov et al. 2017).

In daily life, human get exposed to variety of pollutants such as phthalates and these chemicals appear to play critical roles at chemical-induced epigenetic changes (Anway et al. 2008). One of the most common exposed phthalates, DEHP, was found to be correlated with increased DNA methylation and histone deacetylase 2 interaction toward GLUT4 at pregnant rats with decreased phosphorylation of insulin signaling molecules (Rajesh and Balasubramanian 2014b). Another study examined urinary concentrations of five different phthalate ester metabolites (MBP, MMP, MEHP, MEHHP and MEOHP) and used multiple regression models to reveal the associations between placental DNA methylation and phthalate exposure. At the same study, there were no significant associations were found between placental DNA methylation and urinary concentrations of MBP and MMP however urinary concentrations of MEHHP and MEOHP inversely associated with increased *Igf2* DNA methylation in human placenta (Zhao et al. 2016). Association between phthalates and DNA methylation was further assessed at a study conducted for 3 years in Mexican children. Urinary phthalate concentrations of nine different phthalate metabolites (MEP, MBP, MiBP, MCPP, MBzP, MEHP, MEHHP, MEOHP and MECPP) were measured in mothers at each of the three trimesters of pregnancy and in children at the first peri-adolescent study visit (Bowman et al. 2019). Interestingly, it was found that phthalate exposure revealed sex-specific associations of DNA methylations among Mexican children. Among girls, MBZP exposure was correlated with decreased adiposity and urinary MIBP concentrations were associated with increase in skinfold thickness (Bowman et al. 2019).

A study conducted with 622 adults aged between 18-81 years examined 15 metabolites of 9 phthalates (DMP, DEP, DIBP, DBP, DEHP, DHP, BBP, DINP and DIDP) associated with cytosine-phosphated guanines (CpGs) methylations and the genes within 1 Mb distance to the CpG sites. Methylation marker, cg06890484 in Protein Tyrosine Phosphatase Receptor Type J (PTPRJ) which regulates the insulin signaling pathway by suppressing the insulin sensitivity was found to be associated with both MEHHP and MEOHP (Lu et al. 2020).

There is also growing evidence for the association between phthalate exposure, miRNA expressions and metabolic disorders during gestation (Martínez-Ibarra et al. 2019). A study conducted among Mexican women revealed a significant positive correlation between increased urinary levels of MBZP and expression levels of miR-16-5p in non-diabetic women. In the same study, there was a negative correlation between unadjusted and adjusted urinary levels of MBP and miR-29 level expressions in both diabetic and non-diabetic woman. Moreover, another negative correlation was found between unadjusted MIBP levels and miR-29-3p expression levels ($r = -0.6719$, $p < 0.01$) (Martínez-Ibarra et al. 2019).

Animal models were also used to study the relationship between phthalate exposure and epigenetics of diabetes. Skeletal muscle insulin resistance, an early event of T2DM, was associated with miR200a (Wei et al. 2020). DEHP exposed mice were injected with anti-miR-200a lentivirus and downregulation of insulin signaling genes *Insr* and *Irs1* was suppressed. Insulin dependent pAkt and GLUT4 translocation was also restored with the anti-miR-200a injection in parallel with whole body insulin resistance amelioration (Wei et al. 2020).

Accumulating data demonstrates the relationship between the phthalate exposure and altered epigenetic landscape at diabetes. However, due to the limitations of getting target tissue from diabetes patients, whether epigenetic alterations are cause or correlation still needs to be determined.

Gestational Diabetes and Phthalates

Gestational diabetes (GDM) is a widespread disease revealed in pregnant woman with abnormally elevated blood glucose in the second or third trimester of pregnancy, who has not been diagnosed with diabetes before gestation (ADA 2020). GDM occurs when pregnant women have dysfunctional β-cells that do not meet their increased insulin requirements on a background of chronic insulin resistance (Plows et al. 2018). According to the most recent (2021) International Diabetes Federation (IDF) estimates, global prevalence of hyperglycemia in pregnancy is approximately 16.7% worldwide, representing approximately 21.1 million births annually, and 80.3% were due to GDM (IDF 2021).

The mother undergoes many metabolic and physiological changes during a healthy pregnancy. One of the most important metabolic adaptations during pregnancy is insulin sensitivity promoted by numerous placental hormones. During early gestation, insulin sensitivity increases promoting glucose uptake into fat stores in preparation for energy demands later in pregnancy (Di Cianni et al. 2003, Plows et al. 2018). Chen et al. (2020) examined the toxicological effect of maternal DBP exposure (750 mg/kg bw/day) on development of GDM. STZ, was also treated intraperitoneally to rats at gestational day (GD) 0 with or without DBP on GD 1-3. On GD 1 and 5, the FBG were measured and the insulin levels and OGTT on GD 18. The primary islet β cells were established for *in vitro* experiments to analyze the viability and apoptosis, the expression of phosphorylated signal transducer and activator of transcription 1 (pSTAT1) and Forkhead box protein M1 (FoxM1) of the cells. The researchers reported that DBP exposure with STZ caused higher FBG and lower insulin levels than the other groups. DBP exposure triggered the pSTAT1 expression while FoxM1 was significantly suppressed. The authors concluded that DBP can exacerbate GDM, causing a decline in beta cell viability (Chen et al. 2020).

In addition to the studies showing phthalate exposure in pregnant women (Toft et al. 2012, Preece et al. 2021, He et al. 2019), there are epidemiologic studies revealed the association between phthalate metabolites and GDM (Table 5). In a prospective cohort study by James-Todd et al. (2018), 245 subfertile women, who delivered live births and had data on pregnancy urinary phthalate metabolite concentrations and blood glucose levels, was included to the studyto find out the association between urinary phthalate metabolites and pregnancy glucose levels. The researchers reported that 18% of the pregnant women had glucose levels above 140 mg/dL. MEP and MIBP were found to be associated with higher pregnancy glucose in subfertile women, a population at high risk of glucose intolerance in pregnancy.

In addition to GDM risk factors (such as pre-pregnancy obesity, gestational weight gain (GWG), elevated blood sugar), EDCs are also thought to be among these risks throughout pregnancy (Alonso-Magdalena et al. 2011). For this reason, studies have been conducted to reveal the relationships between phthalate exposure and GDM markers in pregnant women. In a Lifecodes pregnancy cohort study (James-Todd et al. 2016b), it was concluded that higher exposure to MEP may be associated with excessive GWG and impaired glucose tolerance, and higher DEHP exposure was associated with reduced odds of impaired glucose tolerance (James-Todd et al. 2016b). In another study, Fisher et al. (2018) examined the relationship between maternal serum levels of phthalate metabolites and phenols at 10–17 weeks of gestation and glucose homeostasis at 28 weeks of gestation. OGTT were implemented at 28 weeks of gestation. GDM was detected in 47 (20.3%) pregnant women who participated in the study. It was found that MEHP and MCIOP concentration of first trimester in pregnant women without GDM was associated with 120-minute plasma glucose in mid-pregnancy (Fisher et al. 2018). Likewise, another study revealed the relationship between phthalate exposure and gestational blood sugar. 350 pregnant women were measured up to four times throughout pregnancy averaged across pregnancy and log-transformed, adjusted for specific gravity (Noor et al. 2019). Glucose levels of subjects were assessed after 50-g glucose challenge tests to predict GDM at 24–28 weeks of gestation, and categorized as <120 mg/dL, 120–<140 mg/dL and ≥140 mg/dL. MEP concentrations were found to be higher among women who had glucose levels ≥140 mg/dL, not associated with birth weight.

GDM can have long- and short-term consequences for both mother (increased risk of pre-eclampsia, premature rupture of membranes, cesarean section, and preterm delivery) and offspring (higher risk of being macrosomic or large-for-gestational-age) (Xiong et al. 2001). It is stated that phthalates are excreted in very low amounts in meconium, therefore it is a matrix that can be used to determine the exposure of fetuses to phthalates via mother. (Frederiksen et al. 2007). In this respect, Guo et al. (2020) examined the associations between meconium exposure to ten phthalates metabolites (MMP, MEP, MBP, MIBP, MBZP, MEHP, MEHHP, MEOHP, MECPP, MCMHP) in 251 mother–infant pairs and found positive association MIBP, MBP and MEHP levels with GDM only in mothers with male newborns, indicated that meconium exposure to phthalates may adversely affect GDM with a potential gender effect.

Table 5. Summary of the studies assessing the association between phthalate exposure and GDM

Author (Year) Country	Age	N	Sample Matrix/Phthalate Metabolite Analyzed	Outcome
Robledo et al. (2015) USA	>18	72	Urinary/MBP, MIBP, MEHP, MEHHP, MEOHP, MECPP, MCPP, MEP, MBZP	MIBP and MBZP associated lower blood glucose levels
Shapiro et al. (2015) Canada	≥18	2001	Urinary/MEP, MBP, MBZP, MCPP, MEHP, MEHHP, MEOHP, MCHP, MOP, MNP, MMP	No significant associations between phthalate metabolites and impaired glucose tolerance and GDM
James-Todd et al. (2016b) USA	<25, 25-<30, 30-<35, ≥35	350	Urinary/MEP, MBP, MIBP, MBZP, MCPP, MEHP, MECPP, MEHHP, MEOHP	Higher exposure to MEP associated with excessive GWG and impaired glucose tolerance Higher DEHP metabolite exposure associated with reduced odds of impaired glucose tolerance
James-Todd et al. (2018) USA	26-47	245	Urinary/MEHP, MEHHP, MEOHP, MECPP, MCPP, MCOP, MCNP, MBZP, MIBP, MBP	MEP and MIBP concentrations associated with higher pregnancy glucose in subfertile women
Fisher et al. (2018) UK	≥16	2229	Urinary/MEP, MBP, MIBP, MPP, MBZP, MEHP, MEHHP, MEOHP, MECPP, MOP, MCPP, MINP, MHINP, MOINP, MCIOP, MIDP	First trimester MEHP and MCIOP concentration in pregnant women without GDM associated with 120-minute plasma glucose in mid-pregnancy
Shaffer et al. 2019 USA	≥18	705	Urinary/MIBP, MEP, MNBP, MBZP, MCNP, MCOP, MCPP, MEHP, MEHHP, MEOHP, MECPP	The average of T1 and T3 MEP concentration positively associated with GDM
Noor et al. 2019 USA	31.9 (5.4)	350	Urinary/MEP, MBP, MIBP, MBZP, MCCP, MEHP, MEHHP, MEOHP	MEP concentrations were higher among women who had glucose levels ≥140 mg/dL
Martínez-Ibarra et al. (2019) Mexico	24-45	40	Urinary/MBP, MIBP, MBZP, MEHP	Positive correlations between adjusted urinary MBZP and MEHP levels and GDM-related miRNAs Negative correlations between unadjusted and adjusted MBP and unadjusted MIBP concentrations and GDM-related miRNAs

Author (Year) Country	**Age**	**N**	**Sample Matrix/Phthalate Metabolite Analyzed**	**Outcome**
Guo et al. (2020) China	27-31	251	Meconium/MMP, MEP, MBP, MIBP, MBZP, MEHP, MEHHP, MEOHP, MECPP, MCMHP	Positive association MIBP, MBP and MEHP levels with GDM only in mothers with male newborns
Gao et al. (2021) China	≤24.9-35	3273	Urinary/MMP, MEP, MBP, MBZP, MEHP, MEOHP, MEHHP	Most phthalate associated with increased blood glucose and GWG especially in the first trimester Negative relationships with MEHP and MEOHP and FPG during early pregnancy
Wu et al. 2021 Mexico	27.7 (5.5)-27.3(5.6)	618	Urinary/MEHP, MEOHP, MEHHP, MECPP, MECPTP, MONP, MCOP, MCNP, MCPP, MBZP, MHIBP, MIBP, MBP, MHBP, MEP	Higher urinary phthalate metabolite levels related with postpartum concentrations of FBG, plasma insulin, HOMA-IR and % HbA1c. The associations predominantly conducted by MECPTP and the sum of DBP metabolites
Zukin et al. (2021) USA	18-45	415	Urinary/MEP, MBP, MIBP, MZBP, MEHP, MEHHP, MEOHP, MECCP, MCPP, MCOP, MCNP	No association between phthalate metabolites and impaired glucose tolerance, GDM or hyperglycemia, except for an increased odd of excessive GWG

Metabolic changes during pregnancy lead to impaired glucose tolerance, resulting in elevated blood sugar. In response to this, as the pregnancy develops in healthy pregnant women, the need for insulin and insulin production increases. However, glucose intolerance develops in some pregnant women resulting in GDM or impaired glucose tolerance (Tuffnell et al. 2003). In addition to other studies investigating the effects of increased FBG and pregnancy phthalate exposure, there are epidemiological studies that reveal the relationship between impaired glucose tolerance and phthalate exposure in pregnant women (James-Todd et al. 2016b, Fisher et al. 2018, Noor et al. 2019). In The Infant Development and Environment Study (TIDES), the association between 11 urinary phthalate metabolites (MIBP, MEP, MNBP, MBZP, MCNP, MCOP, MCPP, MEHP, MEHHP, MEOHP, MECPP) and GDM, impaired glucose tolerance, and continuous blood glucose concentration during pregnancy was evaluated (Shaffer et al. 2019). The average of first and third trimester MEP concentration was found to be positively associated with GDM.

Women with GDM have a higher risk of developing T2DM later in life than pregnant women without GDM (Sheiner 2020). In addition to the studies in which the relationship between phthalate exposure in pregnant women and markers related to GDM during pregnancy evaluated, there is also a study evaluating the metabolic status of these women beyond pregnancy. Concentrations of 15 urinary phthalate metabolites were measured during the second and third trimesters of 618 pregnant women (Wu et al. 2021). Higher urinary phthalate metabolite levels during pregnancy were found to be related with postpartum concentrations of FBG, plasma insulin, HOMA-IR and % HbA1c. The associations were predominantly conducted by mono-2-ethyl-5-carboxypentyl terephthalate (MECPTP) and the sum of DBP metabolites. Although this study is a cross-sectional study, it was revealed that exposure to phthalates during pregnancy may be associated with metabolic markers even up to 8 years after delivery.

Phthalates are known to activate PPAR which modulates the expression of its target genes and the differentiation of the cells into adipocytes (Rodríguez-Carmona et al. 2019, Desvergne and Wahli 1999). PPARα involves potential changes in lipid deposition and beta cell functioning, with important implications for the insulin-resistant state of pregnancy, and PPARγ is induced during adipocyte differentiation (Evans et al. 2004, Desvergne and Wahli 1999). Excessive GWG during pregnancy is an important risk factor for GDM. There are studies indicating that EDCs are associated with excessive GWG and thus may cause GDM, as these environmental chemicals have been suggested to cause other types of DM (Bellavia et al. 2017, Philips et al. 2020, Rolfo et al. 2020, Rodríguez-Carmona et al. 2019). Based on the Ma'anshan Birth Cohort by Gao et al. (2021), the cumulative risk of multiple phthalate co-exposures was evaluated by using hazard index (HI) includes the outcomes of hypertensive disorders of pregnancy (HDOP), GDM and GWG. MBP, MMP, MEOHP and MEHHP levels revealed that DBP and DEHP exposure were highest among these pregnants. The incidences of HDOP, GDM, and excessive GWG were reported as 5.93%, 13.09%, and 28.95%, respectively. The authors found out that exposure to a single phthalate metabolite or a specific diester during the first trimester of pregnancy elevated blood pressure (BP) and FBG in the third trimester and increased body weight throughout pregnancy. Besides, HI in the first trimester was positively correlated with subsequent BP, FPG, and GWG, HI during the first trimester increased the risks of GDM and excessive GWG in a linear manner thereafter. Noteworthy, the authors concluded that the direct effect of phthalate exposure on FBG and BP of pregnants were related to secondary outcomes of obesogenic effects of certain phthalate exposure that may increase the risks of gestational metabolic syndrome components (Gao et al. 2021). In another study, the authors reported no association between phthalate metabolites and impaired glucose tolerance, GDM or hyperglycemia, except for an increased odd of excessive GWG that is well-known risk factor for GDM (Zukin et al. 2021).

MicroRNAs (miRNAs), which are important in the development of placenta, are epigenetic modifiers involved in the pathogenesis of diseases that occur with pregnancy. Certain miRNAs in the placenta have been associated with pregnancy complications such as pregnancy loss, preeclampsia, intrauterine growth restriction, GDM, obesity, and preterm delivery. These miRNAs may also enter the maternal circulation, saliva, urine, milk and amniotic fluid (Addo et al. 2020). Due to the important role of miRNAs in pregnancy homeostasis and dysregulation of miRNAs may be associated with GDM (Lizárraga and García-Gasca 2021). There are studies showing the relationship between miRNAs and phthalates in pregnancy (LaRocca et al. 2016). Martínez-Ibarra et al. (2019) investigated the relation between urinary MBP, MIBP, MBZP, MEHP and serum levels of GDM risk associated miRNAs (miR-9-5p, miR-16-5p, miR-29a-3p and miR-330-3p) in GDM patients and women without GDM during the second trimester of gestation. Higher levels of miR-9-5p, miR-29a-3p and miR-330-3p of patients with GDM were observed compared to non-diabetic subjects. It was found that 97–100% of urine samples had detectable phthalate concentrations. Besides adjusted MEHP concentrations and miR-29a-3p expression levels, the positive correlations between adjusted urinary MBZP levels and miR-16-5p expression levels were detected. Negative correlations between unadjusted and adjusted MBP concentrations and miR-29a-3p expression levels, as well as unadjusted MIBP concentrations and miR-29a-3p expression levels, were found.

Contrary, some studies showed that there is no relationship between phthalate metabolites and GDM. Shapiro et al. (2015) designed a study in the Maternal–Infant Research on Environmental Chemicals (MIREC) which included women without pre-existing diabetes and with a singleton delivery. When assessing impaired glucose tolerance and GDM, the authors reported no statistically significant associations between phthalate metabolites, BPA or metals, except for arsenic. Besides, Robledo et al. (2015) examined associations between phthalate metabolite concentrations (MBP, MIBP, MEHP, MEHHP, MEOHP, MECPP, MCPP, MEP, MBZP) in urine adjusted by creatinine during early pregnancy and blood glucose levels obtained during GDM screening. Pregnant women with the highest urine concentrations of MIBP and MBZP had lower blood glucose levels at the time of GDM screening compared with pregnant women with the lowest tertile concentrations, after adjusting for urinary creatinine and demographic covariates.

Conclusion

It is evident that exposure to certain phthalates, especially DEHP, DBP and DIBP, is associated with impaired glucose and insulin signaling which are related to diabetes mellitus. PPARs seem to be the main mechanism by which phthalates exert their effects on glucose homeostasis, however, it is still far from being fully understood. There are growing evidence of studies revealing the relationship between phthalate exposure and oxidative stress induced apoptosis at diabetes patients. Phthalates decrease the capacity of antioxidant enzymes and disturb the oxidant/antioxidant balance. Hence a maladaptive response gets triggered by overproduction of superoxide anions and several metabolic and signaling pathways which involved in diabetic complications get affected. Increased levels of oxidants by phthalate exposure leads to apoptotic cell death through mitochondrial membrane potential depolarization and cytochrome c release. Inflammation, another diabetes mediated feature, was also found to be positively associated with urinary phthalate metabolites at DM patients. DNA methylation and histone deacetylase 2 interaction toward GLUT4 was also found to be correlated with phthalate exposure at diabetes suggesting epigenetic modifications also take part in the disease progression. It is clear from epidemiologic studies, metabolites of DEHP and DEP are related with GDM. On the other hand, the mechanism of the phthalate effects during pregnancy needs to be further studied. The underlying mechanism of the association between phthalate exposure, glucose metabolism and insulin action remains to be determined.

DEHP is the most studied phthalate ester. Other phthalate esters should be also studied further to reveal their relationship with these endocrine disruptors and glucose homeostasis. The synergistic effects of phthalates with other phthalates or with other endocrine disruptors have not been analyzed yet. In addition, the possible negative effects of exposure to these substances in the long term and during the critical periods are among the very important issues to be studied. As a conclusion, we cannot clearly state that phthalates are diabetogenic chemicals yet. To highlight their role in the diabetes occurance and progression, further *in vitro, in vivo* and epidemiologic studies should be performed.

References

Abdollahi, M., M. Y. Moridani, O. I. Aruoma, and S. Mostafalou. 2014. "Oxidative stress in aging." *Oxid Med Cell Longev* 2014:876834. doi: 10.1155/2014/876834.

ADA. 2014. "Diagnosis and classification of diabetes mellitus." *Diabetes Care* 37 Suppl 1:S81-90. doi: 10.2337/dc14-S081.

ADA. 2020. "2. Classification and diagnosis of diabetes: standards of medical care in diabetes—2021 American Diabetes Association." *Diabetes Care* 44 (Supplement_1): S15-S33. doi: 10.2337/dc21-S002.

Addo, Kezia A., Niharika Palakodety, Hadley J. Hartwell, Aishani Tingare, and Rebecca C. Fry. 2020. "Placental microRNAs: Responders to environmental chemicals and mediators of pathophysiology of the human placenta." *Toxicology reports* 7:1046-1056. doi: 10.1016/j.toxrep.2020.08.002.

Alonso-Magdalena, P., I. Quesada, and A. Nadal. 2011. "Endocrine disruptors in the etiology of type 2 diabetes mellitus." *Nat Rev Endocrinol* 7 (6):346-53. doi: 10.1038/nrendo.2011.56.

Anway, M. D., S. S. Rekow, and M. K. Skinner. 2008. "Transgenerational epigenetic programming of the embryonic testis transcriptome." *Genomics* 91 (1):30-40. doi: 10.1016/j.ygeno.2007.10.002.

Arif, S., F. Moore, K. Marks, T. Bouckenooghe, C. M. Dayan, R. Planas, M. Vives-Pi, J. Powrie, T. Tree, P. Marchetti, G. C. Huang, E. N. Gurzov, R. Pujol-Borrell, D. L. Eizirik, and M. Peakman. 2011. "Peripheral and islet interleukin-17 pathway activation characterizes human autoimmune diabetes and promotes cytokine-mediated beta-cell death." *Diabetes* 60 (8):2112-9. doi: 10.2337/db10-1643.

Auwerx, J. 1999. "PPARgamma, the ultimate thrifty gene." *Diabetologia* 42 (9):1033-49. doi: 10.1007/s001250051268.

Baralic, K., K. Zivancevic, D. Jorgovanovic, D. Javorac, J. Radovanovic, T. Gojkovic, A. Buha Djordjevic, M. Curcic, Z. Mandinic, Z. Bulat, B. Antonijevic, and D. Dukic-Cosic. 2021. "Probiotic reduced the impact of phthalates and bisphenol A mixture on type 2 diabetes mellitus development: Merging bioinformatics with in vivo analysis." *Food Chem Toxicol* 154:112325. doi: 10.1016/j.fct.2021.112325.

Bellavia, A., R. Hauser, E. W. Seely, J. D. Meeker, K. K. Ferguson, T. F. McElrath, and T. James-Todd. 2017. "Urinary phthalate metabolite concentrations and maternal weight during early pregnancy." *Int J Hyg Environ Health* 220 (8):1347-1355. doi: 10.1016/j.ijheh.2017.09.005.

Benjamin, S., E. Masai, N. Kamimura, K. Takahashi, R. C. Anderson, and P. A. Faisal. 2017. "Phthalates impact human health: Epidemiological evidences and plausible mechanism of action." *J Hazard Mater* 340:360-383. doi: 10.1016/j.jhazmat.2017.06.036.

Bergman, M., M. Abdul-Ghani, R. A. DeFronzo, M. Manco, G. Sesti, T. V. Fiorentino, A. Ceriello, M. Rhee, L. S. Phillips, et. al. 2020. "Review of methods for detecting glycemic disorders." *Diabetes Res Clin Pract* 165:108233. doi: 10.1016/j.diabres.2020.108233.

Bianchi, V. E., and V. Locatelli. 2018. "Testosterone a key factor in gender related metabolic syndrome." *Obesity Reviews* 19 (4):557-575. doi: https://doi.org/10.1111/obr.12633.

Boberg, J., S. Metzdorff, R. Wortziger, M. Axelstad, L. Brokken, A. M. Vinggaard, M. Dalgaard, and C. Nellemann. 2008. "Impact of diisobutyl phthalate and other PPAR agonists on steroidogenesis and plasma insulin and leptin levels in fetal rats." *Toxicology* 250 (2-3):75-81. doi: 10.1016/j.tox.2008.05.020.

Bodin, J., A. Koebach Bølling, A. Wendt, L. Eliasson, R. Becher, F. Kuper, M. Løvik, and U. C. Nygaard. 2015. "Exposure to bisphenol A, but not phthalates, increases spontaneous diabetes type 1 development in NOD mice." *Toxicol Rep* 2:99-110. doi: 10.1016/j.toxrep.2015.02.010.

Bolling, A. K., K. Sripada, R. Becher, and G. Beko. 2020. "Phthalate exposure and allergic diseases: Review of epidemiological and experimental evidence." *Environ Int* 139:105706. doi: 10.1016/j.envint.2020.105706.

Boni-Schnetzler, M., S. Boller, S. Debray, K. Bouzakri, D. T. Meier, R. Prazak, J. Kerr-Conte, F. Pattou, J. A. Ehses, F. C. Schuit, and M. Y. Donath. 2009. "Free fatty acids induce a proinflammatory response in islets via the abundantly expressed interleukin-1 receptor I." *Endocrinology* 150 (12):5218-29. doi: 10.1210/en.2009-0543.

Bowman, A., K. E. Peterson, D. C. Dolinoy, J. D. Meeker, B. N. Sanchez, A. Mercado-Garcia, M. M. Tellez-Rojo, and J. M. Goodrich. 2019. "Phthalate exposures, DNA methylation and adiposity in Mexican children through adolescence." *Front Public Health* 7:162. doi: 10.3389/fpubh.2019.00162.

Bräuner, Elvira V., Cecilie S. Uldbjerg, Youn-Hee Lim, Laura S. Gregersen, Marianna Krause, Hanne Frederiksen, and Anna-Maria Andersson. 2022. "Presence of parabens, phenols and phthalates in paired maternal serum, urine and amniotic fluid."

Environment International 158:106987. doi: https://doi.org/10.1016/j.envint.2021.106987.

Butler, A. E., J. Janson, S. Bonner-Weir, R. Ritzel, R. A. Rizza, and P. C. Butler. 2003. "Beta-cell deficit and increased beta-cell apoptosis in humans with type 2 diabetes." *Diabetes* 52 (1):102-10. doi: 10.2337/diabetes.52.1.102.

Cao, Xu-Liang, Melissa Sparling, Wendy Zhao, and Tye E. Arbuckle. 2021. "GC-MS analysis of phthalates and Di-(2-thylhexyl) adipate in Canadian human milk for exposure assessment of infant population." *Journal of AOAC International* 104 (1): 98-102. doi: 10.1093/jaoacint/qsaa108.

Carlsen, E., A. Giwercman, N. Keiding, and N. E. Skakkebaek. 1992. "Evidence for decreasing quality of semen during past 50 years." *Bmj* 305 (6854):609-13. doi: 10.1136/bmj.305.6854.609.

Casals-Casas, C., J. N. Feige, and B. Desvergne. 2008. "Interference of pollutants with PPARs: endocrine disruption meets metabolism." *Int J Obes (Lond)* 32 Suppl 6:S53-61. doi: 10.1038/ijo.2008.207.

Castro-Correia, C., L. Correia-Sá, S. Norberto, C. Delerue-Matos, V. Domingues, C. Costa-Santos, M. Fontoura, and C. Calhau. 2018. "Phthalates and type 1 diabetes: is there any link?" *Environ Sci Pollut Res Int* 25 (18):17915-17919. doi: 10.1007/s11356-018-1997-z.

Chadt, Alexandra, and Hadi Al-Hasani. 2020. "Glucose transporters in adipose tissue, liver, and skeletal muscle in metabolic health and disease." *Pflügers Archiv - European Journal of Physiology* 472 (9):1273-1298. doi: 10.1007/s00424-020-02417-x.

Chang, W. H., S. Herianto, C. C. Lee, H. Hung, and H. L. Chen. 2021. "The effects of phthalate ester exposure on human health: A review." *Sci Total Environ* 786:147371. doi: 10.1016/j.scitotenv.2021.147371.

Chen, M., S. Zhao, W. H. Guo, Y. P. Zhu, L. Pan, Z. W. Xie, W. L. Sun, and J. T. Jiang. 2020. "Maternal exposure to Di-n-butyl phthalate (DBP) aggravate gestational diabetes mellitus via FoxM1 suppression by pSTAT1 signalling." *Ecotoxicol Environ Saf* 205:111154. doi: 10.1016/j.ecoenv.2020.111154.

Chen, S. Y., J. S. Hwang, F. C. Sung, C. Y. Lin, C. J. Hsieh, P. C. Chen, and T. C. Su. 2017. "Mono-2-ethylhexyl phthalate associated with insulin resistance and lower testosterone levels in a young population." *Environ Pollut* 225:112-117. doi: 10.1016/j.envpol.2017.03.037.

Choi, H. M., H. M. Doss, and K. S. Kim. 2020. "Multifaceted physiological roles of adiponectin in inflammation and diseases." *Int J Mol Sci* 21 (4). doi: 10.3390/ijms21041219.

Chouchani, E. T., V. R. Pell, E. Gaude, D. Aksentijevic, S. Y. Sundier, E. L. Robb, A. Logan, S. M. Nadtochiy, E. N. J. Ord, A. C. Smith, F. Eyassu, R. Shirley, C. H. Hu, A. J. Dare, A. M. James, S. Rogatti, R. C. Hartley, S. Eaton, A. S. H. Costa, P. S. Brookes, S. M. Davidson, M. R. Duchen, K. Saeb-Parsy, M. J. Shattock, A. J. Robinson, L. M. Work, C. Frezza, T. Krieg, and M. P. Murphy. 2014. "Ischaemic accumulation of succinate controls reperfusion injury through mitochondrial ROS." *Nature* 515 (7527):431-435. doi: 10.1038/nature13909.

Cnop, M., N. Welsh, J. C. Jonas, A. Jorns, S. Lenzen, and D. L. Eizirik. 2005. "Mechanisms of pancreatic beta-cell death in type 1 and type 2 diabetes: many differences, few similarities." *Diabetes* 54 Suppl 2:S97-107. doi: 10.2337/diabetes.54.suppl_2.s97.

Cook, Stephen. 2007. "Metabolic Syndrome." In *Pediatric Clinical Advisor (Second Edition)*, edited by Lynn C. Garfunkel, Jeffrey M. Kaczorowski and Cynthia Christy, 371-372. Philadelphia: Mosby.

Dales, R. E., L. M. Kauri, and S. Cakmak. 2018. "The associations between phthalate exposure and insulin resistance, β-cell function and blood glucose control in a population-based sample." *Sci Total Environ* 612:1287-1292. doi: 10.1016/j.scitotenv.2017.09.009.

Dargnat, C., M. Blanchard, M. Chevreuil, and M. J. Teil. 2009. "Occurrence of phthalate esters in the Seine River estuary (France)." *Hydrological Processes* 23 (8):1192-1201. doi: https://doi.org/10.1002/hyp.7245.

Deng, T., Y. Zhang, Y. Wu, P. Ma, J. Duan, W. Qin, X. Yang, and M. Chen. 2018. "Dibutyl phthalate exposure aggravates type 2 diabetes by disrupting the insulin-mediated PI3K/AKT signaling pathway." *Toxicol Lett* 290:1-9. doi: 10.1016/j.toxlet.2018.03.004.

Desdoits-Lethimonier, C., O. Albert, B. Le Bizec, E. Perdu, D. Zalko, F. Courant, L. Lesné, F. Guillé, N. Dejucq-Rainsford, and B. Jégou. 2012. "Human testis steroidogenesis is inhibited by phthalates." *Hum Reprod* 27 (5):1451-9. doi: 10.1093/humrep/des069.

Desvergne, B., and W. Wahli. 1999. "Peroxisome proliferator-activated receptors: nuclear control of metabolism." *Endocr Rev* 20 (5):649-88. doi: 10.1210/edrv.20.5.0380.

Di Cianni, G., R. Miccoli, L. Volpe, C. Lencioni, and S. Del Prato. 2003. "Intermediate metabolism in normal pregnancy and in gestational diabetes." *Diabetes Metab Res Rev* 19 (4):259-70. doi: 10.1002/dmrr.390.

Ding, Y., K. Gao, Y. Liu, G. Mao, K. Chen, X. Qiu, T. Zhao, L. Yang, W. Feng, and X. Wu. 2019. "Transcriptome analysis revealed the mechanism of the metabolic toxicity and susceptibility of di-(2-ethylhexyl)phthalate on adolescent male ICR mice with type 2 diabetes mellitus." *Arch Toxicol* 93 (11):3183-3206. doi: 10.1007/s00204-019-02590-8.

Ding, Yangyang, Tong Xu, Guanghua Mao, Yao Chen, Xuchun Qiu, Liuqing Yang, Ting Zhao, Xiaoxiao Xu, Weiwei Feng, and Xiangyang Wu. 2021. "Di-(2-ethylhexyl) phthalate-induced hepatotoxicity exacerbated type 2 diabetes mellitus (T2DM) in female pubertal T2DM mice." *Food and Chemical Toxicology* 149:112003. doi: https://doi.org/10.1016/j.fct.2021.112003.

Dirinck, E., A. C. Dirtu, T. Geens, A. Covaci, L. Van Gaal, and P. G. Jorens. 2015. "Urinary phthalate metabolites are associated with insulin resistance in obese subjects." *Environ Res* 137:419-23. doi: 10.1016/j.envres.2015.01.010.

Dong, R., S. Zhao, H. Zhang, J. Chen, M. Zhang, M. Wang, M. Wu, S. Li, and B. Chen. 2017. "Sex differences in the association of urinary concentrations of phthalates metabolites with self-reported diabetes and cardiovascular diseases in Shanghai adults." *Int J Environ Res Public Health* 14 (6). doi: 10.3390/ijerph14060598.

Duan, Y., H. Sun, L. Han, and L. Chen. 2019. "Association between phthalate exposure and glycosylated hemoglobin, fasting glucose, and type 2 diabetes mellitus: A case-control study in China." *Sci Total Environ* 670:41-49. doi: 10.1016/j.scitotenv.2019.03.192.

Duan, Y., H. Sun, Y. Yao, L. Han, and L. Chen. 2021. "Perturbation of serum metabolome in relation to type 2 diabetes mellitus and urinary levels of phthalate metabolites and bisphenols." *Environ Int* 155:106609. doi: 10.1016/j.envint.2021.106609.

Duan, Y., L. Wang, L. Han, B. Wang, H. Sun, L. Chen, L. Zhu, and Y. Luo. 2017. "Exposure to phthalates in patients with diabetes and its association with oxidative stress, adiponectin, and inflammatory cytokines." *Environ Int* 109:53-63. doi: 10.1016/j.envint.2017.09.002.

ECHA. 2007. "EUREACH entry 51 and 52 of Annex XVII of the REACH regulation." *O. J. Eur. Commun.* 49 (L396):1-849.

ECHA. 2018. EC (European Commission). Commission Regulation (EU) 2018/2005 of 17 December 2018 Amending Annex XVII to REGULATION (EC) No 1907/2006 of the European Parliament and of the Council Concerning the Registration, Evaluation, Authorisation and Restriction of Chemicals (REACH) as regards Bis(2-ethylhexyl) phthalate (DEHP), dibutyl phthalate (DBP), benzyl butyl phthalate (BBP) and diisobutyl phthalate (DIBP). Available from: https://www.legislation.gov.uk/eur/2018/2005/contents

Ema, M., and E. Miyawaki. 2002. "Effects on development of the reproductive system in male offspring of rats given butyl benzyl phthalate during late pregnancy." *Reprod Toxicol* 16 (1):71-6. doi: 10.1016/s0890-6238(01)00200-3.

Enangue Njembele, A. N., and J. J. Tremblay. 2021. "Mechanisms of MEHP inhibitory action and analysis of potential replacement plasticizers on leydig cell steroidogenesis." *Int J Mol Sci* 22 (21). doi: 10.3390/ijms222111456.

Evans, R. M., G. D. Barish, and Y. X. Wang. 2004. "PPARs and the complex journey to obesity." *Nat Med* 10 (4):355-61. doi: 10.1038/nm1025.

Fénichel, P., and N. Chevalier. 2017. "Environmental endocrine disruptors: New diabetogens?" *C R Biol* 340 (9-10):446-452. doi: 10.1016/j.crvi.2017.07.003.

Ferguson, K. K., R. Loch-Caruso, and J. D. Meeker. 2011. "Urinary phthalate metabolites in relation to biomarkers of inflammation and oxidative stress: NHANES 1999-2006." *Environ Res* 111 (5):718-26. doi: 10.1016/j.envres.2011.02.002.

Ferguson, K. K., R. Loch-Caruso, and J. D. Meeker. 2012. "Exploration of oxidative stress and inflammatory markers in relation to urinary phthalate metabolites: NHANES 1999-2006." *Environ Sci Technol* 46 (1):477-85. doi: 10.1021/es202340b.

Fisher, B. G., H. Frederiksen, A. M. Andersson, A. Juul, A. Thankamony, K. K. Ong, D. B. Dunger, I. A. Hughes, and C. L. Acerini. 2018. "Serum phthalate and triclosan levels have opposing associations with risk factors for gestational diabetes mellitus." *Front Endocrinol (Lausanne)* 9:99. doi: 10.3389/fendo.2018.00099.

Foster, P. M. D. 2005. "Mode of action: Impaired fetal leydig cell function - Effects on male reproductive development produced by certain phthalate esters." *Critical Reviews in Toxicology* 35 (8-9):713-719. doi: 10.1080/10408440591007395.

Foster, P. M. 2006. "Disruption of reproductive development in male rat offspring following in utero exposure to phthalate esters." *Int J Androl* 29 (1):140-7; discussion 181-5. doi: 10.1111/j.1365-2605.2005.00563.x.

Frederiksen, Hanne, Niels E. Skakkebaek, and Anna-Maria Andersson. 2007. "Metabolism of phthalates in humans." *Molecular Nutrition & Food Research* 51 (7):899-911. doi: https://doi.org/10.1002/mnfr.200600243.

Gao, Hui, Bei-bei Zhu, Kun Huang, Yuan-duo Zhu, Shuang-qin Yan, Xiao-yan Wu, Yan Han, Jie Sheng, Hui Cao, Peng Zhu, and Fang-biao Tao. 2021. "Effects of single and combined gestational phthalate exposure on blood pressure, blood glucose and gestational weight gain: A longitudinal analysis." *Environment International* 155: 106677. doi: https://doi.org/10.1016/j.envint.2021.106677.

Gayathri, N. S., C. R. Dhanya, A. R. Indu, and P. A. Kurup. 2004. "Changes in some hormones by low doses of di (2-ethyl hexyl) phthalate (DEHP), a commonly used plasticizer in PVC blood storage bags & medical tubing." *Indian J Med Res* 119 (4):139-44.

Ghoshal, K., and M. Bhattacharyya. 2015. "Adiponectin: Probe of the molecular paradigm associating diabetes and obesity." *World J Diabetes* 6 (1):151-66. doi: 10.4239/wjd.v6.i1.151.

Giulivo, M., M. Lopez de Alda, E. Capri, and D. Barceló. 2016. "Human exposure to endocrine disrupting compounds: Their role in reproductive systems, metabolic syndrome and breast cancer. A review." *Environ Res* 151:251-264. doi: 10.1016/j.envres.2016.07.011.

Goncalves, R. L., C. L. Quinlan, I. V. Perevoshchikova, M. Hey-Mogensen, and M. D. Brand. 2015. "Sites of superoxide and hydrogen peroxide production by muscle mitochondria assessed ex vivo under conditions mimicking rest and exercise." *J Biol Chem* 290 (1):209-27. doi: 10.1074/jbc.M114.619072.

Gore, A. C., V. A. Chappell, S. E. Fenton, J. A. Flaws, A. Nadal, G. S. Prins, J. Toppari, and R. T. Zoeller. 2015. "EDC-2: The Endocrine Society's second scientific statement on endocrine-disrupting chemicals." *Endocr Rev* 36 (6):E1-e150. doi: 10.1210/er.2015-1010.

Gray Jr, L. E., J. Ostby, J. Furr, M. Price, D. N. R. Veeramachaneni, and L. Parks. 2000. "Perinatal exposure to the phthalates DEHP, BBP, and DINP, but not DEP, DMP, or DOTP, alters sexual differentiation of the male rat." *Toxicological Sciences* 58 (2): 350-365. doi: 10.1093/toxsci/58.2.350.

Grundy, Scott M., H. Bryan Brewer, James I. Cleeman, Sidney C. Smith, and Claude Lenfant. 2004. "Definition of metabolic syndrome." *Circulation* 109 (3):433-438. doi: doi:10.1161/01.CIR.0000111245.75752.C6.

Guo, J., M. Wu, X. Gao, J. Chen, S. Li, B. Chen, and R. Dong. 2020. "meconium exposure to phthalates, sex and thyroid hormones, birth size and pregnancy outcomes in 251 mother-infant pairs from Shanghai." *Int J Environ Res Public Health* 17 (21). doi: 10.3390/ijerph17217711.

Halden, R. U. 2010. "Plastics and health risks." *Annu Rev Public Health* 31:179-94. doi: 10.1146/annurev.publhealth.012809.103714.

Halliwell, B., M. V. Clement, and L. H. Long. 2000. "Hydrogen peroxide in the human body." *FEBS Lett* 486 (1):10-3. doi: 10.1016/s0014-5793(00)02197-9.

He, X., J. Zang, P. Liao, Y. Zheng, Y. Lu, Z. Zhu, Y. Shi, and W. Wang. 2019. "Distribution and dietary predictors of urinary phthalate metabolites among pregnant women in

Shanghai, China." *Int J Environ Res Public Health* 16 (8). doi: 10.3390/ijerph16081366.

Heindel, J. J., B. Blumberg, M. Cave, R. Machtinger, A. Mantovani, M. A. Mendez, A. Nadal, P. Palanza, G. Panzica, R. Sargis, L. N. Vandenberg, and F. Vom Saal. 2017. "Metabolism disrupting chemicals and metabolic disorders." *Reprod Toxicol* 68:3-33. doi: 10.1016/j.reprotox.2016.10.001.

Hines, E. P., A. M. Calafat, M. J. Silva, P. Mendola, and S. E. Fenton. 2009. "Concentrations of phthalate metabolites in milk, urine, saliva, and serum of lactating North Carolina women." *Environ Health Perspect* 117 (1):86-92. doi: 10.1289/ehp.11610.

Hiriart, Marcia, Myrian Velasco, Carlos Larqué, and Carlos Manlio Diaz-Garcia. 2014. "Chapter Four - Metabolic Syndrome and Ionic Channels in Pancreatic Beta Cells." In *Vitamins & Hormones*, edited by Gerald Litwack, 87-114. Academic Press.

Hotamisligil, G. S., P. Arner, J. F. Caro, R. L. Atkinson, and B. M. Spiegelman. 1995. "Increased adipose tissue expression of tumor necrosis factor-alpha in human obesity and insulin resistance." *J Clin Invest* 95 (5):2409-15. doi: 10.1172/JCI117936.

Howard, S. G. 2018. "Developmental exposure to endocrine disrupting chemicals and type 1 diabetes mellitus." *Front Endocrinol (Lausanne)* 9:513. doi: 10.3389/fendo.2018.00513.

Howard, S. G. 2019. "Exposure to environmental chemicals and type 1 diabetes: an update." *J Epidemiol Community Health* 73 (6):483-488. doi: 10.1136/jech-2018-210627.

Huang, T., A. R. Saxena, E. Isganaitis, and T. James-Todd. 2014. "Gender and racial/ethnic differences in the associations of urinary phthalate metabolites with markers of diabetes risk: National Health and Nutrition Examination Survey 2001-2008." *Environ Health* 13 (1):6. doi: 10.1186/1476-069x-13-6.

IDF. 2000. IDF *Diabetes Atlas*. Edited by International Diabetes Federation. Brussels, Belgium.

IDF. 2021. IDF *Diabetes Atlas*. Edited by International Diabetes Federation. Brussels, Belgium.

Idriss, H. T., and J. H. Naismith. 2000. "TNF alpha and the TNF receptor superfamily: structure-function relationship(s)." *Microsc Res Tech* 50 (3):184-95. doi: 10.1002/1097-0029(20000801)50:3<184::AID-JEMT2>3.0.CO;2-H.

James-Todd, T. M., Y. H. Chiu, C. Messerlian, L. Mínguez-Alarcón, J. B. Ford, M. Keller, J. Petrozza, P. L. Williams, X. Ye, A. M. Calafat, and R. Hauser. 2018. "Trimester-specific phthalate concentrations and glucose levels among women from a fertility clinic." *Environ Health* 17 (1):55. doi: 10.1186/s12940-018-0399-5.

James-Todd, T. M., T. Huang, E. W. Seely, and A. R. Saxena. 2016a. "The association between phthalates and metabolic syndrome: the National Health and Nutrition Examination Survey 2001-2010." *Environ Health* 15:52. doi: 10.1186/s12940-016-0136-x.

James-Todd, T. M., J. D. Meeker, T. Huang, R. Hauser, K. K. Ferguson, J. W. Rich-Edwards, T. F. McElrath, and E. W. Seely. 2016b. "Pregnancy urinary phthalate metabolite concentrations and gestational diabetes risk factors." *Environ Int* 96:118-126. doi: 10.1016/j.envint.2016.09.009.

James-Todd, T., R. Stahlhut, J. D. Meeker, S. G. Powell, R. Hauser, T. Huang, and J. Rich-Edwards. 2012. "Urinary phthalate metabolite concentrations and diabetes among women in the National Health and Nutrition Examination Survey (NHANES) 2001-2008." *Environ Health Perspect* 120 (9):1307-13. doi: 10.1289/ehp.1104717.

Jepsen, K. F., A. Abildtrup, and S. T. Larsen. 2004. "Monophthalates promote IL-6 and IL-8 production in the human epithelial cell line A549." *Toxicol In Vitro* 18 (3):265-9. doi: 10.1016/j.tiv.2003.09.008.

Jia, Y., T. Liu, L. Zhou, J. Zhu, J. Wu, D. Sun, J. Xu, Q. Wang, H. Chen, F. Xu, Y. Zhang, T. Zhang, H. Liu, and L. Ye. 2016. "Effects of Di-(2-ethylhexyl) phthalate on lipid metabolism by the JAK/STAT pathway in rats." *Int J Environ Res Public Health* 13 (11). doi: 10.3390/ijerph13111085.

Joensen, U. N., N. Jørgensen, M. Meldgaard, H. Frederiksen, A. M. Andersson, T. Menné, J. D. Johansen, B. C. Carlsen, S. Stender, P. B. Szecsi, N. E. Skakkebæk, E. Rajpert-De Meyts, and J. P. Thyssen. 2014. "Associations of filaggrin gene loss-of-function variants with urinary phthalate metabolites and testicular function in young Danish Men." *Environ Health Perspect* 122 (4):345-50. doi: 10.1289/ehp.1306720.

Jones, T. Hugh. 2010. "Effects of testosterone on Type 2 diabetes and components of the metabolic syndrome." *Journal of Diabetes* 2 (3):146-156. doi: https://doi.org/10.1111/j.1753-0407.2010.00085.x.

Kato, Kayoko, Manori J. Silva, Larry L. Needham, and Antonia M. Calafat. 2005. "Determination of 16 phthalate metabolites in urine using automated sample preparation and on-line preconcentration/high-performance liquid chromato-graphy/tandem mass spectrometry." *Analytical Chemistry* 77 (9):2985-2991. doi: 10.1021/ac0481248.

Kern, P. A., M. Saghizadeh, J. M. Ong, R. J. Bosch, R. Deem, and R. B. Simsolo. 1995. "The expression of tumor necrosis factor in human adipose tissue. Regulation by obesity, weight loss, and relationship to lipoprotein lipase." *J Clin Invest* 95 (5):2111-9. doi: 10.1172/JCI117899.

Khan, A. H., and J. E. Pessin. 2002. "Insulin regulation of glucose uptake: a complex interplay of intracellular signalling pathways." *Diabetologia* 45 (11):1475-83. doi: 10.1007/s00125-002-0974-7.

Kim, J. H., H. Y. Park, S. Bae, Y. H. Lim, and Y. C. Hong. 2013. "Diethylhexyl phthalates is associated with insulin resistance via oxidative stress in the elderly: a panel study." *PLoS One* 8 (8):e71392. doi: 10.1371/journal.pone.0071392.

Kim, N. H., D. L. Kim, K. M. Choi, S. H. Baik, and D. S. Choi. 2000. "Serum insulin, proinsulin and proinsulin/insulin ratio in type 2 diabetic patients: as an index of beta-cell function or insulin resistance." *Korean J Intern Med* 15 (3):195-201. doi: 10.3904/kjim.2000.15.3.195.

Korshunov, S. S., V. P. Skulachev, and A. A. Starkov. 1997. "High protonic potential actuates a mechanism of production of reactive oxygen species in mitochondria." *FEBS Lett* 416 (1):15-8. doi: 10.1016/s0014-5793(97)01159-9.

Kruger, T., Y. Cao, S. K. Kjaergaard, L. E. Knudsen, and E. C. Bonefeld-Jorgensen. 2012. "Effects of phthalates on the human corneal endothelial cell line B4G12." *Int J Toxicol* 31 (4):364-71. doi: 10.1177/1091581812449660.

LaRocca, Jessica, Alexandra M. Binder, Thomas F. McElrath, and Karin B. Michels. 2016. "First-trimester urine concentrations of phthalate metabolites and phenols and placenta miRNA expression in a cohort of U.S. women." *Environmental Health Perspectives* 124 (3):380-387. doi: 10.1289/ehp.1408409.

Latini, G. 2005. "Monitoring phthalate exposure in humans." *Clin Chim Acta* 361 (1-2):20-9. doi: 10.1016/j.cccn.2005.05.003.

Latini, G., A. Del Vecchio, M. Massaro, A. Verrotti, and C. De Felice. 2006. "Phthalate exposure and male infertility." *Toxicology* 226 (2-3):90-8. doi: 10.1016/j.tox.2006.07.011.

Li, L., F. Wang, J. Zhang, K. Wang, X. De, L. Li, and Y. Zhang. 2021. "Typical phthalic acid esters induce apoptosis by regulating the PI3K/Akt/Bcl-2 signaling pathway in rat insulinoma cells." *Ecotoxicol Environ Saf* 208:111461. doi: 10.1016/j.ecoenv.2020.111461.

Li, Ming-Chieh, Lidia Mínguez-Alarcón, Andrea Bellavia, Paige L. Williams, Tamarra James-Todd, Russ Hauser, Jorge E. Chavarro, and Yu-Han Chiu. 2019. "Serum beta-carotene modifies the association between phthalate mixtures and insulin resistance: The National Health and Nutrition Examination Survey 2003–2006." *Environmental Research* 178:108729. doi: https://doi.org/10.1016/j.envres.2019.108729.

Lin, Y., J. Wei, Y. Li, J. Chen, Z. Zhou, L. Song, Z. Wei, Z. Lv, X. Chen, W. Xia, and S. Xu. 2011a. "Developmental exposure to di(2-ethylhexyl) phthalate impairs endocrine pancreas and leads to long-term adverse effects on glucose homeostasis in the rat." *Am J Physiol Endocrinol Metab* 301 (3):E527-38. doi: 10.1152/ajpendo.00233.2011.

Lin, Yi, Jie Wei, Yuanyuan Li, Jun Chen, Zhao Zhou, Liqiong Song, Zhengzheng Wei, Ziquan Lv, Xi Chen, Wei Xia, and Shunqing Xu. 2011b. "Developmental exposure to di(2-ethylhexyl) phthalate impairs endocrine pancreas and leads to long-term adverse effects on glucose homeostasis in the rat." *American Journal of Physiology-Endocrinology and Metabolism* 301 (3):E527-E538. doi: 10.1152/ajpendo.00233.2011.

Lind, P. M., B. Zethelius, and L. Lind. 2012. "Circulating levels of phthalate metabolites are associated with prevalent diabetes in the elderly." *Diabetes Care* 35 (7):1519-24. doi: 10.2337/dc11-2396.

Liu, C., X. Feng, Q. Li, Y. Wang, Q. Li, and M. Hua. 2016. "Adiponectin, TNF-alpha and inflammatory cytokines and risk of type 2 diabetes: A systematic review and meta-analysis." *Cytokine* 86:100-109. doi: 10.1016/j.cyto.2016.06.028.

Lizárraga, Dennise, and Alejandra García-Gasca. 2021. "The placenta as a target of epigenetic alterations in women with gestational diabetes mellitus and potential implications for the offspring." *Epigenomes* 5 (2):13. doi: 10.3390/epigenomes5020013.

Lu, X., E. Fraszczyk, T. P. van der Meer, M. van Faassen, V. W. Bloks, I. P. Kema, A. P. van Beek, S. Li, L. Franke, H. J. Westra, Bios Consortium, X. Xu, X. Huo, H. Snieder, B. H. R. Wolffenbuttel, and J. V. van Vliet-Ostaptchouk. 2020. "An epigenome-wide association study identifies multiple DNA methylation markers of exposure to endocrine disruptors." *Environ Int* 144:106016. doi: 10.1016/j.envint.2020.106016.

Lyche, Jan L. 2011. "Chapter 48 - Phthalates." In *Reproductive and Developmental Toxicology*, edited by Ramesh C. Gupta, 637-655. San Diego: Academic Press.

Maedler, K., J. Oberholzer, P. Bucher, G. A. Spinas, and M. Y. Donath. 2003. "Monounsaturated fatty acids prevent the deleterious effects of palmitate and high glucose on human pancreatic beta-cell turnover and function." *Diabetes* 52 (3):726-33. doi: 10.2337/diabetes.52.3.726.

Mahood, I. K., N. Hallmark, C. McKinnell, M. Walker, J. S. Fisher, and R. M. Sharpe. 2005. "Abnormal Leydig Cell aggregation in the fetal testis of rats exposed to di (n-butyl) phthalate and its possible role in testicular dysgenesis." *Endocrinology* 146 (2):613-23. doi: 10.1210/en.2004-0671.

Mangala Priya, V., C. Mayilvanan, N. Akilavalli, P. Rajesh, and K. Balasubramanian. 2014. "Lactational exposure of phthalate impairs insulin signaling in the cardiac muscle of F1 female albino rats." *Cardiovasc Toxicol* 14 (1):10-20. doi: 10.1007/s12012-013-9233-z.

Martinelli, Marcela I, Norberto O Mocchiutti, and Claudio A Bernal. 2006. "Dietary di(2-ethylhexyl)phthalate-impaired glucose metabolism in experimental animals." *Human & Experimental Toxicology* 25 (9):531-538. doi: 10.1191/0960327106het651oa.

Martínez-Ibarra, A., L. D. Martínez-Razo, E. R. Vázquez-Martínez, N. Martínez-Cruz, R. Flores-Ramírez, E. García-Gómez, M. López-López, C. Ortega-González, I. Camacho-Arroyo, and M. Cerbón. 2019. "Unhealthy levels of phthalates and bisphenol A in Mexican pregnant women with gestational diabetes and its association to altered expression of miRNAs involved with metabolic disease." *Int J Mol Sci* 20 (13). doi: 10.3390/ijms20133343.

Milošević, N., M. Milanović, J. Sudji, D. Bosić Živanović, S. Stojanoski, B. Vuković, N. Milić, and M. Medić Stojanoska. 2020. "Could phthalates exposure contribute to the development of metabolic syndrome and liver disease in humans?" *Environ Sci Pollut Res Int* 27 (1):772-784. doi: 10.1007/s11356-019-06831-2.

Mok, Sori, Jae-Eun Lim, Aram Lee, Sungmin Kim, Sunmi Kim, Inae Lee, Younglim Kho, Jeongim Park, Sungkyoon Kim, Kyungho Choi, and Hyo-Bang Moon. 2022. "Within- and between-person variability of urinary phthalate metabolites and bisphenol analogues over seven days: Considerations of biomonitoring study design." *Environmental Research* 209:112885. doi: https://doi.org/10.1016/j.envres.2022.112885.

Mondal, S., and S. Mukherjee. 2020. "Long-term dietary administration of diethyl phthalate triggers loss of insulin sensitivity in two key insulin target tissues of mice." *Hum Exp Toxicol* 39 (7):984-993. doi: 10.1177/0960327120909526.

Monneret, Claude. 2017. "What is an endocrine disruptor?" *Comptes Rendus Biologies* 340 (9):403-405. doi: https://doi.org/10.1016/j.crvi.2017.07.004.

Moran, I., I. Akerman, M. van de Bunt, R. Xie, M. Benazra, T. Nammo, L. Arnes, N. Nakic, J. Garcia-Hurtado, S. Rodriguez-Segui, L. Pasquali, C. Sauty-Colace, A. Beucher, R. Scharfmann, J. van Arensbergen, P. R. Johnson, A. Berry, C. Lee, T. Harkins, V. Gmyr, F. Pattou, J. Kerr-Conte, L. Piemonti, T. Berney, N. Hanley, A. L. Gloyn, L. Sussel, L. Langman, K. L. Brayman, M. Sander, M. I. McCarthy, P. Ravassard, and J. Ferrer. 2012. "Human beta cell transcriptome analysis uncovers lncRNAs that are tissue-specific, dynamically regulated, and abnormally expressed in type 2 diabetes." *Cell Metab* 16 (4):435-48. doi: 10.1016/j.cmet.2012.08.010.

Mykkänen, L., S. M. Haffner, J. Kuusisto, K. Pyörälä, C. N. Hales, and M. Laakso. 1995. "Serum proinsulin levels are disproportionately increased in elderly prediabetic subjects." *Diabetologia* 38 (10):1176-82. doi: 10.1007/bf00422366.

Mylchreest, E., M. Sar, D. G. Wallace, and P. M. D. Foster. 2002. "Fetal testosterone insufficiency and abnormal proliferation of Leydig cells and gonocytes in rats exposed to di(n-butyl) phthalate." *Reproductive Toxicology* 16 (1):19-28. doi: 10.1016/S0890-6238(01)00201-5.

Nam, D. J., Y. Kim, E. H. Yang, H. C. Lee, and J. H. Ryoo. 2020. "Relationship between urinary phthalate metabolites and diabetes: Korean National Environmental Health Survey (KoNEHS) cycle 3 (2015-2017)." *Ann Occup Environ Med* 32:e34. doi: 10.35371/aoem.2020.32.e34.

Nathan, D. M., M. B. Davidson, R. A. DeFronzo, R. J. Heine, R. R. Henry, R. Pratley, and B. Zinman. 2007. "Impaired fasting glucose and impaired glucose tolerance: implications for care." *Diabetes Care* 30 (3):753-9. doi: 10.2337/dc07-9920.

Net, Sopheak, Richard Sempéré, Anne Delmont, Andrea Paluselli, and Baghdad Ouddane. 2015. "Occurrence, fate, behavior and ecotoxicological state of phthalates in different environmental matrices." *Environmental Science & Technology* 49 (7):4019-4035. doi: 10.1021/es505233b.

Nishioka, J., C. Iwahara, M. Kawasaki, F. Yoshizaki, H. Nakayama, K. Takamori, H. Ogawa, and K. Iwabuchi. 2012. "Di-(2-ethylhexyl) phthalate induces production of inflammatory molecules in human macrophages." *Inflamm Res* 61 (1):69-78. doi: 10.1007/s00011-011-0390-x.

Noor, N., K. K. Ferguson, J. D. Meeker, E. W. Seely, R. Hauser, T. James-Todd, and T. F. McElrath. 2019. "Pregnancy phthalate metabolite concentrations and infant birth weight by gradations of maternal glucose tolerance." *Int J Hyg Environ Health* 222 (3):395-401. doi: 10.1016/j.ijheh.2018.12.005.

Olsén, L., L. Lind, and P. M. Lind. 2012. "Associations between circulating levels of bisphenol A and phthalate metabolites and coronary risk in the elderly." *Ecotoxicol Environ Saf* 80:179-83. doi: 10.1016/j.ecoenv.2012.02.023.

Parks, L. G., J. S. Ostby, C. R. Lambright, B. D. Abbott, G. R. Klinefelter, N. J. Barlow, and L. E. Gray Jr. 2000. "The plasticizer diethylhexyl phthalate induces malformations by decreasing fetal testosterone synthesis during sexual differentiation in the male rat." *Toxicological Sciences* 58 (2):339-349. doi: 10.1093/toxsci/58.2.339.

Parsanathan, R., A. Maria Joseph, and B. Karundevi. 2019. "Postnatal exposure to di-(2-ethylhexyl)phthalate alters cardiac insulin signaling molecules and GLUT4(Ser488) phosphorylation in male rat offspring." *J Cell Biochem* 120 (4):5802-5812. doi: 10.1002/jcb.27866.

Perera, F., and J. Herbstman. 2011. "Prenatal environmental exposures, epigenetics, and disease." *Reprod Toxicol* 31 (3):363-73. doi: 10.1016/j.reprotox.2010.12.055.

Philips, E. M., S. Santos, E. A. P. Steegers, A. G. Asimakopoulos, K. Kannan, L. Trasande, and V. W. V. Jaddoe. 2020. "Maternal bisphenol and phthalate urine concentrations and weight gain during pregnancy." *Environ Int* 135:105342. doi: 10.1016/j.envint.2019.105342.

Piecha, R., S. Svacina, M. Maly, K. Vrbik, Z. Lacinova, M. Haluzik, J. Pavlouskova, A. Vavrous, D. Matejkova, D. Mullerova, M. Mraz, and M. Matoulek. 2016. "Urine levels of phthalate metabolites and bisphenol A in relation to main metabolic syndrome components: dyslipidemia, hypertension and type 2 diabetes. a pilot study." *Cent Eur J Public Health* 24 (4):297-301. doi: 10.21101/cejph.a4704.

Plows, J. F., J. L. Stanley, P. N. Baker, C. M. Reynolds, and M. H. Vickers. 2018. "The pathophysiology of gestational diabetes mellitus." *Int J Mol Sci* 19 (11). doi: 10.3390/ijms19113342.

Preece, A. S., H. Shu, M. Knutz, A. M. Krais, G. Bekö, and C. G. Bornehag. 2021. "Indoor phthalate exposure and contributions to total intake among pregnant women in the SELMA study." *Indoor Air* 31 (5):1495-1508. doi: 10.1111/ina.12813.

Qi, C., Y. Zhu, and J. K. Reddy. 2000. "Peroxisome proliferator-activated receptors, coactivators, and downstream targets." *Cell Biochem Biophys* 32 Spring:187-204. doi: 10.1385/cbb:32:1-3:187.

Rajagopal, G., R. S. Bhaskaran, and B. Karundevi. 2019a. "Developmental exposure to DEHP alters hepatic glucose uptake and transcriptional regulation of GLUT2 in rat male offspring." *Toxicology* 413:56-64. doi: 10.1016/j.tox.2018.12.004.

Rajagopal, G., R. S. Bhaskaran, and B. Karundevi. 2019b. "Maternal di-(2-ethylhexyl) phthalate exposure alters hepatic insulin signal transduction and glucoregulatory events in rat F(1) male offspring." *J Appl Toxicol* 39 (5):751-763. doi: 10.1002/jat.3764.

Rajesh, P., and K. Balasubramanian. 2014a. "Di(2-ethylhexyl)phthalate exposure impairs insulin receptor and glucose transporter 4 gene expression in L6 myotubes." *Hum Exp Toxicol* 33 (7):685-700. doi: 10.1177/0960327113506238.

Rajesh, P., and K. Balasubramanian. 2014b. "Phthalate exposure in utero causes epigenetic changes and impairs insulin signalling." *J Endocrinol* 223 (1):47-66. doi: 10.1530/joe-14-0111.

Rajesh, P., and K. Balasubramanian. 2015. "Gestational exposure to di(2-ethylhexyl) phthalate (DEHP) impairs pancreatic β-cell function in F1 rat offspring." *Toxicol Lett* 232 (1):46-57. doi: 10.1016/j.toxlet.2014.09.025.

Rajesh, P., S. Sathish, C. Srinivasan, J. Selvaraj, and K. Balasubramanian. 2013. "Phthalate is associated with insulin resistance in adipose tissue of male rat: role of antioxidant vitamins." *J Cell Biochem* 114 (3):558-69. doi: 10.1002/jcb.24399.

Rajeshwari S G, A. A. Choudhry, A. Gururaja, and K. Prabhu. 2014. "Correlation of Plasma Lipid Profile with Salivary Oxidative Stress Markers in Type II Diabetes Mellitus Patients." *J Clin Diagn Res* 8 (6):CC08-10. doi: 10.7860/JCDR/2014/8233.4451.

Rask-Madsen, C., Q. Li, B. Freund, D. Feather, R. Abramov, I. H. Wu, K. Chen, J. Yamamoto-Hiraoka, J. Goldenbogen, K. B. Sotiropoulos, A. Clermont, P. Geraldes, C. Dall'Osso, A. J. Wagers, P. L. Huang, M. Rekhter, R. Scalia, C. R. Kahn, and G. L. King. 2010. "Loss of insulin signaling in vascular endothelial cells accelerates atherosclerosis in apolipoprotein E null mice." *Cell Metab* 11 (5):379-89. doi: 10.1016/j.cmet.2010.03.013.

Rodríguez-Carmona, Yanelli, Alejandra Cantoral, Belem Trejo-Valdivia, Martha M. Téllez-Rojo, Katherine Svensson, Karen E. Peterson, John D. Meeker, Lourdes Schnaas, Maritsa Solano, and Deborah J. Watkins. 2019. "Phthalate exposure during pregnancy and long-term weight gain in women." *Environmental research* 169:26-32. doi: 10.1016/j.envres.2018.10.014.

Rolfo, A., A. M. Nuzzo, R. De Amicis, L. Moretti, S. Bertoli, and A. Leone. 2020. "Fetal-maternal exposure to endocrine disruptors: correlation with diet intake and pregnancy outcomes." *Nutrients* 12 (6). doi: 10.3390/nu12061744.

Rorsman, P., and M. Braun. 2013. "Regulation of insulin secretion in human pancreatic islets." *Annu Rev Physiol* 75:155-79. doi: 10.1146/annurev-physiol-030212-183754.

Saengkaew, Tansit, Chutima Jantarat, Wichit Nosoognoen, and Vichit Supornsilchai. 2017. "Association between urinary phthalates and metabolic abnormalities in obese Thai children and adolescents." *Journal of Pediatric Endocrinology and Metabolism* 30 (9):931-938. doi: doi:10.1515/jpem-2017-0172.

Saillenfait, A. M., J. P. Sabaté, A. Robert, B. Cossec, A. C. Roudot, F. Denis, and M. Burgart. 2013. "Adverse effects of diisooctyl phthalate on the male rat reproductive development following prenatal exposure." *Reprod Toxicol* 42:192-202. doi: 10.1016/j.reprotox.2013.09.004.

Saillenfait, A. M., J. P. Sabaté, and F. Gallissot. 2008. "Diisobutyl phthalate impairs the androgen-dependent reproductive development of the male rat." *Reprod Toxicol* 26 (2):107-15. doi: 10.1016/j.reprotox.2008.07.006.

Sánchez-Avila, Juan, Jordi Bonet, Gemma Velasco, and Silvia Lacorte. 2009. "Determination and occurrence of phthalates, alkylphenols, bisphenol A, PBDEs, PCBs and PAHs in an industrial sewage grid discharging to a Municipal Wastewater Treatment Plant." *Science of The Total Environment* 407 (13):4157-4167. doi: https://doi.org/10.1016/j.scitotenv.2009.03.016.

Sauter, N. S., F. T. Schulthess, R. Galasso, L. W. Castellani, and K. Maedler. 2008. "The antiinflammatory cytokine interleukin-1 receptor antagonist protects from high-fat diet-induced hyperglycemia." *Endocrinology* 149 (5):2208-18. doi: 10.1210/en.2007-1059.

Schwartz, D., and F. Collins. 2007. "Medicine. Environmental biology and human disease." *Science* 316 (5825):695-6. doi: 10.1126/science.1141331.

Serrano, S. E., J. Braun, L. Trasande, R. Dills, and S. Sathyanarayana. 2014. "Phthalates and diet: a review of the food monitoring and epidemiology data." *Environ Health* 13 (1):43. doi: 10.1186/1476-069x-13-43.

Shaffer, R. M., K. K. Ferguson, L. Sheppard, T. James-Todd, S. Butts, S. Chandrasekaran, S. H. Swan, E. S. Barrett, R. Nguyen, N. Bush, T. F. McElrath, and S. Sathyanarayana. 2019. "Maternal urinary phthalate metabolites in relation to gestational diabetes and glucose intolerance during pregnancy." *Environ Int* 123:588-596. doi: 10.1016/j.envint.2018.12.021.

Shapiro, G. D., L. Dodds, T. E. Arbuckle, J. Ashley-Martin, W. Fraser, M. Fisher, S. Taback, E. Keely, M. F. Bouchard, P. Monnier, R. Dallaire, A. Morisset, and A. S. Ettinger. 2015. "Exposure to phthalates, bisphenol A and metals in pregnancy and the association with impaired glucose tolerance and gestational diabetes mellitus: The MIREC study." *Environ Int* 83:63-71. doi: 10.1016/j.envint.2015.05.016.

She, Y., L. Jiang, L. Zheng, H. Zuo, M. Chen, X. Sun, Q. Li, C. Geng, G. Yang, L. Jiang, and X. Liu. 2017. "The role of oxidative stress in DNA damage in pancreatic beta cells induced by di-(2-ethylhexyl) phthalate." *Chem Biol Interact* 265:8-15. doi: 10.1016/j.cbi.2017.01.015.

Shea, K. M., and Health American Academy of Pediatrics Committee on Environmental. 2003. "Pediatric exposure and potential toxicity of phthalate plasticizers." *Pediatrics* 111 (6 Pt 1):1467-74. doi: 10.1542/peds.111.6.1467.

Sheiner, Eyal. 2020. "Gestational diabetes mellitus: long-term consequences for the mother and child grand challenge: how to move on towards secondary prevention?" *Frontiers in Clinical Diabetes and Healthcare* 1. doi: 10.3389/fcdhc. 2020.546256.

Shen, Dan, Hao Li, Rui Zhou, Meng-jie Liu, Hong Yu, and Dong-Fang Wu. 2018. "Pioglitazone attenuates aging-related disorders in aged apolipoprotein E deficient mice." *Experimental Gerontology* 102:101-108. doi: https://doi.org/10.1016/j.exger. 2017.12.002.

Sherwani, S. I., H. A. Khan, A. Ekhzaimy, A. Masood, and M. K. Sakharkar. 2016. "Significance of HbA1c Test in diagnosis and prognosis of diabetic patients." *Biomark Insights* 11:95-104. doi: 10.4137/bmi.S38440.

Shi, L., L. Jiang, X. Zhang, G. Yang, C. Zhang, X. Yao, X. Wu, M. Fu, X. Sun, and X. Liu. 2020. "Pyrroloquinoline quinone protected autophagy-dependent apoptosis induced by mono(2-ethylhexyl) phthalate in INS-1 cells." *Hum Exp Toxicol* 39 (2):194-211. doi: 10.1177/0960327119882983.

Shi, Y. Q., G. Q. Fu, J. Zhao, S. Z. Cheng, Y. Li, L. N. Yi, Z. Li, L. Zhang, Z. B. Zhang, J. Dai, and D. Y. Zhang. 2019. "Di(2-ethylhexyl)phthalate induces reproductive toxicity via JAZF1/TR4 pathway and oxidative stress in pubertal male rats." *Toxicol Ind Health* 35 (3):228-238. doi: 10.1177/0748233718824911.

Silva, Manori J., Ella Samandar, James L. Preau, John A. Reidy, Larry L. Needham, and Antonia M. Calafat. 2007. "Quantification of 22 phthalate metabolites in human urine." *Journal of Chromatography B* 860 (1):106-112. doi: https://doi.org/10.1016/j.jchromb.2007.10.023.

Song, Y., E. L. Chou, A. Baecker, N. C. You, Y. Song, Q. Sun, and S. Liu. 2016. "Endocrine-disrupting chemicals, risk of type 2 diabetes, and diabetes-related metabolic traits: A systematic review and meta-analysis." *J Diabetes* 8 (4):516-32. doi: 10.1111/1753-0407.12325.

Srinivasan, Chinnapaiyan, Adam Ismail Khan, Venkataraman Balaji, Jayaraman Selvaraj, and Karundevi Balasubramanian. 2011. "Diethyl hexyl phthalate-induced changes in insulin signaling molecules and the protective role of antioxidant vitamins in gastrocnemius muscle of adult male rat." *Toxicology and Applied Pharmacology* 257 (2):155-164. doi: https://doi.org/10.1016/j.taap.2011.08.022.

Stahlhut, R. W., E. van Wijngaarden, T. D. Dye, S. Cook, and S. H. Swan. 2007. "Concentrations of urinary phthalate metabolites are associated with increased waist circumference and insulin resistance in adult U.S. males." *Environ Health Perspect* 115 (6):876-82. doi: 10.1289/ehp.9882.

Stitzel, M. L., P. Sethupathy, D. S. Pearson, P. S. Chines, L. Song, M. R. Erdos, R. Welch, S. C. Parker, A. P. Boyle, L. J. Scott, Nisc Comparative Sequencing Program, E. H. Margulies, M. Boehnke, T. S. Furey, G. E. Crawford, and F. S. Collins. 2010. "Global epigenomic analysis of primary human pancreatic islets provides insights into type 2 diabetes susceptibility loci." *Cell Metab* 12 (5):443-55. doi: 10.1016/j.cmet.2010. 09.012.

Strakovsky, R. S., S. Lezmi, I. Shkoda, J. A. Flaws, W. G. Helferich, and Y. X. Pan. 2015. "In utero growth restriction and catch-up adipogenesis after developmental di (2-ethylhexyl) phthalate exposure cause glucose intolerance in adult male rats following a high-fat dietary challenge." *J Nutr Biochem* 26 (11):1208-20. doi: 10.1016/j.jnutbio.2015.05.012.

Street, Maria Elisabeth, Sabrina Angelini, Sergio Bernasconi, Ernesto Burgio, Alessandra Cassio, Cecilia Catellani, Francesca Cirillo, Annalisa Deodati, Enrica Fabbrizi, Vassilios Fanos, Giancarlo Gargano, Enzo Grossi, Lorenzo Iughetti, Pietro Lazzeroni, Alberto Mantovani, Lucia Migliore, Paola Palanza, Giancarlo Panzica, Anna Maria Papini, Stefano Parmigiani, Barbara Predieri, Chiara Sartori, Gabriele Tridenti, and Sergio Amarri. 2018. "Current knowledge on endocrine disrupting chemicals (edcs) from animal biology to humans, from pregnancy to adulthood: highlights from a National Italian Meeting." *International Journal of Molecular Sciences* 19 (6):1647. doi: 10.3390/ijms19061647.

Su, Zhiguang, Yuhua Li, Jessica C. James, Alan H. Matsumoto, Gregory A. Helm, Aldons J. Lusis, and Weibin Shi. 2006. "Genetic linkage of hyperglycemia, body weight and serum amyloid-P in an intercross between C57BL/6 and C3H apolipoprotein E-deficient mice." *Human Molecular Genetics* 15 (10):1650-1658. doi: 10.1093/hmg/ddl088.

Svensson, K., R. U. Hernández-Ramírez, A. Burguete-García, M. E. Cebrián, A. M. Calafat, L. L. Needham, L. Claudio, and L. López-Carrillo. 2011. "Phthalate exposure associated with self-reported diabetes among Mexican women." *Environ Res* 111 (6):792-6. doi: 10.1016/j.envres.2011.05.015.

Thannickal, V. J., and B. L. Fanburg. 2000. "Reactive oxygen species in cell signaling." *Am J Physiol Lung Cell Mol Physiol* 279 (6):L1005-28. doi: 10.1152/ajplung.2000.279.6.L1005.

Thomaidou, S., A. Zaldumbide, and B. O. Roep. 2018. "Islet stress, degradation and autoimmunity." *Diabetes Obes Metab* 20 Suppl 2:88-94. doi: 10.1111/dom.13387.

Thomas, H. E., R. Darwiche, J. A. Corbett, and T. W. Kay. 2002. "Interleukin-1 plus gamma-interferon-induced pancreatic beta-cell dysfunction is mediated by beta-cell nitric oxide production." *Diabetes* 51 (2):311-6. doi: 10.2337/diabetes.51.2.311.

Toft, G., B. A. Jönsson, C. H. Lindh, T. K. Jensen, N. H. Hjollund, A. Vested, and J. P. Bonde. 2012. "Association between pregnancy loss and urinary phthalate levels around the time of conception." *Environ Health Perspect* 120 (3):458-63. doi: 10.1289/ehp.1103552.

Tong, H. V., N. K. Luu, H. A. Son, N. V. Hoan, T. T. Hung, T. P. Velavan, and N. L. Toan. 2017. "Adiponectin and pro-inflammatory cytokines are modulated in Vietnamese patients with type 2 diabetes mellitus." *J Diabetes Investig* 8 (3):295-305. doi: 10.1111/jdi.12579.

Toppari, J., J. C. Larsen, P. Christiansen, A. Giwercman, P. Grandjean, L. J. Guillette, Jr., B. Jégou, T. K. Jensen, P. Jouannet, N. Keiding, H. Leffers, J. A. McLachlan, O. Meyer, J. Müller, E. Rajpert-De Meyts, T. Scheike, R. Sharpe, J. Sumpter, and N. E. Skakkebaek. 1996. "Male reproductive health and environmental xenoestrogens." *Environ Health Perspect* 104 Suppl 4 (Suppl 4):741-803. doi: 10.1289/ehp.96104s4741.

Trasande, L., A. J. Spanier, S. Sathyanarayana, T. M. Attina, and J. Blustein. 2013. "Urinary phthalates and increased insulin resistance in adolescents." *Pediatrics* 132 (3):e646-55. doi: 10.1542/peds.2012-4022.

Tuffnell, D. J., J. West, and S. A. Walkinshaw. 2003. "Treatments for gestational diabetes and impaired glucose tolerance in pregnancy." *Cochrane Database Syst Rev* (3):Cd00 3395. doi: 10.1002/14651858.Cd003395.

van Dam, R. M., W. C. Willett, E. B. Rimm, M. J. Stampfer, and F. B. Hu. 2002. "Dietary fat and meat intake in relation to risk of type 2 diabetes in men." *Diabetes Care* 25 (3):417-24. doi: 10.2337/diacare.25.3.417.

Ventrice, P., D. Ventrice, E. Russo, and G. De Sarro. 2013. "Phthalates: European regulation, chemistry, pharmacokinetic and related toxicity." *Environ Toxicol Pharmacol* 36 (1):88-96. doi: 10.1016/j.etap.2013.03.014.

Venturelli, A. C., K. B. Meyer, S. V. Fischer, D. H. Kita, R. A. Philipsen, R. N. Morais, and A. J. Martino Andrade. 2019. "Effects of in utero and lactational exposure to phthalates on reproductive development and glycemic homeostasis in rats." *Toxicology* 421:30-40. doi: 10.1016/j.tox.2019.03.008.

Venturelli, A. C., S. V. Fischer, R. Nogueira de Morais, S. Grassiolli, and A. J. Martino Andrade. 2015. "Effects of exposure to Di-(2-ethylhexyl) phthalate (DEHP) during lactation and puberty on sexual maturation and glycemic homeostasis in males rats." *Clin Nutr ESPEN* 10 (1):e5-e12. doi: 10.1016/j.clnme.2014.10.002.

Volkov, P., K. Bacos, J. K. Ofori, J. L. Esguerra, L. Eliasson, T. Ronn, and C. Ling. 2017. "Whole-genome bisulfite sequencing of human pancreatic islets reveals novel differentially methylated regions in type 2 diabetes pathogenesis." *Diabetes* 66 (4):10 74-1085. doi: 10.2337/db16-0996.

Wang, Jing, Jinquan Li, Kashif Rafiq Zahid, Kun Wang, Yan Qian, Ping Ma, Shumao Ding, Xu Yang, and Xianliang Wang. 2016. "Adverse effect of DEHP exposure on the serum insulin level of Balb/c mice." *Molecular & Cellular Toxicology* 12 (1):83-91. doi: 10.1007/s13273-016-0011-4.

Wang, Yu, Hongkai Zhu, and Kurunthachalam Kannan. 2019. "A review of biomonitoring of phthalate exposures." *Toxics* 7 (2):21.

Waterland, R. A. 2006. "Epigenetic mechanisms and gastrointestinal development." *J Pediatr* 149 (5 Suppl):S137-42. doi: 10.1016/j.jpeds.2006.06.064.

Wei, J., Q. Hao, C. Chen, J. Li, X. Han, Z. Lei, T. Wang, Y. Wang, X. You, X. Chen, H. Li, Y. Ding, W. Huang, Y. Hu, S. Lin, H. Shen, and Y. Lin. 2020. "Epigenetic repression of miR-17 contributed to di(2-ethylhexyl) phthalate-triggered insulin resistance by targeting Keap1-Nrf2/miR-200a axis in skeletal muscle." *Theranostics* 10 (20):9230-9248. doi: 10.7150/thno.45253.

World Health Organization. 2019. *Classification of Diabetes Mellitus*. Available from https://www.who.int/publications/i/item/classification-of-diabetes-mellitus.

Wren, J. D., and H. R. Garner. 2005. "Data-mining analysis suggests an epigenetic pathogenesis for type 2 diabetes." *J Biomed Biotechnol* 2005 (2):104-12. doi: 10.11 55/JBB.2005.104.

Wu, H., A. C. Just, E. Colicino, A. M. Calafat, E. Oken, J. M. Braun, N. McRae, A. Cantoral, I. Pantic, M. L. Pizano-Zárate, M. C. Tolentino, R. O. Wright, M. M. Téllez-Rojo, A. A. Baccarelli, and A. L. Deierlein. 2021. "The associations of phthalate biomarkers during pregnancy with later glycemia and lipid profiles." *Environ Int* 155:106612. doi: 10.1016/j.envint.2021.106612.

Wu, Haotian, Alexandra Olmsted, David E. Cantonwine, Shahin Shahsavari, Tayyab Rahil, Cynthia Sites, and J. Richard Pilsner. 2017. "Urinary phthalate and phthalate alternative metabolites and isoprostane among couples undergoing fertility treatment." *Environmental research* 153:1-7. doi: 10.1016/j.envres.2016.11.003.

Xiong, X., L. D. Saunders, F. L. Wang, and N. N. Demianczuk. 2001. "Gestational diabetes mellitus: prevalence, risk factors, maternal and infant outcomes." *International Journal of Gynecology & Obstetrics* 75 (3):221-228. doi: https://doi.org/10.1016/S0020-7292(01)00496-9.

Yang, Jinzeng. 2014. "Chapter Five - Enhanced skeletal muscle for effective glucose homeostasis." In *Progress in Molecular Biology and Translational Science*, edited by Ya-Xiong Tao, 133-163. Academic Press.

Yoon, K. H., S. H. Ko, J. H. Cho, J. M. Lee, Y. B. Ahn, K. H. Song, S. J. Yoo, M. I. Kang, B. Y. Cha, K. W. Lee, H. Y. Son, S. K. Kang, H. S. Kim, I. K. Lee, and S. Bonner-Weir. 2003. "Selective beta-cell loss and alpha-cell expansion in patients with type 2 diabetes mellitus in Korea." *J Clin Endocrinol Metab* 88 (5):2300-8. doi: 10.1210/jc.2002-020735.

Zhang, J., C. A. Powell, M. K. Kay, M. H. Park, S. Meruvu, R. Sonkar, and M. Choudhury. 2020. "A moderate physiological dose of benzyl butyl phthalate exacerbates the high fat diet-induced diabesity in male mice." *Toxicol Res (Camb)* 9 (4):353-370. doi: 10.1093/toxres/tfaa037.

Zhang, W., X. Y. Shen, W. W. Zhang, H. Chen, W. P. Xu, and W. Wei. 2017. "Di-(2-ethylhexyl) phthalate could disrupt the insulin signaling pathway in liver of SD rats and L02 cells via PPARγ." *Toxicol Appl Pharmacol* 316:17-26. doi: 10.1016/j.taap.2016.12.010.

Zhang, Y., W. Zhang, X. Fu, F. Zhou, H. Yu, and X. Na. 2018. "Transcriptomics and metabonomics analyses of maternal DEHP exposure on male offspring." *Environ Sci Pollut Res Int* 25 (26):26322-26329. doi: 10.1007/s11356-018-2596-8.

Zhao, Yan, Jiao Chen, Xiu Wang, Qi Song, Hui-Hui Xu, and Yun-Hui Zhang. 2016. "Third trimester phthalate exposure is associated with DNA methylation of growth-related genes in human placenta." *Scientific Reports* 6 (1):33449. doi: 10.1038/srep33449.

Zhong, S. R., H. H. Yang, C. H. Liao, D. H. Yang, S. K. Tu, C. L. Hung, and C. C. Liao. 2021. "Association between low serum testosterone and the development of metabolic syndrome in elderly Taiwanese men." *Diabetes Metab Syndr Obes* 14:99-106. doi: 10.2147/dmso.S282832.

Zhou, L., H. Chen, Q. Xu, X. Han, Y. Zhao, X. Song, T. Zhao, and L. Ye. 2019. "The effect of di-2-ethylhexyl phthalate on inflammation and lipid metabolic disorder in rats." *Ecotoxicol Environ Saf* 170:391-398. doi: 10.1016/j.ecoenv.2018.12.009.

Zhou, W., M. H. Chen, and W. Shi. 2015. "Influence of phthalates on glucose homeostasis and atherosclerosis in hyperlipidemic mice." *BMC Endocr Disord* 15:13. doi: 10.1186/s12902-015-0015-4.

Zukin, H., B. Eskenazi, N. Holland, and K. G. Harley. 2021. "Prenatal exposure to phthalates and maternal metabolic outcomes in a high-risk pregnant Latina population." *Environ Res* 194:110712. doi: 10.1016/j.envres.2021.110712.

Chapter 6

Reproductive and Developmental Effects of Phthalates

Gözde Karabulut[1] and Nurhayat Barlas[2,*]
[1]Dumlupınar University, Faculty of Science,
Department of Biology, Kütahya, Turkey
[2]Hacettepe University, Science Faculty,
Department of Biology, Ankara, Turkey

Abstract

The endocrine disrupting chemicals were associated with the abnormalities of normal reproductive function and hormone signaling. Phthalates are common environmental chemicals with endocrine interference and currently one of the most widely used plasticizers. Since these chemicals are prevalent in plastics, personal care products, and insecticides, humans and wildlife are exposed to these chemicals every day. Since phthalates have been found to have deleterious impacts on both male and female fertility in humans and animal models according to the literature, the potential adverse effects of prenatal or adult exposure to phthalates on the reproductive health of future generations has made it an important issue for researchers. Various animal and human studies of phthalate exposure have clearly demonstrated that sperm concentration, motility, and/or morphology have a deleterious effect on semen quality. These phthalates may have estrogenic and/or anti-androgenic impacts that disrupt the hypothalamic-pituitary-gonadal axis (HPGA), damage to sperm DNA, or cause changes in sperm epigenetics. The basic properties and knowledge of the potential impacts of phthalates on reproductive systems for male and female are covered in this chapter.

---

* Corresponding Author's Email: barlas@hacettepe.edu.tr.

In: Phthalates: Environmental and Health Effects
Editors: Müfide Aydoğan Ahbab and Nurhayat Barlas
ISBN: 978-1-68507-970-3

Keywords: Phthalates, reproduction, toxicant; plasticizers, health impact

Introduction

People are exposed to multiple chemicals, plasticizers, and heavy metals in their living environments. These exposures have been shown to cause reproductive toxicity for both men and women, according to dose and duration of the exposure to these chemicals. Phthalates, a group of these chemicals, are known to be both estrogenic and anti-androgenic (Diamanti-Kandarakis et al. 2009). From 1950 to 2015, approximately 8300 million metric tons of plastics were produced (Geyer et al. 2017) and the rate of production has been increasing, reaching 368 million metric tons (annually) in 2019 (Plastics Europe, 2020). Plastic production is expected to more than double in the next 20 years and nearly quadruple by 2050 (WEF 2016).

Production of phthalate esters (PE) is expected to be between 6 and 8 million tons per year globally (Seyoum and Pradhan 2019), with more than 3 million tons used by various industrial businesses (Zhang et al. 2021). In 2020, phthalates accounted for more than 55% of global plasticizer consumption (IHS 2021). The phthalates are easily dissociated and released into the environment since they are not securely attached to the plastic matrix (Talsness et al. 2009). Many drugs produced and in use include dimethyl phthalate (DMP), diethyl phthalate (DEP), cellulose acetate phthalate (CAP), polyvinyl acetate phthalate (PVAP) and dibutyl phthalate (DBP) (Hauser et al. 2004, Bahadar et al. 2014).

Phthalates can also contaminate waters and accumulate in plants (Saeidnia and Abdolahi 2013). In addition, babies are exposed to di-isononyl phthalate (DINP) because of the presence of this phthalate in toys used as teether (Bogen et al. 2001). Entry 52 of Annex XVII of the Registration, Evaluation, Authorization and Restriction of Chemicals Regulation restricts the use of DINP in toys and childcare articles, which can be placed in the mouth by children (ECHA 2018).

Phthalate esters consist of a di-ester group that has an acidhead of the two ester side chains (NICNAS 2008) and the chemical structures of common phthalate diesters are shown in Figure 1. This includes 3 groups: low-molecular weight phthalates, high-molecular weight phthalates and transitional phthalates. Diethyl phthalate (DEP), di-methyl phthalate (DMP), di-isobutyl phthalate (DIBP), di-alkyl phthalate (DAP), and di-methylethyl phthalate (DMEP) are examples of low weight phthalates. Dibutyl phthalate

(DBP), di-isononyl phthalates (DINP), di-isodosyl phthalates (DIDP) and di-nonyl phthalate (DNP) are examples of high weight phthalates. Benzyl butyl phthalate (BBP), and di-(2-ethylhexyl) phthalates (DEHP) are presented as transitional phthalates. DMP phthalate type has been employed in hair spray to prevent hair rigidity whilst DEP is used as a fastener and solvent in fragrances. In nail polishes, DBP-style transition phthalates are present both to prevent cracks and as solvents (Hubinger 2010).

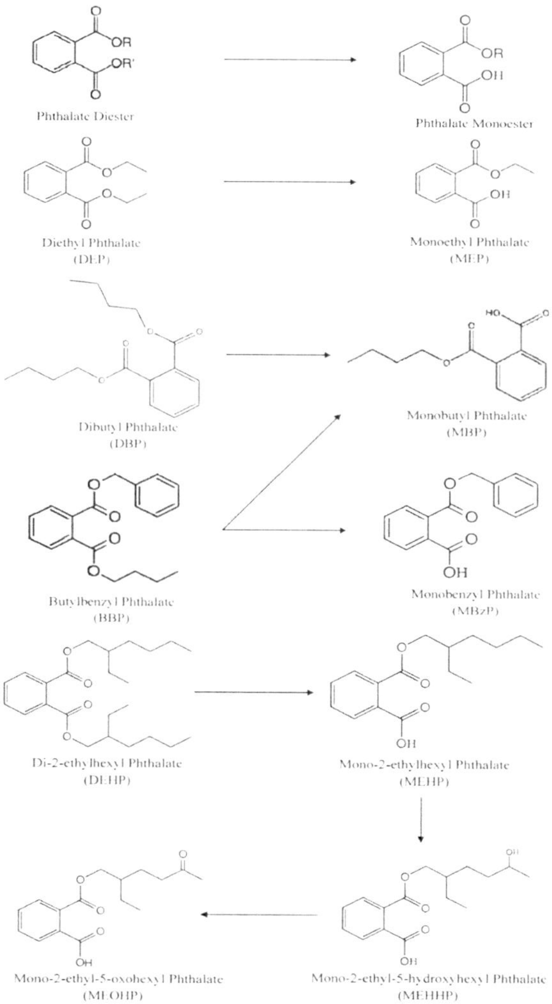

Figure 1. The general chemical structures of phthalate diesters and major metabolites (Kay et al. 2013).

This chapter has been prepared to explain the toxic consequences of such frequent use of phthalates and to provide literature information on both experimental and clinical studies.

Characterization of Phthalates

The glands of endocrine system in human body regulate metabolic events with the hormones they secrete. The hormones act as chemical messengers, and derive from steroids (progesterone, estrogens, and androgens), amino acids (melatonin, epinephrine, and thyroxine), and peptides (glucagon, oxytocin, and insulin) (Pincus et al. 2017).

Since phthalates are soluble in fat, they immediately enter the bloodstream and are separated into their metabolites. These metabolites are glucuronide, oxidative and hydrolytic conjugates. These plasticizers are considered endocrine disrupting chemicals because they act as antagonist and agonist ligands and inhibit chemical signaling of hormones (Kabir et al. 2015). The biological half-life of these chemicals is crucial for endocrine disrupting effects to occur. As a result of chemical interference, more than one abnormality occurs such as infertility, precocious puberty, insulin resistance, type II diabetes, and obesity (Meeker et al. 2009b, Kamrin 2009).

Male Reproductive Health Effects

Testicular dysgenesis syndrome is one of the most important and well-known damage to the male reproductive system by phthalates, and the manifestations of the syndrome are cryptorchidism, hypospadias, and undescended testicles (Johnson et al. 2012). This syndrome is also known as phthalate syndrome. Besides these effects, phthalates may cause changes in anogenital distance (AGD), decrease in sperm count and quality, infertility, and decrease in testosterone hormone (Swan 2008). Exposure to phthalates at developmental stages may cause deterioration in sperm quality in the future. This section discusses the impacts of phthalates on the male reproductive system.

Effects of Phthalates on Testosterone

The main male sex hormone, testosterone (T), is necessary for the development of the male reproductive system. This hormone also promotes secondary male sexual properties like body hair, bone density and voice intensification (NASEM 2017). Deficiency in the level of this hormone causes infertility and abnormal sex characteristics.

Growth and activity of the reproductive system involves different genes and these genes are generated by the HPG axis (Acevedo-Rodriguez et al. 2018). This axis controls the functioning of reproductive hormones by negative and positive feedback mechanisms. Steroidogenesis and its control are the main task of this axis. Cholesterol is the precursor molecule of steroidogenic hormones produced by the catalysis of enzymes involved in steroidogenesis such as P450 and hydroxysteroid dehydrogenase (HSD). Sex hormones such as testosterone, dihydrotestosterone, and progesterone, are synthesized by these enzymes (Miller and Auchus 2011).

Phthalates have been shown in rodent studies to have a negative effect on male testicular function. DiNP exposed male rats had multi-nucleated gonocytes, whereas DBP exposed rats had lower spermatogenesis and more cord disruptions after birth (Li et al. 2015, Aly et al. 2016). From day 12 to day 21 GD (gestational day) of pregnancy, pregnant Sprague-Dawley rats were given a control vehicle (corn oil) or DINP (10, 100, 500, and 1000 mg/kg) by gavage (Li et al. 2015). Testicular testosterone production, fetal Leydig cell count and distribution, as well as testicular gene and protein expression levels, were all measured at GD 21.5. DINP caused fetal Leydig cell aggregation in a dose-dependent manner, with a low observed adverse effect level (LOAEL) of 10 mg/kg bw/day, and a LOAEL of 100 mg/kg bw/day in multinucleated germ cells. DINP enhanced the size of fetal Leydig cells at a dose of 10 mg/kg bw/day, but reduced the gene expression and protein levels of insulin-like 3 and 3-hydroxysteroid dehydrogenase. At a dose of 1000 mg/kg bw/day, DINP inhibits testicular testosterone levels. The findings revealed that fetal steroid-producing gene expression in Leydig cells, germ cell multinucleation, and Leydig cell aggregation are affected by DINP exposure in utero. Adult male albino rats were given DBP orally for 15 days at dosages of 0, 200, 400, or 600 mg/kg bw/day in the study by Aly et al. (2016). The weight of the testicles, the number of sperm, and the motility of the sperm were all significantly reduced. DBP treatment decreased testicular lactate dehydrogenase activity, serum follicle-stimulating hormone and testosterone levels. DBP medication lowered serum total antioxidant capacity as well as the activity of enzymes such as superoxide dismutase, catalase, and glutathione reductase. These findings revealed oxidative stress as a possible mechanism for DBP-induced testicular damage and subsequent testosterone secretion reduction.

DEHP has been caused an increase in the population of Leydig cells, which is linked to chronically elevated serum luteinizing hormone (LH) and testosterone (T) levels (Akingbemi et al. 2004). Again, it has been shown that puberty is delayed in male rats administered DEHP (Ge et al. 2007). Male Long-Evans rat pups have been exposed to low or high doses of DEHP, using the androgen-driven foreskin separation process as an indicator of puberty time. Starting from the 21st day after birth, rats were treated with DEHP doses of 0, 10, 500 or 750 mg/kg body weight for 28 days. Compared with the control serum testosterone and seminal vesicle weight, the 10 mg/kg bw/day DEHP administration dose also significantly increased serum testosterone (T) levels and seminal vesicle weight, while the 750 mg/kg bw/day dose group, decreased serum testosterone, testes and body weight (Ge et al. 2007). Compared with dibutyl phthalate (DBP), the number of prostate cells in male rats increased before birth (Scarano et al. 2009). In this study, pregnant rats were divided into two experimental groups as a control and treatment groups. The females in the treatment group received DBP (100 mg/kg bw/day) from the 12th day of pregnancy to the 21st day after delivery, and the control group received corn oil. The animals were euthanized in adulthood (90 days old). The serum and testicular testosterone levels and prostate weight between the two groups were comparable. In the treatment group, the relative proportions of epithelial and interstitial compartments of prostate increased, while luminal compartments decreased. In the treatment group, disseminated inflammatory infiltration in the stroma and prostate intraepithelial neoplasia (PIN) were observed. In another study, phthalates reduced testosterone levels and inhibited androgen activity (Radke et al. 2018). In addition, DEHP caused DNA damage in blood lymphocytes and sperm and concrete negative effects on the reproductive system in rats from the pre-pubertal period to the pubertal period (Karabulut and Barlas 2018). Tail intensity increased significantly at the end of the experiment, compared to a control group in the dose groups of 100 mg/kg bw/day ($p < 0.032$), 200 mg/kg bw/day ($p = 0.019$), and 400 mg/kg bw/day ($p = 0.012$). Testosterone levels were also lower in all exposed groups than in the control group (Karabulut and Barlas 2018). In these studies, the damage caused by phthalate exposure before and after birth on the male reproductive system has been revealed."

Phthalates are plasticizers that can be found in medical devices, furniture, baby bottles, and toys. There are results that hormonal regulation is disrupted in the babies of people exposed to phthalates before birth (Qian et al. 2020). In *in vitro* studies, MEHP has been shown to reduce testosterone hormone levels in human testicular explants (Chauvigné et al. 2009). Exposure to some phthalates was linked to delayed development of puberty, a delayed development of pubic hair and testis and lower serum testosterone levels in young children. In boys, urine monobutyl phthalate (MBP) levels negatively correlated with testicular volume, and 2-ethyl-5-hydroxyhexyl (MEHHP) and 2-ethyl-5-oxohexyl (MEOHP) associated with the pubic hair stage. The probability of entering puberty has been reduced by 43% to 51%. In girls, the levels of mono(2-ethylhexyl) phthalate (MEHP), MEHHP, and MEOHP and the sum of these levels are positively correlated with breast stage, and this association is stronger in girls with high body fat proportion (BF%) The probability of entering the puberty increased by 29% to 50% (Shi et al. 2015).

BBOP (bis (2-butoxyethyl) phthalate) is a one-of-a-kind phthalate having oxygen atoms in its carbon backbone. Its reproductive and developmental toxicity is poorly understood. The aim of Liu et al. (2021)'s study was to see how BBOP affected the development of fetal Leydig cells in rats after intrauterine exposure. Pregnant Sprague Dawley rats were randomly separated into six groups and given BBOP (0, 10, 100, 250, 500, and 1000 mg/kg bw/day) from GD 14 to 21. Seven of the eight dams in the 1000 mg/kg BBOP group died before giving birth. In the 500 mg/kg BBOP group, twelve of the twenty rats had no litter. The body weight of GD 21 female and male progeny, as well as serum testosterone levels and male fetal anogenital distance, were significantly lowered by BBOP at 500mg/kg group. At 500 mg/kg bw/day, BBOP boosted the proliferation and quantity of fetal Leydig cells, but at 250 and 500 mg/kg, it induced aberrant aggregation. The relationship between INSL3 and testosterone levels and phthalates has been shown (Chang et al. 2015). In a study, MEHP and MBP concentrations were found to be increases in the blood of 74 men who were occupationally exposed to DBP and DEHP (Pan et al. 2006). In addition, an inverse correlation was found between estradiol, testosterone, and free androgen indices and MEHP (Meeker et al. 2009a).

Rats exposed to DEHP in utero had decreased fetal testicular testosterone, according to a meta-analysis published by the National Academy of Sciences in the United States (NAS 2017), however the results were not consistent in humans (NAS 2017). In breast milk studies, MBP exposure was found to be negatively related to the free testosterone ($r = -0.22$, $P = 0.033$), and other phthalate monoesters had comparable effects, but they were not significant (Main et al. 2006). In urine samples from 155 pregnant women collected in the third trimester, monobenzyl phthalate (MBzP), monoethylhexyl phthalate (MEHP), mono-(2-ethyl-5-hydroxyhexyl) phthalate (5OH-MEHP), mono-methyl phthalate (MMP), and monoethyl phthalate (MEP) were found, but there was no link to hormones (Lin et al. 2011). Finally, there is no indication that phthalate metabolites in newborn boys are linked to steroid hormones. As a result of the mixed results, the link between phthalate exposure and reduced fetal testosterone has been deemed questionable.

The link between prenatal phthalate exposure and reproductive damage in adult male offspring was investigated further. According to Hart et al. (2018), DiNP metabolite concentrations in the mother's serum at 18 and 34 weeks of pregnancy were negatively correlated with testicular volume in young adult offspring (about 20 years) but positively connected with serum total testosterone levels. The complicated connections between numerous hormone axes, including the hypothalamic-pituitary gonadal axis, growth factors, and thyroid hormones, can explain these contradictory findings.

DEHP and its metabolite MEHP were shown to be the most prevalent phthalate in the urine of mothers during pregnancy in two investigations from Taiwan and Japan (Lin et al. 2011, Araki et al. 2014). Furthermore, in a study by Main et al. (2006), they analyzed individual breast milk samples collected as additive aliquots during 1–3 months postnatally (n = 130; 62 cryptorchid/68 healthy boys) for phthalate monoesters (MMP), (MEP), (MBP), (MBzP), (MEHP), mono-isononyl phthalate (miNP), mono-isononyl phthalate (miNP) and testosterone. In another Taiwanese investigation, both mother and child urinary DEHP metabolites were analyzed, and higher prenatal DEHP concentrations were linked to lower levels of progesterone in females (Wen et al. 2017). The researchers discovered that phthalate exposure reduces testosterone, progesterone, and the T/E2 ratio, implying that CYP19 was increased. Increased levels of estradiol in children and high levels of testosterone and DHEA sulfate were linked to higher prenatal exposure to phthalate metabolites in girls aged 8 to 13 (Watkins et al. 2017a, Watkins et al. 2017b).

The levels of reactive oxygen species (ROS) increase when people are exposed to contaminants in the environment leading to oxidative stress (Mourabit et al. 2019). One of the causes of male infertility due to environmental stimulation is oxidative stress (Menezo et al. 2016). ROS can potentially cause male reproductive failure by disrupting the epigenetic states of sperm (Sharma et al. 2019). Excessive accumulation of ROS in testicular cells of rats was observed after exposure to DEHP (Yi et al. 2018). It is also caused the expression of redox sensitive miRNAs (miR-181a upregulation and miR-126p 3p downregulation), which has meant enzymes related to the synthesis of testosterone, disruption of synthesis and serum tests for the reduction of estrone level (Helmy et al. 2020). In another study, the activity of antioxidant enzymes in the brain and testes in the DEHP provided groups was statistically not significant compared with the control group, except for the 400 mg/kg/day DEHP exposed groups. DEHP may alter trace elements and mineral levels while the blood-brain and testis-blood barrier as well as the short-term exposure to DEHP may disrupt antioxidant enzymes (Aydemir et al. 2019).

DEHP (0, 0.5, 50 or 500 mg/kg bw/day) was administered orally to 5-week-old male mice for 35 days. Exposure to DEHP at a dose of 500 mg/kg bw/day resulted in a reduction in testicular weight and sperm count in mice. In mice treated with DEHP at a dose of 500 mg/kg bw/day, the number of stage VII-VIII mature seminiferous tubules decreased, and the number of stage IX-XII immature tubules increased. Multiple apoptotic germ cells have been identified in the seminiferous tubules of mice exposed to 50 and 500 mg/kg bw/day of DEHP (Zhu et al. 2021).

These findings were regarded as indication that phthalate-induced ROS alterations in testicular cells can cause redox-sensitive epigenetic modifications to shift and contribute to male reproductive disruption.

The Studies on Semen Quality with Phthalate Exposure

In about half of male infertility cases, insemination is difficult and most cases are unexplained (Vander Borght and Wyns, 2018). When it comes to getting pregnant, sperm quality is crucial. DEHP exposure has been linked to apoptosis, the formation of reactive oxygen species (ROS), and sperm aneuploidy in studies (Jurewicz et al. 2013). The baseline sample of 473 (94%) males, and of whom 378 (80%) men submitted for their second sample in the next month, were acquired from urine and semen. 14 monoester metabolites of the phthalate diesters were examined in urine samples by high performance liquid chromatography combined with tandem mass spectrometry. Analyzed 34 sperm quality criteria were general, motility, morphology, sperm head and structure of sperm chromatin (Bloom et al. 2015). According to Hauser et al. (2007), urinary MEP and MEHP levels are associated with sperm DNA damage. The relationship between the urinary levels of phthalate metabolite concentrations and the motility and morphology of sperm, sperm aneuploidy and sperm chromatin was investigated. Therefore, the decrease in sperm motility is related to the level of major urinary phthalate metabolites (Jurewicz et al. 2013, Cai et al. 2015).

Many Chinese researches revealed that phthalate exposure has addressed the negative effects on sperm quality. The elevated MBP ratio discovered in the samples of 1040 Chinese men in infertility clinic was linked to reduce sperm concentration (Wang et al. 2015a). To higher exposure to MEHP and MBZP caused the abnormal sperm percentage, sperm motility parameter and decreased sperm volume (Wang et al. 2016a). For old Chinese men, urine with high MEP content was associated with impaired sperm percentage (Wang et al. 2018). MEP and MnBP that are hydrolytic metabolites have been associated with damage to sperm DNA, while DEHP oxidative metabolites and MBzP have been related to HDS and MiNP with sperm morphologies (Axelsson et al. 2015).

There are two Meta-analyzes of the effect of phthalates on semen quality (Cai et al. 2015, Radke et al. 2018). The first, published in 2015, analyzed 14 researches and discovered that urine MBP and MBzP were linked to lower sperm concentration. Motility was reversed to MBP and MEHP (Cai et al. 2015). A meta-analysis of 15 studies from Radke et al. (2018) concluded that increased DBP exposure was linked to lower semen quality, particularly sperm concentration, with a robust relationship, but there was a weaker relationship between semen quality and DEHP for increased sperm concentration.

Two studies examined post-exposure maternal phthalate and sperm quality in male children (Axelsson et al. 2015, Hart et al. 2018). Among 112 adolescent males in Sweden, DiNP metabolites were detected in maternal serum after 12 weeks of gestation, and sperm quality was checked. High prenatal DEHP and DiNP exposures were related to testicular size and sperm volume and sperm concentration. These researchers reported that maternal levels of certain metabolites, prenatal exposure to DiNP and DEHP seemed negatively associated with the reproductive function of these adolescent men (Axelsson et al. 2015). In 185 young Australian men, maternal serum concentrations of monoisononyl phthalate (MiNP), DEHP, and DiNP metabolites were found to be negative correlated with testicular volume. These two studies demonstrate that DEHP and DiNP exposure during pregnancy may influence testicular development and consequently adult testicular size. DBP suppresses the AKT, which contributes to reduced sperm quantity and motility, by boosting PTEN (Phosphatase and tensin homolog) expression via miR-29b-targeted DNMT3b-mediated PTEN demethylation, according to *in vitro* studies in GC-1 and GC-2 cells (Li et al. 2019). Multiple phthalate exposures during the perinatal period activated methylation of sterol regulatory elements that bind to the transcription factor testis 1 (Srebf1) and down-regulated of Srebf2 methylation in rat adipose tissue that affected steroid hormones synthesis in a tissue-specific manner (Li et al. 2019).

In general, there has been a well-established link between more exposure to phthalate and lower quality of semen, particularly semen concentration.

The Studies on Anogenital Distance and Hypospadias with Phthalate Exposure

Anogenital Distance (AGD) is the distance between the anus and genitalia that indicates in utero androgenic action throughout the reproductive system's development (Kita et al. 2016). Furthermore, AGD is a measure of fetal testosterone synthesis by the testis; rats prenatally exposed to certain phthalates had lower AGD (Braun et al. 2013).

In a systematic evaluation of human epidemiological evidence, Radke et al. (2018) found moderate evidence of the inverse relationship between AGD and DEHP and DBP exposure with mostly consistent results in five research studies. DINP, BBP, DIBP and DEP were only shown in a smidgeon. In a study revealed that the AGD of male fetuses in the DHP and DCHP treatment groups decreased compared to control group. Moreover, the ratio of AGD to body weight also decreased in high dose DHP and all DCHP treated groups (Ahbab and Barlas, 2015).

Swan (2008) discovered an inverse relationship between maternal urine DEHP exposure, AGD, and penile size. Prenatal exposure to DEHP was substantially related with shorter AGD, according to a recent review (Quian et al. 2020) and meta-analysis (Zarean et al. 2019), which comprised 10 research. Monobutyl phthalate (MBP), monoethyl phthalate (MEP), and monoibutyl phthalate (MiBP) in urine are also associated with AGD.

Wagner et al. (2011) found that children born to mothers with occupational exposure to phthalates had a higher incidence of cryptorchidism. Conducted a three-year prospective study was in two maternity hospitals screening newborns for boys with a gestational age ≥34 weeks. Information concerning the kid and the parents was collected using medical records or self-fulfilled questionnaires (medical history, pregnancy and lifestyle). Of the 6.246 children, 102 were born of cryptorchidism (1.6 percent, including 95). However, 10 percent had a secondary recurrence (repeating coding theory) for

12 months, which warrants long-term follow up. These researchers reported that cryptorchidism at birth was associated with instrumental delivery, inguinal hernia and urogenital malformations, particularly micropenis and paternal history of cryptorchidism.

Swan et al. (2008) found that among 119 boys with both testicular localization and pre-existing phthalate concentrations, higher concentrations of the DEHP metabolite were essentially associated with a higher risk of cryptorchidism. No other phthalate metabolites associated with testicular prolapse have been identified. On the other hand, anti-androgen EDCs are relevant to investigations for hypospadias. In a case-control study of 471 hypospadias and 490 randomly selected contraceptives, an occupational exposure matrix showed an increased risk of hypospadias from phthalate exposure (OR = 3.12; 95 percent confidence range, 1.04–11.46) (Ormond et al. 2009).

Carran et al. (2012) found that the incidence of hypospadias and cryptorchidism was higher in the children of New Zealand soldiers who served in Malaya (1948-1960) and were rubbed on their clothes with DBP daily as an acaricide to combat tick-borne typhus in the jungle. On the other side, some study has identified a relationship between phthalates and cryptorchidism and hypospadias. There is no connection to the prevalence of cryptorchidism and hypospadias, according to Chevrier et al. (2012). Similarly, no link was established between phthalate monoester levels and cryptorchidism in a sample of 62 cryptorchid and 68 healthy boys (Main et al. 2006). Vrijheld et al. observed no link between phthalate exposure and the frequency of hypospadias even after controlled for a social level, year of birth, location and mother age (Vrijheid et al. 2003).

In a large follow-up study conducted in Australia, Nassar et al. (2010) found no association between phthalate exposure and the occurrence of hypospadias, while women exposed to phthalates more often had a son with hypnotism (OR 1.2; 95% CI 0.8–1.7). In amniotic fluid samples from 270 cases of cryptorchidism, 75 cases and 300 control group patients, scientists analyzed metabolites of DEHP and DiNP (n=645) as well as steroid hormones (n = 545, etc.) and found that neither of those metabolites were consistently associated with hypocrisy or cryptorchidism. The authors argued that phthalate and its metabolites could be related to cryptorchidism and hypocrisy on the basis of testosterone and INSL3 (Jensen et al. 2015).

Female Reproductive Health Effects

There is substantial evidence that phthalates are toxic to male reproduction when compared to female reproduction. Crain et al. (2008) investigated the potential role of endocrine disruptors in female reproductive disorders and concluded that endocrine disruptors contribute to a wide range of human female reproductive abnormalities, emphasizing the importance of early life-stage exposures. As a result, female reproduction is thought to be less sensitive to phthalates than male reproduction; however, several studies have shown that some phthalates may also have an impact on female reproduction (Repouskou et al. 2021).

The Studies on Precocious Puberty with Phthalate Exposure

Puberty is a complicated transitional period in which children's growth accelerates and secondary sexual features develop. It is a time of physical and psychological growth. The onset and progression of puberty are influenced by a number of genetic, environmental, and nutritional elements (Kiess et al. 2016).

In a Taiwanese study, greater DEHP concentrations in maternal urine were linked to smaller uteruses in girls aged 8 to 11, whereas higher butyl benzyl phthalate (BBzP) concentrations were linked to increased bone age/chronological age ratio in girls aged 8 to 11 (Su et al. 2015). Greater DEHP in utero exposure was linked to earlier pubic hair development and delayed breast development in Mexican girls aged 8–13 years (Watkins et al. 2017a), whereas higher DEHP in utero exposure was linked to delayed pubic hair development in males aged 8–14 years (Watkins et al. 2017b). Higher urine phthalate metabolites were linked to a later onset of puberty in American girls aged 6–8 years old, both cross-sectional at baseline and after 2 or 5 years of follow-up (Wolff et al. 2010, Wolff et al. 2014, Wolff et al. 2017).

Increased phthalate concentrations, on the other hand, delayed puberty in Danish girls (5–19 years of age) in a cross-sectional study, but not in boys (6–19 years of age) (Mieritz et al. 2012, Frederiksen et al. 2012). However, increased DBP exposure was linked to early puberty in males but not in girls during a 5-year follow-up (Mouritsen et al. 2013). Finally, after a year and a half of follow-up, a Taiwanese study looked at phthalates in the urine of 9-year-olds and found that DBP slowed pubic hair growth in boys, while exposure to with DBP, DMP, DEP and DEHP accelerated breasts and first period in girls (Zhang et al. 2015).

Prenatal exposures to phthalate combinations or mixtures of numerous EDCs have also been shown to cause reproductive abnormalities in female mouse offspring, including changes in sex organs, puberty onset, and infertility (Zhou et al. 2017a).

The Studies on Endometriosis with Phthalate Exposure

Endometriosis is one of the most frequent causes of female infertility, accounting for 30 to 50 percent of all cases of difficulty or inability to conceive (Young et al. 2016). Even though there are various causes for the sickness, current evidence suggests that environmental contaminants may play a part in its development. Because endometriosis is an estrogen-dependent disease, some studies have looked into the potential link between phthalate exposure and endometriosis. According to *in vitro* studies, phthalates, specifically DEHP, improved the survival and resistance of endometrial stromal cells under stressful conditions (Kim et al. 2010, Wang et al. 2012).

The uterus is a female reproductive organ regulated by the hypothalamic-pituitary axis (HPA), providing the environment for embryo implantation, continuation of pregnancy, and delivery. Endocrine disruptors can impact uterine structure and function, leading to disease, like endometriosis and fibroids, depending on several human and animal studies. Endometriosis is a gynecological illness that involves the development of complex glandular tissues or stroma outside of the uterine canal and affects 10-15% of fertile women and up to 50% of women suffering from infertility and/or severe pelvic pain (Bergman et al. 2013).

According to Gore et al. (2015) women with severe endometriosis have elevated levels of mono (2-ethylhexyl) phthalate (MEHP), di (2-ethylhexyl) phthalate (DEHP), and mono butyl phthalate (MBP). In the United States, however, a population-based case-control research found no link between increased endometriosis risk and increased risk exposure (Crain et al. 2008). Recent transversal exposure studies have shown that MBP has a positive connection with a higher fibroid risk, but that MEHP derivatives are reversely linked with tumors. Further research has discovered a link between MEHP exposure and the GSTM1 null genotype and fibroids.

Many human case-control studies focused on phthalate metabolite plasma concentrations in relation to endometriosis (Cobellius et al. 2003, Reddy et al.

2006), particularly in relation to DEHP exposures. Endometriosis, and urine phthalate metabolites, which are more sensitive indicators of phthalate diester exposure, have lately been investigated by researchers (Louis et al. 2013). There were no significant variations in urine levels of distinct phthalate metabolites between controls and endometriosis patients with verified histological diagnosis in a case-control study (Fernandez et al. 2019).

The Studies on Abnormalities of Pregnancy with Phthalate Exposure

When exposed to phthalates during pregnancy, fetal development is impaired, which can result in significant and even permanent harmful effects in babies and children (Watkins et al. 2017a).

Prenatal DEHP exposure altered gene expression and DNA methylation in male rats (Sekaran and Jagadeesan 2015), whereas maternal DEHP exposure resulted in hypomethylation of the Igf2r (insulin-like growth factor 2 receptor) and Peg3 (paternally-expressed gene 3) genes in F1 and F2 mice, both of which are important for germ cell proliferation driven by estrogen signaling. Furthermore, phthalate exposure is linked to epigenetic and gene expression alterations mediated by nuclear receptor signaling. These effects were associated with decreased expression of oocyte specific genes such as LIM homeobox 8 (*Lhx8*), factor in the germline alpha (*Figla*), spermatogenesis and oogenesis helix-loop-helix (*Sohlh2*), and newborn ovary homeobox (*Nobox*) (Zhang et al. 2014).

In rats exposed to MEHP, apoptosis and the nuclear factor B (NFB) pathway were activated (Giammona et al. 2002). The initial line of defense against MEHP-induced apoptosis is the interaction of NF-B with the Pi3k/Akt signal pathway. The impact of phthalates on metabolism and reproductive systems has been repeatedly examined using rodent models (Rogers et al. 2008). They discover that Akt kinase activity increases in the testes of postnatal day 28 wild-type mice after exposure to 500 mg/kg mono-(2-ethylhexyl) phthalate (MEHP), and that Akt1 deficiency causes germ cell apoptosis to occur prematurely.

In GD11.5 XX embryos, DEHP has been demonstrated to boost the expression of the genes Forkhead Box L2 (Foxl2), R-Spondin1 (Rspo1), Wnt Family Member 4 (Wnt4), and -catenin (Ctnnb1), which are needed for the development of the mouse bipotential gonad towards the ovary (Wang et al. 2015b, Wang et al. 2016b). In prepubertal females from the previous study,

Foxl2 levels were higher and Follistatin (Fst) levels were lower, while the expression of the first-step steroidogenic enzymes StAR and Cyp11A1 was significantly lower, indicating disturbed granulosa cell differentiation, follicular growth, and estrogen production (Wang et al. 2016b).

The expression of steroidogenic enzymes, follicle stimulating hormone (FSH) and estradiol (E2) levels, and estrous onset /cyclicity in adult offspring were all significantly affected. The researchers stated that in utero exposure to DEHP resulted in reduced estrogen levels at proestrus. Theca cell layer thickness was decreased starting at 50 mg DEHP/kg bw/day dose. Follicle-stimulating hormone levels were significantly increased at proestrus and estrus (Meltzer et al. 2015).

Moyer et al. (2012) reported that pregnant C57/Bl6 mice were exposed via oral gavage to corn oil, 100, 500, or 1000 mg/kg MEHP from gestational days 17–19, reproductive lifespan decreased by one month in the highest F1 exposure group. Also, they were observed that in F1 females exhibited delayed estrous onset at the two higher exposures and prolonged estrus in all MEHP-exposed females. Adult rodents who were exposed to DEHP while in the womb developed ovarian histopathology. To evaluate the effects of DEHP in adult female progeny, pregnant dams were gavage with oil containing 1, 20, 50, or 300 mg/kg bw/day of DEHP from gestational day 14 until birth. Rat follicles have been found to have a thinner theca cell layer (Meltzer et al. 2015). Dams of pregnant F0 rats were exposed to 0, 0.05, 5 mg/kg bw/day DEHP in the diet from 0.5 gestational day until the end of the lactation cycle. The incidence of adult reproductive disease was observed in the F1, F2 and F3 progeny and DEHP induced imbalance and decreased primordial follicular reserve in mice (Pocar et al. 2017). CD1-pregnant mice were given either corn oil (vehicle control) or DEHP (20 and 200 mg/kg bw/day and 500 and 750 mg/kg bw/day) from day 11 of gestation until delivery. F1 females mate with untreated males to produce the F2 generation, and F2 females mate with untreated males to produce the F3 generation. These changes lead to lower pregnancy rates, increased ovarian aging, and shorter reproductive times (Brehm et al. 2018).

Phthalates can cause transgenerational reproductive problems in F2 or F3 offspring if they are exposed to them during pregnancy. DEHP increased the size of F3 generation rats' litters while decreasing the expression of steroidogenesis and folliculogenesis-related genes in F2 and F3 generation mice. According to further studies, epidermal growth factor receptor (EGFR) is a major candidate gene that mediates the relationship between phthalate exposure and early placental function (Grindler et al. 2018). Thus, phthalates may influence the regular operation of the placenta by altering the expression of placental genes through epigenetic control.

Chiang et al. (2019) conducted in a short time study in adult 39-40 days old CD1 female mice who have been exposed to diisononyl phthalate (DiNP). They fed them orally for 10 days with DiNP concentrations ranging from 20mg/kg bw/day to 200 mg/kg bw/day. They found that 10 days of adult DiNP exposure had not only a short-term but long-term effect on the reproductive lives of these mice. DiNP affected the distribution of ovarian follicular population and sex steroid hormone levels (including E2, P4, T and FSH) at multiple time points, but did not prevent (B) (immediately after dosing, 3, 6 and 9 months after use) (Chiang et al. 2020). Furthermore, the researchers discovered that adult exposure to DiNP resulted in long-term negative effects (12, 15 and 18 months after taking the DiNP). In addition to alterations in follicular population, hormone levels, and estrous cycle (increased number of males), DiNP lowered fertility, increased miscarriage, and altered the sex ratio of progeny (Chiang et al. 2020).

A case-control study was performed that included 150 miscarriages and 150 matched controls for normal pregnancies. The levels of phthalate exposure in the two groups were compared by analyzing 13 phthalate metabolites in urine samples. To assess the relationship between serum hormone levels and phthalate exposure, blood samples were taken, and Yi et al. (2016) discovered that monomethyl phthalate (MMP) level of case group was significantly higher than the control group, and that the level of MMP and stillbirth were strongly related to dose response. Phthalate exposure has been found to reduce litter size and number, decrease viability of live embryos or offspring, and increase rates of miscarriage, post-implantation loss, and uptake in uterus in rat and mouse models (Saillenfait et al. 2006, Mankidy et al. 2013).

Also, animal experiments have shown that DEHP exposure alters the levels of gene expression and protein synthesis during the oestrus cycle in mice, as well as folliculogenesis and estrogen synthesis (Hannon et al. 2014). DEHP may also block angiogenic proteins such as placental growth factor and soluble fms-like tyrosine kinase-1, according to another idea (Mu et al. 2015). Therefore, placental growth or function during pregnancy can be affected by phthalates. Moreover, the oxidative stress associated with MBzP, MBP and MiBP has been shown which can lead to a lack of pregnancy.

In summary, there is a lot of research to support the idea that exposure to phthalates can lead to abnormal pregnancies, such as miscarriages. Therefore, exposure to phthalates should be minimized in pregnant and lactating women.

Other Reproductive System Disorders

Phthalates are frequently connected to other areas of reproductive health and/or have detrimental consequences. While animal studies of individual phthalate exposure can assist identify biological endpoints, temporal frames, and dose-dependent consequences for each phthalate, they fall short of simulating real-world settings in which organisms are exposed to many hazardous chemicals at the same time. Furthermore, failing to assess the impact of many exposures may lead to the overlooking of important dangers to human health (Kortenkamp et al. 2018).

If the mixture acts independently for all components that target a single endpoint, the additive may be the reason of the mixture. This is not often the case with a variety of endpoints affected by phthalates and other endocrine disruptors. Various phthalates in a mixture could have different/independent toxicity patterns, such as a binding to the same receptor that could affect the same or comparable results. As a result, they may have cumulative (i.e., growing with each addition) or synergistic effects (resulting from possible biochemical interactions between the components of the mixture). Comparatives of individual compounds versus compounds (Howdeshell et al. 2008, Kortenkamp et al. 2020) demonstrated that their combined action can have medical implications at lower concentrations, meaning that they act as a dose additive (when they are of a common mode of action).

The reduction of fetal testosterone production associated with male reproductive system defects is one of the best-known examples of phthalate dose-additive effects. This case has been seen in individual phthalates exposed rats. In utero, combined exposure to the DBP and DEHP is more likely to lead to hormone depletion than single exposures (Howdeshell et al. 2008, Martino-Andrade et al. 2009). Similarly, the dose addition pattern (Hannas et al. 2011) is followed by the reduction in fetal testosterone with a mixture of nine phthalates. Another comparison investigation in male rats; the overall effect was the mean of the individual effects on fetal Leydig cells (FLC) at levels of 3 beta-hydroxysteroid dehydrogenase 1 (*Hsd3b1*) (Hu et al. 2018). The results showed that the gestational (GD12-20) exposure of DEP + DEHP resulted in synergistic and/or dose-additive effects on the development of fetal Leydig cell. The lowest observed adverse-effect levels (LOAEL) for fetal Leydig cell (aggregation and cell size), and *StAR* expressions were of 10 mg/kg and, lower than when these chemicals were exposed alone (Hu et al. 2018).

When compared to the individual drugs, combined exposure at the lower dose of 10 mg/kg resulted in greater aggregation for fetal Leydig cells (FLC).

The combination treatment, on the other hand, had a synergistic impact in reducing FLC numbers and *StAR* expression, lowering the effective dose by more than 10-fold. In a study, researchers stated that in female rats, 520 and 780 mg/kg dose of five phthalate mixtures (BBP, DBP, DEHP, DIBP and DPEP) gestational exposure caused uterine agenesis or aplasia in PND120, absent vaginal opening and canal agenesis (Hannas et al. 2013).

The applicability of the mixture's individual ingredients to typical human exposure is an important issue in animal studies. In studies dams were exposed to a mixture of phthalates and their metabolites are frequently discovered in the urine of pregnant women (Zhou et al. 2017, Li et al. 2020, Brehm et al. 2020). Brehm et al. (2020) tested the hypothesis that prenatal exposure to a mixture of phthalates accelerates biomarkers of reproductive aging in multiple generations of female mice. Pregnant CD-1 mice were orally dosed with vehicle control or a phthalate mixture (20 μg/kg/day-500 mg/kg/day) daily from gestational day 10 to birth. Adult F1 females born to these dams were used to create the F2 and F3 generations by mating them with unexposed males. At 13 months, estrous cyclicity was monitored and ovaries and sera were collected for analysis. In the F1 generation, the mixture decreased testosterone and inhibin B levels, but increased follicle-stimulating hormone and luteinizing hormone levels compared to control. In the F2 generation, the phthalate mixture decreased the percent of antral follicles and testosterone hormone levels compared to control. In the F3 generation, prenatal exposure to the phthalate mixture increased ovarian weight, increased the time in metaestrus/diestrus, altered follicle numbers, and decreased the levels of luteinizing hormone compared to control.

Li et al. (2020) tested prenatal exposure to an environmentally relevant phthalate mixture would lead to changes in uterine morphology and function in mice in a multi-generational manner. To test this hypothesis, pregnant CD-1 dams were orally dosed with vehicle or a phthalate mixture (20 μg/kg/day, 200 μg/kg/day, 200 mg/kg/day, and 500 mg/kg/day) from gestational day 10.5 to parturition. The mixture contained 35% diethyl phthalate, 21% di-(2-ethylhexyl) phthalate, 15% dibutyl phthalate, 15% diisononyl phthalate, 8% diisobutyl phthalate, and 5% benzylbutyl phthalate. The F1 pups were maintained and mated to produce two more generations (F2 and F3). At the age of 13 months, all females were euthanized, and tissue samples were collected in diestrus. The results showed that exposure to a phthalate mixture caused a decrease in progesterone levels in the treated groups in the F2 generation. The 200 mg/kg bw/day treatment group showed a decreased and increased luminal epithelial cell proliferation in the F1 and F2 generations respectively. In addition, these mice in the F2 generation had reduced *Hand2* expression in the sub-epithelial stroma compared to the controls (Li et al. 2020). A higher incidence of multilayered luminal epithelium and large dilated endometrial glands were observed in the phthalate mixture exposed groups in all generations. The mixture also caused a higher incidence of smooth muscle actin expression and collagen deposition in the endometrium compared to controls.

Zhou et al. (2017b) hypothesized that prenatal exposure to the phthalate mixture induces multigenerational and transgenerational effects on female reproduction. Pregnant CD-1 dams were orally dosed with vehicle (tocopherol-stripped corn oil) or a phthalate mixture (20 and 200 μg/kg/day, 200 and 500 mg/kg/day) daily from gestational day 10 to birth. F2 and F3 females were subjected to tissue collections and fertility tests. Zhou et al. (2017b) reported that prenatal phthalate mixture exposure increased uterine weight, anogenital distance, and body weight; induced cystic ovaries; and caused fertility complications in the F2 generation. It also increased uterine weight, decreased anogenital distance, and caused fertility complications in the F3 generation. These data suggest that prenatal exposure to the phthalate mixture induces multigenerational and transgenerational effects on female reproduction.

Various reproductive difficulties, such as altered AGD, gene expression, hormone levels, and ovarian histopathology, were detected in female mouse progeny, consistent with accelerated reproductive senescence. Some of the adversities were also observed in the F2 and F3 generations, implying epigenetic impacts (Zhou et al. 2017a). In another study, pregnant C57/Bl6 mice were exposed *via* oral gavage to corn oil, 100, 500, or 1000 mg/kg MEHP from gestational days 17–19. Reproductive lifespan was decreased by one month in the highest F1 exposure group (9.8 ± 0.4 *versus* 11.1 ± 0.6 months in control F1 females). F1 females exhibited delayed estrous onset at the two higher exposures and prolonged estrus was observed in all MEHP-exposed females (Moyer and Hixon 2012).

A mixture of four phthalate monoesters: mono-butyl phthalate (MBP), mono-benzyl phthalate (MBzP), mono-ethylhexyl phthalate (MEHP), and mono-isononyl phthalate (MIHP), in accordance with the usage of human-relevant exposures to mixes of EDCs were exposed to mice. These monoesters were chosen from a large number of compounds analyzed in the serum and urine of a human pregnancy cohort, the Swedish Environmental Longitudinal, Mother and Child, Asthma and Allergy (SELMA) (Bornehag et al. 2012), during the first and second trimesters of pregnancy, based on their association with decreased anogenital distance (AGD) in the baby boys (Bornehag et al. 2015). On PND21 and in maturity in male and female offspring exposed to this mixture, typical reproductive endpoints described from single phthalate investigations were also characterized (Repouskou et al. 2019).

AGD decrease, gonadal histopathology, disrupted steroidogenesis-related gene expression, reduced gametogenesis, and T/E2 serum levels were among the mixed effects. At doses of 0.26, 2.6, or 13.1 mg/kg, the aberrations were generally identified. In mice gestationally exposed just to DEHP, a multitude of affected endpoints has been seen (Ungewitter et al. 2017, Barakat et al. 2017, Pocar et al. 2017), whereas other single phthalates elicit effects at greater exposure ranges (e.g., DBP at roughly 100 mg/kg) (Motohashi et al. 2016, Ma et al. 2017). As a result, when phthalates are mixed, their effective doses are reduced.

As for mice, which were exposed to mixtures of different phthalates (DEHP, benzyl butyl phthalate (BBzP), DBP, and two alkyl phenols), antral follicle development was inhibited, and the number of antral follicles were reduced (Patino-García et al. 2020). Other studies on mice have prevailed similar results, involving reduced number of follicles after DEHP exposure (Hannon et al. 2015). Female mice exposed to DEHP had changed peroxisome proliferator-activated receptor-gamma (PPAR) and prostaglandin levels, indicating that DEHP can damage primordial germ cells, germ cell survival, and meiotic development, as well as an increase in follicular atresia pregnancy (Mirihagalle et al. 2019).

Since phthalates relate to dysregulation of the HPG axis, interaction with steroidogenic enzymes and hormones are seen (Hannon and Flaws 2015, Hlisníková et al. 2020). Exposure to DEHP in rats revealed decrease in testosterone, FSH and LH levels (Ha et al. 2016). Furthermore, studies have shown that prenatal DEHP exposure reduced E2 levels in rats (Martinez-Arguelles et al. 2011, Meltzer et al. 2015). Prenatal DHEP exposure, on the other hand, resulted in higher levels of E2 in female mice (Brehm et al. 2018). The effect of toxicity on intersexual differences may differ depending on the animal, sex, exposure length, isoforms of biotransformation enzymes, and enzyme activity, according to several studies on mice and rats (Johnson et al. 2012). These findings suggested that hormonal and steroidogenic enzymes may affect the HPG axis following phthalate exposure.

To explore the intergenerational testicular injury and the influence on offspring gut microbiota of the widely used phthalate di-butylphthalate (DBP), Zhang et al. (2022) conducted a prenatal DBP exposure experiment with microbiota sequencing. They finally explained the gestational DBP exposure-induced gut dysbacteriosis, which is one of the mechanisms of testicular injury in the offspring.

Phthalates can disrupt and modify gene expression, apoptosis, cell proliferation, and gonadal cells by interfering with epigenetic, genomic, and non-epigenetic mechanisms of action (Acevedo-Rodriguez et al. 2018). As a result of postnatal DEHP exposures, female rats demonstrate an increase in postnatal BBzP exposure of the GnRH receptor (GNRHR) (Liu et al. 2019) and the LH receptor (LHR) (Somasundaram et al. 2016), as well as upregulation of the FSH receptor (FSHR) in male rats. DEHP can cause prostate cancer in addition to disrupting testosterone synthesis and sperm production (Lv et al. 2019).

DEHP was observed to increase prostate carcinogenesis susceptibility, which could be due to a significant reduction in DNA methylation of the prostate stem cell antigen *(Psca)* gene in all CpG sites of the prostate tissue (Xia et al. 2018). Zhou et al. (2017) dosed pregnant CD-1 mice (F0) with a combination of phthalates containing 35 percent DEP, 21 percent DEHP, 15 percent DBP, 15 percent DiNP, 8 percent DIBP, and 5 percent BzBP from gestational day 10 till birth. In the F3 generation of CD-1 mice, this mixture reduced anogenital distance at PND 21 (200 mg/kg bw/day), increased uterine weight at PND 60 (200 mg/kg bw/day), and decreased ovarian weight at PND 60 (200 mg/kg bw/day). The mixture also reduced the percentage of females who delivered live pups (500 mg/kg bw/day) and some fertility indices in the F3 generation during breeding trials. The success of females in becoming pregnant, maintaining a pregnancy, and/or delivering pups were among the fertility indices. Furthermore, the mixture (200 mg/kg bw/day) slowed the time to pregnancy in the F3 generation but had no effect on puberty. Finally, in the F4 generation, the mixture (500 mg/kg bw/day) reduced pup numbers. The findings of this study imply that transgenerational exposure to phthalate mixtures can have a deleterious impact on female fertility (Zhou et al. 2017).

Ovarian carcinoma is one of the most common gynecologic tumors and the primary cause of death from gynecologic malignancies (Kang et al. 2012). Most ovarian cells, including germ cells, granulosa, and stromal cells, can become cancerous, although the majority of tumors come from the ovarian surface epithelium. Although the pathogenesis of ovarian cancer is yet unknown, research suggests that estrogen hormone play a role in its progression. ERa levels are higher in human ovarian cancer cells than in benign tumors and normal ovaries. Normal and altered ovarian cells both express ERa and ERb, with ERb being abundant in granulosa cells and ERa being abundant in theca and interstitial cells. Estrogens may then influence ovarian cell proliferation and death and generate a hormonal milieu that aids tumor growth (Gao et al. 2015). EDC exposure might, obviously, mirror the effects of estrogen in ovarian cells. In murine ovarian cells, di-n-butyl phthalate (DnBP; 0.1 mM) elevated *Cdk4, Ccne1, Ccnd2, ESR1, Bcl2* genes (Peretz et al. 2012), and downregulated (at 40 nM) p21 and *CASP3* genes (Ptak et al. 2013).

Conclusion

Phthalates are found in all parts of nature and are daily exposed by food, inhalation, medication, clothes, and personal care products. Furthermore, they have the ability to infiltrate practically every area of the body. Phthalates and their metabolites are endocrine disrupting chemicals that act as agonist or antagonist ligands and disturb the chemical signaling of endocrine hormones. Defective endocrine signaling disrupts normal physiological processes in both genders, including babies. Such abnormalities include sex anomalies, type 2 diabetes, overweight, and obesity. Given the magnitude of phthalate toxicity, better alternatives should be implemented as soon as possible to protect future generations from such fatal toxicants.

Chronic phthalate-like exposure problems such as impaired fertility, neural development disorder, cardiovascular disease, and reproductive system disorders have raised growing interest and concern. In humans it is essential to understand phthalate mechanisms because it clarifies their effects, gives a mean to prevent hormone agonism and adversity, hormonal synthesis and/or clearance, and modification in the expression of hormonal receptors. Estrogen, androgen and thyroid hormones and their receptors are prominent targets, while non-steroidal hormone abnormalities are also documented. These are shared goals. This shows how some phthalates impact the receptors of steroid hormones, whereas others are not steroid hormones. According to study, the impacts on the phthalate body have also been associated with epigenetic and immunological systems (Kay et al. 2013).

The reproductive systems of humans and rodents exposed to phthalates are not the same. In addition, differences in dosage, occupational or environmental exposure, sample size, protocol type and critical stages of development have been revealed in various clinical and cross-sectional studies. Phthalates work synergistically with other toxicants in a toxicant mixture. As a result, determining the source and impact of a phthalate can be difficult. The study of phthalates is critical because the effects of exposure may differ depending on the toxicant. These effects can occur all at once or gradually over time, and they can be passed down to future generations. As a result of numerous experimental studies, we have made remarkable progress in identifying and understanding the biological function of phthalates (Hlisníková et al. 2020).

Phthalates have been studied for their ability to influence apoptosis, cell cycle, and epigenetic regulation in addition to their traditional function (agonism and antagonism with hormone and nuclear receptors). Epidemiological and clinical studies have failed to provide compelling evidence of the impact of endocrine receptors on human health. Each study has its own set of flaws and methods, as well as different types of exposure, exposure time frames, age groups, and other variables that make direct comparison and contrast difficult. Poor sperm quality, testicular dysgenesis, testicular cancer, infertility, endometriosis, and miscarriage in general have all been linked to phthalate exposure.

References

Acevedo-Rodriguez, A., Kauffman, A. S, Cherrington, B. D, Borges, C. S., Roepke, T. A. and Laconi, M. 2018. "Emerging insights into hypothalamic-pituitary-gonadal axis regulation and interaction with stress signaling." *Journal of Neuroendocrinology* 30:e12590.

Ahbab, Aydoğan, M and Barlas, N. 2015. "Influence of in utero di-n-hexyl phthalate and dicyclohexyl phthalate on fetal testicular development in rats." *Toxicology Letters* 233(2): 125-137.

Akingbemi, B. T., Ge, R., Klinefelter, G. R., Zirkin, B. R. and Hardy, M. P. 2004. "Phthalate-induced Leydig cell hyperplasia is associated with multiple endocrine disturbances." *Proceedings of the National Academy of Sciences* 101(3): 775-780.

Aly, H. A., Hassan, M. H., El-Beshbishy, H. A., Alahdal, A. M. and Osman, A. M. M. 2016. "Dibutyl phthalate induces oxidative stress and impairs spermatogenesis in adult rats." *Toxicology and Industrial Health* 32(8): 1467-1477.

Araki, A., Mitsui, T., Goudarzi, H., Nakajima, T., Miyashita, C. and Itoh, S. 2017. "Prenatal di-(2-ethylhexyl) phthalate exposure and disruption of adrenal androgens and glucocorticoids levels in cord blood: The Hokkaido Study." *Science of the Total Environment* 581-582:297–304.

Araki, A., Mitsui, T., Miyashita, C., Nakajima, T., Naito, H. and Ito, S. 2014. "Association between maternal exposure to di(2-ethylhexyl) phthalate and reproductive hormone levels in fetal blood: The Hokkaido Study on Environment and Children's Health." *PLoS One* 9(10):e109039.

Axelsson, J., Rylander, L., Rignell-Hydbom, A, Jönsson, B. A., Lindh, C. H. and Giwercman, A. 2015. "Phthalate exposure and reproductive parameters in young men from the general Swedish population." *Environment International* 85: 54-60.

Axelsson, J., Rylander, L., Rignell-Hydbom, A., Lindh, C. H., Jonsson, B. A. and Giwercman, A. 2015. "Prenatal phthalate exposure and reproductive function in young men." *Environmental Research* 138:264–70.

Aydemir, D., Karabulut, G., Gok, M., Barlas, N. and Ulusu, N. N. 2019. "Data the DEHP induced changes on the trace element and mineral levels in the brain and testis tissues of rats." *Data in Brief* 26: 104526.

Bahadar, H., Maqbool, F. and Abdollahi, M. 2014. "Consumption of phthalates coated pharmaceutical tablets: An unnoticed threat." *International Journal of Pharmacology* 10(2): 78-81.

Barakat, R., Lin, P. C. P., Rattan, S., Brehm, E., Canisso, I. F., Abosalum, M. E. and Ko, C. 2017. "Prenatal exposure to DEHP induces premature reproductive senescence in male mice." *Toxicological Sciences* 156(1): 96-108.

Benjamin, S., Masai, E., Kamimura, N., Takahashi, K., Anderson, R. C. and Faisal, P. A. 2017. "Phthalates impact human health: epidemiological evidences and plausible mechanism of action." *Journal of Hazardous Materials* 340: 360-383.

Bergman, Å., Heindel, J. J., Jobling, S., Kidd, K. Zoeller, T. R. 2013. "State of the science of endocrine disrupting chemicals." *World Health Organization.*

Bloom, M. S., Whitcomb, B. W., Chen, Z., Ye, A., Kannan, K. and Buck Louis, G. M. 2015. "Associations between urinary phthalate concentrations and semen quality parameters in a general population." *Human Reproduction* 30(11): 2645-2657.

Bogen, K. T., Boekelheide, K., Cunningham, M. L., Jackson, B. A., Peters, J. M., Reddy, J. K. Zeise, L. 2001. "Report to the US consumer product safety commis-sion by the chronic hazard advisory panel on di-isononyl phthalate." *Bethesda.*

Bornehag, C. G., Carlstedt, F., Jönsson, B. A., Lindh, C. H., Jensen, T. K., Bodin, A. and Swan, S. H. 2015. "Prenatal phthalate exposures and anogenital distance in Swedish boys." *Environmental Health Perspectives* 123(1): 101-107.

Bornehag, C. G., Moniruzzaman, S., Larsson, M., Lindström, C. B., Hasselgren, M., Bodin, A. and Janson, S. 2012. "The SELMA study: a birth cohort study in Sweden following more than 2000 mother–child pairs." *Pediatric and Perinatal Epidemiology* 26(5): 456-467.

Braun, J. M., Sathyanarayana, S., Hauser, R. 2013. "Phthalate exposure and children's health." *Current Opinion in Pediatrics 25*(2): 247.

Brehm, E., Rattan, S., Gao, L. and Flaws, J. A. 2018. "Prenatal exposure to di (2-ethylhexyl) phthalate causes long-term transgenerational effects on female reproduction in mice." *Endocrinology* 159(2): 795-809.

Brehm, E., Zhou, C., Gao, L. and Flaws, J. A. 2020. "Prenatal exposure to an environmentally relevant phthalate mixture accelerates biomarkers of reproductive aging in a multiple and transgenerational manner in female mice." *Reproductive Toxicology* 98: 260-268.

Cai, H., Zheng, W., Zheng, P., Wang, S., Tan, H., He, G. and Qu, W. 2015. "Human urinary/seminal phthalates or their metabolite levels and semen quality: a meta-analysis." *Environmental Research* 142: 486-494.

Carran, M. and Shaw, I. C. 2012. "New Zealand Malayan war veterans' exposure to dibutylphthalate is associated with an increased incidence of cryptorchidism, hypospadias and breast cancer in their children." *The New Zealand Medical Journal* 125(1358): 52-63.

Chang, W. H., Li, S. S., Wu, M. H., Pan, H. A. and Lee, C. C. 2015. "Phthalates might interfere with testicular function by reducing testosterone and insulin-like factor 3 levels." *Human Reproduction* 30(11): 2658-2670.

Chauvigné, F., Menuet, A., Lesné, L., Chagnon, M. C., Chevrier, C., Regnier, J. F., and Jégou, B. 2009. "Time-and dose-related effects of di-(2-ethylhexyl) phthalate and its main metabolites on the function of the rat fetal testis in vitro." *Environmental Health* Services 17(4): 515–521.

Chiang, C., and Flaws, J. A. 2019. "Subchronic exposure to di (2-ethylhexyl) phthalate and diisononyl phthalate during adulthood has immediate and long-term reproductive consequences in female mice." *Toxicological Sciences* 168(2): 620-631.

Chiang, C., Lewis, L. R., Borkowski, G., and Flaws, J. A. 2020. "Exposure to di (2-ethylhexyl) phthalate and diisononyl phthalate during adulthood disrupts hormones and ovarian folliculogenesis throughout the prime reproductive life of the mouse." *Toxicology and Applied Pharmacology* 393: 114952.

Cobellis, L., Latini, G., Felice, C. D., Razzi, S., Paris, I., Ruggieri, F. and Petraglia, F. 2003. "High plasma concentrations of di-(2-ethylhexyl)-phthalate in women with endometriosis." *Human Reproduction* 18(7): 1512-1515.

Crain, D. A., Janssen, S. J., Edwards, T. M., Heindel, J., Ho, S. M., Hunt, P. and Guillette Jr, L. J. 2008. "Female reproductive disorders: the roles of endocrine-disrupting compounds and developmental timing." *Fertility and Sterility* 90(4): 911-940.

Dadvand, P., de Nazelle, A., Triguero-Mas, M., Schembari, A., Cirach, M., Amoly, E. and Nieuwenhuijsen, M. 2012. "Surrounding greenness and exposure to air pollution during pregnancy: an analysis of personal monitoring data." *Environ-mental Health Perspectives* 120(9): 1286-1290.

Diamanti-Kandarakis, E., Bourguignon, J. P., Giudice, L. C., Hauser, R., Prins, G. S., Soto, A. M. and Gore, A. C. 2009. "Endocrine-disrupting chemicals: an Endocrine Society scientific statement." *Endocrine Reviews* 30(4): 293-342.

Donaire-Gonzalez D, Curto A, Valentín A, Andrusaityte S, Basagaña X, Casas M, Chatzi L, de Bont J, de Castro M, Dedele A, Granum B, Grazuleviciene R, Kampouri M, Lyon-Caen S, Manzano-Salgado CB, Aasvang GM, McEachan R, Meinhard-Kjellstad CH, Michalaki E, Pañella P, Petraviciene I, Schwarze PE, Slama R, Robinson O, Tamayo-Uria I, Vafeiadi M, Waiblinger D, Wright J, Vrijheid M. and Nieuwenhuijsen MJ. 2019. "Personal assessment of the external exposome during pregnancy and childhood in Europe." *Environmental Research* 74:95–104.

ECHA 2018. EC (European Commission). Commission Regulation (EU) 2018/2005 of 17 December 2018 Amending Annex XVII to REGULATION (EC) No 1907/2006 of the European Parliament and of the Council Concerning the Registration, Evaluation, Authorisation and Restriction of Chemicals (REACH) as regards Bis(2-ethylhexyl) Phthalate (DEHP), Dibutyl Phthalate (DBP), Benzyl Butyl Phthalate (BBP) and Diisobutyl Phthalate (DIBP). *Official Journal of the European Union.*

Fernandez, M. A. M., Cardeal, Z. L., Carneiro, M. M. and André, L. C. 2019. "Study of possible association between endometriosis and phthalate and bisphenol A by biomarkers analysis." *Journal of Pharmaceutical and Biomedical Analysis* 172: 238-242.

Frederiksen, H., Sørensen, K., Mouritsen, A., Aksglaede, L., Hagen, C. P., Petersen, J. H. and Juul, A. 2012. "High urinary phthalate concentration associated with delayed pubarche in girls." *International Journal of Andrology,* 35(3): 216-226.

Gao, H., Yang, B. J., Li, N., Feng, L. M., Shi, X. Y., Zhao, W. H. and Liu, S. J. 2015. "Bisphenol A and hormone-associated cancers: current progress and perspectives." *Medicine* 94(1): e211.

Gao, H., Zhu, Y. D., Xu, Y. Y., Zhang, Y. W., Yao, H. Y., Sheng, J. and Tao, F. B. 2017a. "Season-dependent concentrations of urinary phthalate metabolites among Chinese pregnant women: Repeated measures analysis." *Environment Internat-ional* 104: 110-117.

Gao, H., Zhang, Y. W., Huang, K., Yan, S. Q., Mao, L. J., Ge, X. and Tao, F. B. 2017b. "Urinary concentrations of phthalate metabolites in early pregnancy associated with clinical pregnancy loss in Chinese women." *Scientific Reports* 7(1): 1-7.

Ge, R. S., Chen, G. R., Dong, Q., Akingbemi, B., Sottas, C. M., Santos, M. and Hardy, M. P. 2007. "Biphasic effects of postnatal exposure to diethylhexylphthalate on the timing of puberty in male rats." *Journal of Andrology* 28(4): 513-520.

Geyer, R., Jambeck, J. R. and Law, K. L. 2017. "Production, use, and fate of all plastics ever made." *Science Advances* 3(7), e1700782.

Giammona, C. J., Sawhney, P., Chandrasekaran, Y. and Richburg, J. H. 2002. "Death receptor response in rodent testis after mono-(2-ethylhexyl) phthalate exposure." *Toxicology and Applied Pharmacology* 185(2): 119-127.

Gore, A. C., Chappell, V. A., Fenton, S. E., Flaws, J. A., Nadal, A., Prins, G. S. Zoeller, R. T. 2015. "EDC-2: the Endocrine Society's second scientific statement on endocrine-disrupting chemicals." *Endocrine Reviews* 36(6): E1-E150.

Grindler, N. M., Vanderlinden, L., Karthikraj, R., Kannan, K., Teal, S., Polotsky, A. J. and Jansson, T. 2018. "Exposure to phthalate, an endocrine disrupting chemical, alters the first trimester placental methylome and transcriptome in women." *Scientific Reports.* 8(1): 1-9.

Ha, M., Guan, X., Wei, L., Li, P., Yang, M. and Liu, C. 2016. "Di-(2-ethylhexyl) phthalate inhibits testosterone level through disturbed hypothalamic–pituitary–testis axis and ERK-mediated 5α-Reductase 2." *Science of the Total Environment* 563: 566-575.

Hannas, B. R., Lambright, C. S., Furr, J., Howdeshell, K. L., Wilson, V. S. and Gray Jr, L. E. 2011. "Dose-response assessment of fetal testosterone production and gene expression levels in rat testes following in utero exposure to diethylhexyl phthalate, diisobutyl phthalate, diisoheptyl phthalate, and diisononyl phthalate." *Toxicological Sciences* 123(1): 206-216.

Hannas, B. R., Howdeshell, K. L., Furr, J. and Gray Jr, L. E. 2013. "In utero phthalate effects in the female rat: a model for MRKH syndrome." *Toxicology Letters* 223(3): 315-321.

Hannon, P. R., Peretz, J. and Flaws, J. A. 2014. "Daily exposure to Di (2-ethyl-hexyl) phthalate alters estrous cyclicity and accelerates primordial follicle recruitment potentially via dysregulation of the phosphatidylinositol 3-kinase signaling pathway in adult mice." *Biology of Reproduction* 90(6): 136-1.

Hannon, P. R. and Flaws, J. A. 2015. "The effects of phthalates on the ovary." *Frontiers in Endocrinology* 6: 8.

Hannon, P. R., Brannick, K. E., Wang, W., Gupta, R. K. and Flaws, J. A. 2015. "Di (2-ethylhexyl) phthalate inhibits antral follicle growth, induces atresia, and inhibits steroid hormone production in cultured mouse antral follicles." *Toxicology and Applied Pharmacology* 284(1): 42-53.

Hart, R. J., Frederiksen, H., Doherty, D. A., Keelan, J. A., Skakkebaek, N. E., Minaee, N. S. and Main, K. M. 2018. "The possible impact of antenatal exposure to ubiquitous phthalates upon male reproductive function at 20 years of age." *Frontiers in Endocrinology* 9: 288.

Hauser, R., Duty, S., Godfrey-Bailey, L. and Calafat, A. M. 2004. "Medications as a source of human exposure to phthalates." *Environmental Health Perspectives* 112(6): 751-753.

Hauser, R., Meeker, J. D., Singh, N. P., Silva, M. J., Ryan, L., Duty, S. and Calafat, A. M. 2007. "DNA damage in human sperm is related to urinary levels of phthalate monoester and oxidative metabolites." *Human Reproduction* 22(3): 688-695.

Helmy, H. S., Senousy, M. A., El-Sahar, A. E., Sayed, R. H., Saad, M. A. and Elbaz, E. M. 2020. "Aberrations of miR-126-3p, miR-181a and sirtuin1 network mediate Di-(2-ethylhexyl) phthalate-induced testicular damage in rats: The protective role of hesperidin." *Toxicology* 433: 152406.

Hlisníková, H., Petrovičová, I., Kolena, B., Šidlovská, M., Sirotkin, A., 2020. "Effects and Mechanisms of Phthalates' Action on Reproductive Processes and Reproductive Health: A Literature Review." *Int J Environ Res Public Health.* 17(18): 6811.Howdeshell, K. L., Wilson, V. S., Furr, J., Lambright, C. R., Rider, C. V., Blystone, C. R. and Gray Jr, L. E. 2008. "A mixture of five phthalate esters inhibits fetal testicular testosterone production in the Sprague-dawley rat in a cumulative, dose-additive manner." *Toxicological Sciences* 105(1): 153-165.

Howdeshell, K. L., Hotchkiss, A. K. Gray Jr, L. E. 2017. "Cumulative effects of antiandrogenic chemical mixtures and their relevance to human health risk assessment." *International Journal of Hygiene and Environmental Health* 220(2): 179-188.

Hu, G., Li, J., Shan, Y., Li, X., Zhu, Q., Li, H. and Ge, R. S. 2018. "In utero combined di-(2-ethylhexyl) phthalate and diethyl phthalate exposure cumulatively impairs rat fetal Leydig cell development." *Toxicology* 395, 23-33.

Huang, P. C., Tsai, E. M., Li, W. F., Liao, P. C., Chung, M. C., Wang, Y. H. and Wang, S. L. 2010. "Association between phthalate exposure and glutathione S-transferase M1 polymorphism in adenomyosis, leiomyoma and endometriosis." *Human Reproduction* 25(4): 986-994.

Hubinger, J. C. 2010. "A survey of phthalate esters in consumer cosmetic products." *Journal of Cosmetic Science*, 61(6): 457-465.

Itoh, H., Iwasaki, M., Hanaoka, T., Sasaki, H., Tanaka, T. and Tsugane, S. 2009. "Urinary phthalate monoesters and endometriosis in infertile Japanese women." *Science of the Total Environment* 408(1): 37-42.

Jensen, M. S., Anand-Ivell, R., Nørgaard-Pedersen, B., Jönsson, B. A., Bonde, J. P., Hougaard, D. M. and Toft, G. 2015. "Amniotic fluid phthalate levels and male fetal gonad function." *Epidemiology* 26(1): 91-99.

Johnson, K. J., Heger, N. E. and Boekelheide, K. 2012. "Of mice and men (and rats): phthalate-induced fetal testis endocrine disruption is species-dependent." *Toxicological Sciences* 129(2): 235-248.

Jukic, A. M., Calafat, A. M., McConnaughey, D. R., Longnecker, M. P., Hoppin, J. A., Weinberg, C. R. and Baird, D. D. 2016. "Urinary concentrations of phthalate metabolites and bisphenol A and associations with follicular-phase length, luteal-phase length, fecundability, and early pregnancy loss." *Environmental Health Perspectives* 124(3): 321-328.

Jurewicz, J., Radwan, M., Sobala, W., Ligocka, D., Radwan, P., Bochenek, M. and Hanke, W. 2013. "Human urinary phthalate metabolites level and main semen parameters, sperm chromatin structure, sperm aneuploidy and reproductive hormones." *Reproductive Toxicology* 42: 232-241.

Kabir, E. R., Rahman, M. S. and Rahman, I. 2015. "A review on endocrine disruptors and their possible impacts on human health." *Environmental Toxicology and Pharmacology* 40(1): 241-258.

Kamrin, M. A. 2009. "Phthalate risks, phthalate regulation, and public health: a review." *Journal of Toxicology and Environmental Health, Part B* 12(2): 157-174.

Kang, N. H., Hwang, K. A., Kim, T. H., Hyun, S. H., Jeung, E. B. and Choi, K. C. 2012. "Induced growth of BG-1 ovarian cancer cells by 17β-estradiol or various endocrine disrupting chemicals was reversed by resveratrol via downregulation of cell cycle progression." *Molecular Medicine Reports* 6(1): 151-156.

Karabulut, G. and Barlas, N. 2018. "Genotoxic, histologic, immunohistochemical, morphometric and hormonal effects of di-(2-ethylhexyl)-phthalate (DEHP) on reproductive systems in pre-pubertal male rats." *Toxicology Research* 7(5): 859-873.

Kay, V. R., Chambers, C. and Foster, W. G. 2013. "Reproductive and develop-mental effects of phthalate diesters in females." *Critical Reviews in Toxicology* 43(3): 200-219.

Kiess, W., Hoppmann, J., Gesing, J., Penke, M., Körner, A., Kratzsch, J. and Pfaeffle, R. 2016. "Puberty–genes, environment and clinical issues." *Journal of Pediatric Endocrinology and Metabolism* 29(11): 1229-1231.

Kim, Y. H., Kim, S. H., Lee, H. W., Chae, H. D., Kim, C. H. and Kang, B. M. 2010. "Increased viability of endometrial cells by in vitro treatment with di-(2-ethylhexyl) phthalate." *Fertility and sterility* 94(6): 2413-2416.

Kita, D. H., Meyer, K. B., Venturelli, A. C., Adams, R., Machado, D. L., Morais, R. N. and Martino-Andrade, A. J. 2016. "Manipulation of pre and postnatal andro-gen environments and anogenital distance in rats." *Toxicology* 368: 152-161.

Kortenkamp, A. and Faust, M. 2018. "Regulate to reduce chemical mixture risk." *Science* 361(6399): 224-226.

Kortenkamp, A. 2020. "Which chemicals should be grouped together for mixture risk assessments of male reproductive disorders?" *Molecular and Cellular Endocrinology* 499: 110581.

Li, K., Liszka, M., Zhou, C., Brehm, E., Flaws, J. A. and Nowak, R. A. 2020. "Prenatal exposure to a phthalate mixture leads to multigenerational and trans-generational effects on uterine morphology and function in mice." *Reproductive Toxicology* 93: 178-190.

Li, L., Bu, T., Su, H., Chen, Z., Liang, Y., Zhang, G. and Ge, R. S. 2015. "In utero exposure to diisononyl phthalate caused testicular dysgenesis of rat fetal testis." *Toxicology Letters* 232(2): 466-474.

Li, R., Yu, C., Gao, R., Liu, X., Lu, J., Zhao, L. and He, J. 2012. "Effects of DEHP on endometrial receptivity and embryo implantation in pregnant mice." *Journal of Hazardous Materials* 241: 231-240.

Li, R., Xing, Q. W., Wu, X. L., Zhang, L., Tang, M., Tang, J. Y. and Qin, Z. Q. 2019. "Di-n-butyl phthalate epigenetically induces reproductive toxicity via the PTEN/AKT pathway." *Cell Death & Disease* 10(4): 1-16.

Liao, K. W., Kuo, P. L., Huang, H. B., Chang, J. W., Chiang, H. C. and Huang, P. C. 2018. "Increased risk of phthalates exposure for recurrent pregnancy loss in reproductive-aged women." *Environmental Pollution* 241: 969-977.

Lin, L. C., Wang, S. L., Chang, Y. C., Huang, P. C., Cheng, J. T., Su, P. H. and Liao, P. C. 2011. "Associations between maternal phthalate exposure and cord sex hormones in human infants." *Chemosphere* 83(8): 1192-1199.

Lind, P. M., Risérus, U., Salihovic, S., van Bavel, B. and Lind, L. 2013. "An environmental wide association study (EWAS) approach to the metabolic syndrome." *Environment International* 55: 1-8.

Liu, F. F., Liu, G. Z., Zhu, Z. L., Wang, S. C. and Zhao, F. F. 2019. "Interactions between microplastics and phthalate esters as affected by microplastics charac-teristics and solution chemistry." *Chemosphere* 214: 688-694.

Liu, M., Chen, H., Dai, H., Zhou, L., Wang, Y., Xin, X. Ge, R. S. 2021. "Effects of bis (2-butoxyethyl) phthalate exposure in utero on the development of fetal Leydig cells in rats." *Toxicology Letters* 351: 65–77.

Louis, G. M. B., Sundaram, R., Schisterman, E. F., Sweeney, A. M., Lynch, C. D., Gore-Langton, R. E. and Barr, D. B. 2013. "Persistent environmental pollutants and couple fecundity: the LIFE study." *Environmental Health Perspectives* 121(2): 231-236.

Lv, Y., Fang, Y., Chen, P., Duan, Y., Huang, T., Ma, L. and Ge, R. S. 2019. "Dicy-clohexyl phthalate blocks Leydig cell regeneration in adult rat testis." *Toxicology* 411: 60-70.

Ma, T., Yin, X., Han, R., Ding, J., Zhang, H., Han, X. and Li, D. 2017. "Effects of in utero exposure to di-n-butyl phthalate on testicular development in rat." *International Journal of Environmental Research and Public Health* 14(10): 1284.

Magdouli, S., Daghrir, R., Brar, S. K., Drogui, P. and Tyagi, R. D. 2013. "Di 2-ethylhexylphtalate in the aquatic and terrestrial environment: a critical review." *Journal of Environmental Management,* 127: 36-49.

Main, K. M., Mortensen, G. K., Kaleva, M. M., Boisen, K. A., Damgaard, I. N., Chellakooty, M. and Skakkebæk, N. E. 2006. "Human breast milk contamination with phthalates and alterations of endogenous reproductive hormones in infants three months of age." *Environmental Health Perspectives* 114(2): 270-276.

Mankidy, R., Wiseman, S., Ma, H. and Giesy, J. P. 2013. "Biological impact of phthalates." *Toxicology Letters* 217(1): 50-58.

Markit, I. H. S. 2021. "Plasticizers: chemical economics handbook." https://ihsmarkit.com/products/plasticizers-chemical-economics-handbook.html.

Martinez-Arguelles, D. B., Guichard, T., Culty, M., Zirkin, B. R. and Papadopoulos, V. 2011. "In utero exposure to the antiandrogen di-(2-ethylhexyl) phthalate decreases adrenal aldosterone production in the adult rat." *Biology of Reproduction* 85(1): 51-61.

Martino-Andrade, A. J., Morais, R. N., Botelho, G. G., Muller, G., Grande, S. W., Carpentieri, G. B. and Dalsenter, P. R. 2009. "Coadministration of active phthalates results in disruption of foetal testicular function in rats." *International Journal of Andrology* 32(6): 704-712.

Masuyama, H., Hiramatsu, Y., Kodama, J. I. and Kudo, T. 2003. "Expression and potential roles of pregnane X receptor in endometrial cancer." *The Journal of Clinical Endocrinology & Metabolism* 88(9): 4446-4454.

Meeker, J. D., Calafat, A. M. and Hauser, R. 2009a. "Urinary metabolites of di (2-ethylhexyl) phthalate are associated with decreased steroid hormone levels in adult men." *Journal of Andrology* 30(3): 287-297.

Meeker, J. D., Sathyanarayana, S. and Swan, S. H. 2009b. "Phthalates and other additives in plastics: human exposure and associated health outcomes." *Philosoph-ical Transactions of the Royal Society B: Biological Sciences* 364(1526): 2097-2113.

Meltzer, D., Martinez–Arguelles, D. B., Campioli, E., Lee, S. and Papadopoulos, V. 2015. "In utero exposure to the endocrine disruptor di (2-ethylhexyl) phthalate targets ovarian theca cells and steroidogenesis in the adult female rat." *Repro-ductive toxicology* 51: 47-56.

Menezo, Y. J., Silvestris, E., Dale, B. and Elder, K. 2016. "Oxidative stress and alterations in DNA methylation: two sides of the same coin in reproduction." *Reproductive Biomedicine Online* 33(6): 668-683.

Mieritz, M. G., Frederiksen, H., Sørensen, K., Aksglaede, L., Mouritsen, A., Hagen, C. P. and Juul, A. 2012. "Urinary phthalate excretion in 555 healthy Danish boys with and without pubertal gynaecomastia." *International Journal of Andro-logy* 35(3): 227-235.

Miller, W. L. and Auchus, R. J. 2011. "The molecular biology, biochemistry, and physiology of human steroidogenesis and its disorders." *Endocrine Reviews* 32(1): 81-151.

Mirihagalle, S., You, T., Suh, L., Patel, C., Gao, L., Rattan, S. and Qiao, H. 2019. "Prenatal exposure to di-(2-ethylhexyl) phthalate and high-fat diet synergistically disrupts mouse fetal oogenesis and affects folliculogenesis." *Biology of Repro-duction* 100(6): 1561-1570.

Motohashi, M., Wempe, M. F., Mutou, T., Okayama, Y., Kansaku, N., Takahashi, H. and Wakui, S. 2016. "In utero-exposed di (n-butyl) phthalate induce dose dependent, age-related changes of morphology and testosterone-biosynthesis enzymes/associated proteins of Leydig cell mitochondria in rats." *The Journal of Toxicological Sciences* 41(2): 195-206.

Mourabit, S., Fitzgerald, J. A., Ellis, R. P., Takesono, A., Porteus, C. S., Trznadel, M. and Tyler, C. R. 2019. "New insights into organ-specific oxidative stress mechanisms using a novel biosensor zebrafish." *Environment International* 133: 105138.

Mouritsen, A., Frederiksen, H., Sørensen, K., Aksglaede, L., Hagen, C., Skakkebaek, N. E. and Juul, A. 2013. "Urinary phthalates from 168 girls and boys measured twice a year during a 5-year period: associations with adrenal androgen levels and puberty." *The Journal of Clinical Endocrinology & Metabolism* 98(9): 3755-3764.

Moyer, B. and Hixon, M. L. 2012. "Reproductive effects in F1 adult females exposed in utero to moderate to high doses of mono-2-ethylhexylphthalate (MEHP)." *Reproductive Toxicology* 34(1): 43-50.

Mu, D., Gao, F., Fan, Z., Shen, H., Peng, H. and Hu, J. 2015. "Levels of phthalate metabolites in urine of pregnant women and risk of clinical pregnancy loss." *Environmental Science & Technology* 49(17): 10651-10657.

Nassar, N., Abeywardana, P., Barker, A. and Bower, C. 2010. "Parental occupational exposure to potential endocrine disrupting chemicals and risk of hypospadias in infants." *Occupational and Environmental Medicine* 67(9): 585-589.

National Academies of Sciences 2017. "National Academies of Sciences, Engineering, and Medicine. Division on Earth and Life Studies, Board on Environmental Studies and Toxicology, & Committee on Endocrine-Related Low-Dose Toxicity. Application of systematic review methods in an overall strategy for evaluating low-dose toxicity from endocrine active chemicals." *National Acad-emies Press (US).*

NICNAS 2008. "Existing chemical hazards assessment report. Diisotridecyl phthalate.2008." Available on https://www.industrialchemicals.gov.au/sites/default/files/Diisotridecyl%20phthalate%20DITDP.pdf

Ormond, G., Nieuwenhuijsen, M. J., Nelson, P., Toledano, M. B., Iszatt, N., Geneletti, S. and Elliott, P. 2009. "Endocrine disruptors in the workplace, hair spray, folate supplementation, and risk of hypospadias: case–control study." *Environmental Health Perspectives* 117(2): 303-307.

Pan, G., Hanaoka, T., Yoshimura, M., Zhang, S., Wang, P., Tsukino, H. and Takahashi, K. 2006. "Decreased serum free testosterone in workers exposed to high levels of di-n-butyl phthalate (DBP) and di-2-ethylhexyl phthalate (DEHP): a cross-sectional study in China." *Environmental Health Perspectives* 114(11): 1643-1648.

Patel, C. J., Rehkopf, D. H., Leppert, J. T., Bortz, W. M., Cullen, M. R., Chertow, G. M. and Ioannidis, J. P. 2013. "Systematic evaluation of environmental and behavioural factors associated with all-cause mortality in the United States National Health and Nutrition Examination Survey." *International Journal of Epidemiology* 42(6): 1795-1810.

Patel, C. J., Yang, T., Hu, Z., Wen, Q., Sung, J., El-Sayed, Y. Y,, Cohen, H., Gould, J., Stevenson, D. K., Shaw, G. M., Ling, X. B. and Butte, A. J. 2014. "Investigation of maternal environmental exposures in association with self-reported preterm birth." *Reproductive Toxicology* 45:1–7.

Patel, C. J., Manrai, A. K., Corona, E. and Kohane, I. S. 2017. "Systematic correlation of environmental exposure and physiological and self-reported behaviour factors with leukocyte telomere length." *International Journal of Epidemiology* 46(1): 44-56.

Patiño-García, D., Cruz-Fernandes, L., Buñay, J., Orellana, R. and Moreno, R. D. 2020. "Daily exposure to phthalates and alkylphenols alters miR biogenesis and expression in mice ovaries." *Journal of Molecular Endocrinology* 65(4): 175-186.

Peretz, J., Craig, Z. R. and Flaws, J. A. 2012. "Bisphenol A inhibits follicle growth and induces atresia in cultured mouse antral follicles independently of the genomic estrogenic pathway." *Biology of Reproduction* 87(3): 63-1.

Phthalate Hazard Compendium 2008. "A summary of physicochemical and human health hazard data for 24 ortho-phthalate chemicals. Existing Chemical Hazard Assessment Report." *Phthalate Hazard Compendium, June 2008. National Industrial Chemicals Notification and Assessment Scheme, Australia.*

Piferrer, F. 2013. "Epigenetics of sex determination and gonadogenesis." *Develop-mental Dynamics* 242(4): 360-370.

Pincus, G., Thimann, K. V. and Astwood, E. B. (Eds.). 2017. "The hormones: physiology, chemistry, and applications." *Elsevier.*

Plastics Europe, 2020. "Plastics-the facts: An analysis of European plastics production, demand and waste." Available from https://plasticseurope.org/knowled ge-hub/plastics-the-facts-2020/

Pocar, P., Fiandanese, N., Berrini, A., Secchi, C. and Borromeo, V. 2017. "Maternal exposure to di (2-ethylhexyl) phthalate (DEHP) promotes the transgenerational inheritance of adult-onset reproductive dysfunctions through the female germline in mice." *Toxicology and Applied Pharmacology* 322: 113-121.

Ptak, A., Rak-Mardyła, A. and Gregoraszczuk, E. L. 2013. "Cooperation of bisphenol A and leptin in inhibition of caspase-3 expression and activity in OVCAR-3 ovarian cancer cells." *Toxicology in Vitro* 27(6): 1937-1943.

Qian, Y., Shao, H., Ying, X., Huang, W. and Hua, Y. 2020. "The endocrine disruption of prenatal phthalate exposure in mother and offspring." *Frontiers in Public Health* 8: 366.

Radke, E. G., Braun, J. M., Meeker, J. D. and Cooper, G. S. 2018. "Phthalate exposure and male reproductive outcomes: a systematic review of the human epidemiological evidence." *Environment International* 121: 764-793.

Reddy, B. S., Rozati, R., Reddy, B. V. R. and Raman, N. V. V. 2006. "General gynaecology: Association of phthalate esters with endometriosis in Indian women." *BJOG: An International Journal of Obstetrics & Gynaecology* 113(5): 515-520.

Repouskou, A., Panagiotidou, E., Panagopoulou, L., Bisting, P. L., Tuck, A. R., Sjödin, M. O. and Kitraki, E. 2019. "Gestational exposure to an epidemiologically defined mixture of phthalates leads to gonadal dysfunction in mouse offspring of both sexes." *Scientific Reports* 9(1): 1-17.

Repouskou, A., Stamatakis, A. and Kitraki, E. 2021. "In utero exposure to phthalates and reproductive toxicity in rodents." *Best Practice & Research Clinical Endocrinology & Metabolism* 35(5): 101512.

Rogers, R., Ouellet, G., Brown, C., Moyer, B., Rasoulpour, T. and Hixon, M. 2008. "Cross-talk between the akt and nf-κb signaling pathways inhibits mehp-induced germ cell apoptosis". *Toxicological Sciences* 106(2): 497-508.

Saeidnia, S. and Abdollahi, M. 2013. "Are medicinal plants polluted with phthalates?." *DARU Journal of Pharmaceutical Sciences* 21(1): 1-3.

Saillenfait, A. M., Sabate, J. P. and Gallissot, F. 2006. "Developmental toxic effects of diisobutyl phthalate, the methyl-branched analogue of di-n-butyl phthalate, administered by gavage to rats." *Toxicology Letters* 165(1): 39-46.

Scarano, W. R., de Toledo, F. C., Guerra, M. T., de Campos, S. G. P., Júnior, L. A. J., Felisbino, S. L. and Kempinas, W. D. G. 2009. "Long-term effects of develop-mental exposure to di-n-butyl-phthalate (DBP) on rat prostate: proliferative and inflammatory disorders and a possible role of androgens." *Toxicology* 262(3): 215-223.

Schettler, T. E. D. 2006. "Human exposure to phthalates via consumer products." *International Journal of Andrology* 29(1): 134-139.

Sekaran, S. and Jagadeesan, A. 2015. "In utero exposure to phthalate down-regulates critical genes in Leydig cells of F1 male progeny." *Journal of Cellular Biochemistry* 116(7): 1466-1477.

Sever, R. and Glass, C. K. 2013. "Signaling by nuclear receptors." *Cold Spring Harbor Perspectives in Biology* 5(3): a016709.

Seyoum, A. and Pradhan, A. 2019. "Effect of phthalates on development, reproduction, fat metabolism and lifespan in Daphnia magna." *Science of the Total Environment* 654: 969-977.

Sharma, P., Ghanghas, P., Kaushal, N., Kaur, J. and Kaur, P. 2019. "Epigenetics and oxidative stress: A twin-edged sword in spermatogenesis." *Andrologia* 51(11): e13432.

Shi, H., Cao, Y., Shen, Q., Zhao, Y., Zhang, Z. and Zhang, Y. 2015. "Association between urinary phthalates and pubertal timing in Chinese adolescents." *Journal of Epidemiology* 25(9): 574-82.

Shoaito, H., Petit, J., Chissey, A., Auzeil, N., Guibourdenche, J., Gil, S. and Degrelle, S. A. 2019. "The role of peroxisome proliferator–activated receptor gamma (ppar γ) in mono (2-ethylhexyl) phthalate (mehp)-mediated cytotrophoblast differentiation". *Environmental Health Perspectives* 127(2): 027003.

Singh, S. and Li, S. S. L. 2012. "Epigenetic effects of environmental chemicals bisphenol A and phthalates." *International Journal of Molecular Sciences,* 13(8): 10143-10153.

Somasundaram, D. B., Manokaran, K., Selvanesan, B. C. and Bhaskaran, R. S. 2017. "Impact of di-(2-ethylhexyl) phthalate on the uterus of adult Wistar rats." *Human and Experimental Toxicology* 36(6): 565-572.

Su, P. H., Chang, C. K., Lin, C. Y., Chen, H. Y., Liao, P. C., Hsiung, C. A. and Wang, S. L. 2015. "Prenatal exposure to phthalate ester and pubertal development in a birth cohort in central Taiwan: a 12-year follow-up study." *Environmental Research* 136: 324-330.

Swan, S.H. 2008. "Environmental phthalate exposure in relation to reproductive outcomes and other health endpoints in humans." *Environmental Research* 108 (2):177-84.

Talsness, C. E., Andrade, A. J., Kuriyama, S. N., Taylor, J. A. and Vom Saal, F. S. 2009. "Components of plastic: experimental studies in animals and relevance for human health." *Philosophical Transactions of the Royal Society B: Biological Sciences* 364(1526): 2079-2096.

Ungewitter, E., Rotgers, E., Bantukul, T., Kawakami, Y., Kissling, G. E. and Yao, H. H. C. 2017. "From the cover: Teratogenic effects of in utero exposure to di-(2-ethylhexyl)-phthalate (DEHP) in B6: 129S4 mice." *Toxicological Sciences* 157(1): 8-19.

Upson, K., Sathyanarayana, S., De Roos, A. J., Thompson, M. L., Scholes, D., Dills, R. and Holt, V. L. 2013. "Phthalates and risk of endometriosis." *Environ-mental Research* 126: 91-97.

Vander Borght, M. and Wyns, C. 2018. "Fertility and infertility: Definition and epidemiology." *Clinical Biochemistry* 62: 2-10.

Vercellini, P., Viganò, P., Somigliana, E. and Fedele, L. 2014. "Endometriosis: pathogenesis and treatment." *Nature Reviews Endocrinology* 10(5): 261-275.

Vrijheid, M., Armstrong, B., Dolk, H., Van Tongeren, M. and Botting, B. 2003. "Risk of hypospadias in relation to maternal occupational exposure to potential endocrine disrupting chemicals." *Occupational and Environmental Medicine* 60(8): 543-550.

Wagner-Mahler, K., Kurzenne, J. Y., Delattre, I., Bérard, E., Mas, J. C., Bornebush, L. and Brucker-Davis, F. 2011. "Prospective study on the prevalence and associated risk factors of cryptorchidism in 6246 newborn boys from Nice area, France." *International Journal of Andrology* 34(5pt2): e499-e510.

Wang, W., Craig, Z. R., Basavarajappa, M. S., Gupta, R. K. and Flaws, J. A. 2012. "Di (2-ethylhexyl) phthalate inhibits growth of mouse ovarian antral follicles through an oxidative stress pathway." *Toxicology and Applied Pharmacology* 258(2): 288-295.

Wang, Y., Liu, W., Yang, Q, Yu, M., Zhang, Z. 2015b. "Di (2-ethylhexyl) phthalate exposure during pregnancy disturbs temporal sex determination regulation in mice offspring." *Toxicology* 336: 10-6.

Wang, Y., Yang, Q., Liu, W., Yu, M., Zhang, Z., Cui, X. 2016b. "DEHP exposure in utero disturbs sex determination and is potentially linked with precocious puberty in female mice." *Toxicology and Applied Pharmacology*. 15; 307:123-129.

Wang, Y. X., You, L., Zeng, Q., Sun, Y., Huang, Y. H., Wang, C. 2015a. "Phthalate exposure and human semen quality: results from an infertility clinic in China." *Environmental Research* 142:1–9.

Wang, Y. X., Zeng, Q, Sun, Y., Yang, P., Wang, P. and Li, J. 2016a. "Semen phthalate metabolites, semen quality parameters and serum reproductive hormones: a cross-sectional study in China." *Environmental Pollution* 211: 173–82.

Wang, Y. X., Zhou, B., Chen, Y. J., Liu, C., Huang, L. L., Liao, J. Q. and Pan, A. 2018. "Thyroid function, phthalate exposure and semen quality: Exploring associations and mediation effects in reproductive-aged men." *Environment International* 116: 278-285.

Watkins, D. J., Sánchez, B. N., Téllez-Rojo, M. M., Lee, J. M., Mercado-García, A., Blank-Goldenberg, C. and Meeker, J. D. 2017. "Phthalate and bisphenol A exposure during in utero windows of susceptibility in relation to reproductive hormones and pubertal development in girls." *Environmental Research* 159: 143-151.

Watkins, D. J., Sánchez, B. N., Téllez-Rojo, M. M., Lee, J. M., Mercado-García, A., Blank-Goldenberg, C. and Meeker, J. D. 2017. "Impact of phthalate and BPA exposure during in utero windows of susceptibility on reproductive hormones and sexual maturation in peripubertal males." *Environmental Health* 16(1): 1-10.

Wen, H. J., Sie, L., Su, P. H., Chuang, C. J., Chen, H. Y., Sun, C. W. and Wang, S. L. J. 2017. "Prenatal and childhood exposure to phthalate diesters and sex steroid hormones in 2-, 5-, 8-, and 11-year-old children: a pilot study of the Taiwan Maternal and Infant Cohort Study." *Journal of Epidemiology* 27(11): 516-523.

Weuve, J., Hauser, R., Calafat, A. M., Missmer, S. A. and Wise, L. A. 2010. "Association of exposure to phthalates with endometriosis and uterine leiomyo-mata: findings from NHANES, 1999–2004." *Environmental Health Perspectives* 118(6): 825-832.

Wierman, M. E. 2007. "Sex steroid effects at target tissues: mechanisms of action." *Advances in Physiology Education,* 31(1): 26-33.

Wolff, M. S., Teitelbaum, S. L., McGovern, K., Windham, G. C., Pinney, S. M., Galvez, M. and Breast Cancer and Environment Research Program. 2014. "Phthalate exposure and pubertal development in a longitudinal study of US girls." *Human Reproduction* 29(7): 1558-1566.

Wolff, M. S., Pajak, A., Pinney, S. M., Windham, G. C., Galvez, M., Rybak, M. and Teitelbaum, S. L. 2017. "Associations of urinary phthalate and phenol biomarkers with menarche in a multiethnic cohort of young girls." *Reproductive Toxicology* 67: 56-64.

Wolff, M. S., Teitelbaum, S. L., Pinney, S. M., Windham, G., Liao, L., Biro, F. and Breast Cancer and Environment Research Centers. 2010. "Investigation of relationships between urinary biomarkers of phytoestrogens, phthalates, and phenols and pubertal stages in girls." *Environmental Health Perspectives* 118(7): 1039-1046.

World Economic Forum 2016. *The New Plastic Economy, Rethinking the future of plastics.* 1-36.

Xia, B., Zhu, Q., Zhao, Y., Ge, W., Zhao, Y., Song, Q. and Zhang, Y. 2018. "Phthalate exposure and childhood overweight and obesity: urinary metabolomic evidence." *Environment International,* 121: 159-168.

Xie, F., Chen, X., Weng, S., Xia, T., Sun, X., Luo, T. and Li, P. 2019. "Effects of two environmental endocrine disruptors' di-n-butyl phthalate (DBP) and mono-n-butyl phthalate (MBP) on human sperm functions *in vitro*." *Reproductive Toxicol-ogy* 83: 1-7.

Xin, W. A. N. G., Li-xin, S. H. A. N. G. and Nan, W. U. 2011. "Effect of di-(2-ethylexyl) phthalate on embryo implantation in early pregnancy and fetus development during medium and late pregnancy in rat." *中国公共卫生* 27(5): 597-599.

Yi, H., Gu, H., Zhou, T., Chen, Y., Wang, G., Jin, Y. and Zhang, L. 2016. "A pilot study on association between phthalate exposure and missed miscarriage." *European Review for Medical and Pharmacological Sciences* 20(9): 1894-1902.

Yi, W. E. I., Xiang-Liang, T., Yu, Z., Bin, L., Lian-Ju, S., Chun-Lan, L. And Guang-Hui, W. E. I. 2018. "DEHP exposure destroys blood-testis barrier (BTB) integrity of immature testes through excessive ROS-mediated autophagy." *Genes & Diseases* 5(3): 263-274.

Young, K. Fisher, J. Kirkman, M. 2016. "Endometriosis and fertility: women's accounts of healthcare." *Human Reproduction,* 31 (3): 554–562.

Zarean, M., Keikha, M., Feizi, A., Kazemitabaee, M. and Kelishadi, R. 2019. "The role of exposure to phthalates in variations of anogenital distance: A systematic review and meta-analysis." *Environmental Pollution* 247: 172-179.

Zhang, T., Li, L., Qin, X. S., Zhou, Y., Zhang, X. F., Wang, L. Q. and Shen, W. 2014. "Di(2-ethylhexyl) phthalate and bisphenol A exposure impairs mouse prim-ordial follicle assembly in vitro." *Environmental and Molecular Mutagenesis* 55(4): 343-353.

Zhang, T., Zhou, X., Zhang, X., Ren, X., Wu, J., Wang, Z. and Wang, Z. 2022. "Gut microbiota may contribute to the postnatal male reproductive abnormalities induced by prenatal dibutyl phthalate exposure." *Chemosphere* 287: 132046.

Zhang, Y., Cao, Y., Shi, H., Jiang, X., Zhao, Y., Fang, X. and Xie, C. 2015. "Could exposure to phthalates speed up or delay pubertal onset and development? A 1.5-year follow-up of a school-based population." *Environment International* 83, 41-49.

Zhang, Y., Jiao, Y., Li, Z., Tao, Y. and Yang, Y. 2021. "Hazards of phthalates (PAEs) exposure: A review of aquatic animal toxicology studies." *Science of The Total Environment* 771, 145418.

Zhou, C., Gao, L. and Flaws, J. A. 2017. "Exposure to an environmentally relevant phthalate mixture causes transgenerational effects on female reproduction in mice." *Endocrinology* 158(6): 1739-1754.

Zhou, C., Gao, L. and Flaws, J. A. 2017. "Prenatal exposure to an environmentally relevant phthalate mixture disrupts reproduction in F1 female mice." *Toxicology and Applied Pharmacology* 318: 49-57.

Zhu, B. B., Zhang, Z. C., Li, J., Gao, X. X., Chen, Y. H., Wang, H. and Xu, D. X. 2021. "Di-(2-ethylhexyl) phthalate induces testicular endoplasmic reticulum stress and germ cell apoptosis in adolescent mice." *Environmental Science and Pollution Research* 28(17): 21696-21705.

Chapter 7

Impact of Phthalates on Oxidative Stress Metabolism: A Key Mechanism Contributes to the Disease Pathogenesis

Duygu Aydemir and Nuriye Nuray Ulusu*
Koc University, School of Medicine,
Department of Medical Biochemistry,
Sariyer, Istanbul, Turkey and
Koç University Research Center for Translational Medicine,
Sariyer, Istanbul, Turkey

Abstract

Endocrine-disrupting chemicals (EDCs) are xenobiotics found in almost all types of industrial products such as toys, pharmaceuticals, cosmetics, food wrappings, furniture, paints, solvents, plasticizer, and households. Phthalates are the most used chemicals in the industry belonging to the EDCs family. Di(2-ethylhexyl) phthalate (DEHP), di-isononyl phthalate (DiNP), di-n-octyl phthalate (DnOP), diethyl phthalate (DEP), dibutyl phthalate (DBP), dimethyl phthalate (DMP), di-n-butyl phthalate (DnBP), benzyl butyl phthalate (BzBP), di-isobutyl phthalate (DiBP) and di-isodecyl phthalate (DiDP) belong to the phthalate family and cause adverse health effects by altering hormone metabolism on human and wildlife. Phthalates have different mechanisms to alter hormone metabolism, including mimicking or antagonizing hormones, altering hormone synthesis, dysregulation of hormone transport, and activation/repression of hormone receptors. Phthalates are metabolized by skin esterases, gut, liver, and kidneys; however, metabolized products of phthalates are very harmful, and some parts of phthalates accumulate

* Corresponding Author's Email: nulusu@ku.edu.tr.

In: Phthalates: Environmental and Health Effects
Editors: Müfide Aydoğan Ahbab and Nurhayat Barlas
ISBN: 978-1-68507-970-3

in the body without being metabolized. Besides impaired hormone metabolism, phthalates alter oxidative stress metabolism via reducing antioxidant defense, interfering with detoxification pathways, and altering energy metabolism. Peroxisome-proliferator-activated receptors (PPARs) comprise three subtypes (PPARα, δ, and γ) and main regulators of carbohydrate, protein, and oxidative stress metabolisms. Phthalates can bind to PPAR receptors and activate them, causing elevated levels of oxidative stress in the cell. Besides, phthalates may interfere with antioxidant enzymes, including glucose-6-phosphate dehydrogenase (G6PD), 6-phosphogluconate dehydrogenase (6PGD), glutathione s-transferase (GST), glutathione reductase (GR), superoxide dismutase (SOD), catalase (CAT), thioredoxin family, and glutathione peroxidase (GPx) leading to the impaired redox balance in the cell. Oxidative stress is characterized by reduced antioxidant defense and enhanced reactive oxygen species (ROS) contributing to the pathogenesis of various diseases, including diabetes mellitus (DM), cancer, obesity, metabolic syndrome, infertility, cardiovascular diseases, and cancer. This chapter discusses the impact of phthalates on the oxidative stress metabolism involved in the pathogenesis of various diseases, including fertility, metabolic syndrome, diabetes mellitus, cardiovascular diseases, and cancer.

Keywords: phthalates, oxidative stress, antioxidant defense, detoxification, disease pathogenesis

Introduction

Endocrine-disrupting chemicals (EDCs) are a group of xenobiotics found in various types of industrial products, including pesticides, detergents, paints, food additives, flame retardants, cosmetics, heavy metals, solvents, plasticizers, surfactants, packaging materials, furniture, toys, and households (Aydemir et al. 2018). EDCs can be classified as naturally found chemicals and synthetic (non-natural) chemicals that interfere with the endocrine system of humans or animals by interfering with the hormone metabolism (Gore et al. 2019, Diamanti-Kandarakis et al. 2009). EDCs exert their adverse effect on the hormone metabolism via different mechanisms such as mimicking or antagonizing hormones, altering hormone synthesis, dysregulation of hormone transport, and activation/repression of hormone receptors (Aydemir et al. 2018). Thus, EDCs have enormous adverse effects on human health, including impairment in the reproductive system of female and male individuals, hormone-sensitive cancers, thyroid dysfunction, cardiovascular diseases, infertility, asthma, congenital disabilities, dysregulation in the neurodevelopment and neuroendocrine system, obesity, metabolic disorder, diabetes, cancers, childhood diseases, and developmental impairments (Gore et al. 2015, Braun 2017, Aydemir et al. 2019a). EDCs cause metabolic alterations by affecting cytosolic and mitochondrial pathways such as glucose uptake, gluconeogenesis, insulin tolerance, pentose phosphate pathway (PPP), lipid metabolism, fatty acid beta-oxidation, basal metabolic rate, detoxification, xenobiotic receptors, drug metabolism, and oxidative stress (Cai et al. 2021, Küblbeck et al. 2020).

Phthalates belonging to the EDCs family are the most used chemical as a plasticizer in various industrial products, including cosmetics, packaging materials, medical devices, paints, households, pharmaceuticals, pesticides, toys, personal-care products, agricultural adjuvants, solvents, and textile products. Di(2-ethylhexyl) phthalate (DEHP), di-isononyl phthalate (DiNP), di-n-octyl phthalate (DnOP), diethyl phthalate (DEP), dibutyl phthalate (DBP), dimethyl phthalate (DMP), di-n-butyl phthalate (DnBP), benzyl butyl phthalate (BzBP), di-isobutyl phthalate (DiBP) and di-isodecyl phthalate (DiDP) belong to the phthalate family used in various types of industrial products (Serrano et al. 2014). Since phthalates have non-covalent bonds, they are easily released from materials. After exposure, phthalates are metabolized by liver, kidney, gut, and skin esterases into harmful monoester metabolites such as mono-n-methyl phthalate (MnMP), mono-ethyl phthalate (MEP), mono-isobutyl phthalate (MiBP), mono-n-butyl phthalate (MnBP), mono-(3-carboxypropyl) phthalate (MCPP), mono-carboxyoctyl phthalate (MCOP), mono-carboxynonyl phthalate (MCNP), mono-(2-ethyl-5-hydroxyhexyl) phthalate (MEHHP), mono-(2-ethyl-5-carboxypentyl) phthalate (MECPP), mono-benzyl phthalate (MBzP), mono-2-ethylhexyl phthalate (MEHP) and mono-(2-ethyl-5-oxohexyl) phthalate (MEOHP) (Wallner et al. 2016).

Phthalates are hydrolyzed into their monoesters and metabolized by P450 enzymes into oxidative molecules; however, some parts of them accumulate in the body over time, causing adverse health effects (Dutta et al. 2020, Aydemir et al. 2018, Aydemir, et al. 2020a). Detoxification of phthalates and accumulation of their metabolites are associated with elevated levels of oxidative stress contributing to the pathogenesis of various diseases, including obesity, cancer, metabolic syndrome, and infertility. We have previously reported that exposure to EDCs such as phthalates and parabens induce tissue damage via elevated levels of oxidative stress (Aydemir et al. 2018, 2019a, 2019b, 2019c, 2020a). Oxidative stress can be described as the impairment in the balance between antioxidant defense and reactive oxygen species (ROS) that alter both cytosolic and mitochondrial homeostasis (Ozcan et al. 2021). Thus, investigating and understanding the role of phthalate-induced oxidative stress in disease pathogenesis is vital for preventing diseases and alterations in humans in the future.

Correlation of the Oxidative Stress Metabolism with Detoxification Process

EDCs are metabolized and excreted via detoxification metabolism, including oxidation, reduction, conjugation, and hydrolysis reactions responsible for converting lipophilic and hydrophobic compounds into hydrophilic forms to excrete metabolites from the biological systems (Blanco-Castañeda et al. 2020, Hakkola et al. 1998). Alterations in the detoxification metabolism lead to the accumulation of harmful and toxic compounds and reaching them at lethal concentrations in the organism (Kato et al. 2006, Petrakis et al. 2017b). Detoxification metabolism uses various enzymes that can be grouped as phase I; bioactivation, phase II; conjugation, phase III; transportation, depending on their role during the detoxification process. Indicated enzymes conjugate with the molecules and transform them into more water-soluble forms to be excreted or inactivated easily. The main aim of the detoxification pathway is to metabolize xenobiotics into the less toxic molecule to prevent oxidative damage in the cell (Croom 2012; Reinen and Vermeulen 2014, Yee, 2012). Enzymes involved in this pathway required key antioxidant molecules such as glutathione, thioredoxin, glucuronic acid, and sulfate (Frohlich et al. 2008, Hodges & Minich, 2015, Lin et al. 2016, Zhang et al. 2013).

Glutathione is the major antioxidant molecule in the cell and exists in two forms reduced glutathione (GSH) and oxidized glutathione (GSSG) (Aydemir and Ulusu 2020b, Aydemir et al. 2019a-d). GSH, desired form in the cell, is responsible for the bioconjugation reactions and used by glutathione s-transferase enzyme (GST), where GSSG is converted into GSH by glutathione reductase (GR) enzymes (Aydemir et al. 2020a). Maintenance and homeostasis of GSH/GSSG ratio are crucial for the cell's antioxidant defense and considered a significant biomarker for oxidative stress status (Forman, Zhang, and Rinna 2009a). NADPH and thioredoxin are essential in reducing glutathione disulfide to the sulfhydryl form. Glutathione s-transferase enzymes are multi-functional, and these enzymes can catalyze glutathione conjugation with xenobiotics, electrophiles, or reactive species then formed product, glutathione -s conjugate would be easily excreted from the cell. EDCs exposure may lead to the decrease in the cytosolic concentrations of GSH, causing various diseases because of impaired oxidative stress metabolism (Cooper and Hanigan 2018, Forman et al. 2009, Kondolot et al. 2016, Tandogan et al. 2011a, 2011b, Tandoğan and Ulusu 2007, Tandogan and Ulusu 2010, Ulusu et al. 2003a).

Reduction of the GSH to their reduced form is under the control of $NADP^+$ reducing enzymes. NADP+ reducing enzymes are found in the cytosol and mitochondria in animals and human malate dehydrogenase, isocitrate dehydrogenase, 10-formyltetrahyfrofolate dehydrogenase, methylenetetra-hydrofolate reductase, glucose-6-phosphate dehydrogenase (G6PD), and 6-phosphogluconate dehydrogenase (6PGD). G6PD and 6PGD enzymes are crucial for oxidative stress metabolism since they synthesize NADPH used by GR enzyme for the conversion of GSSG to GSH (Kondolot et al. 2016, Tandogan et al. 2011b, Gök et al. 2016, Moolna and Bowsher 2010, Fernandez-Marcos and Nóbrega-Pereira 2016, Saccoccia et al. 2014). EDCs, including DEHP and butylparaben, can lead impairment in the G6PD and 6PGD enzyme activities resulting in the altered oxidative stress metabolism and pentose phosphate pathway (PPP) (Aydemir et al. 2019a-e).

Peroxiredoxin enzymes are one of the essential classes of enzymes that have crucial in the antioxidant system, and they can reduce hydrogen peroxide to water. These enzymes use thioredoxin (Trx) for their catalytic activity. Thioredoxin reductase enzymes are from the reductase family. They can reduce oxidized form of thioredoxin to reduced form, and thioredoxins are also crucial detoxification reactions of many xenobiotics (Saccoccia et al. 2014). Thioredoxin reductase and glutathione peroxidase (GPx) enzymes contain selenium, and the antioxidant property of selenium comes from the essential role of these enzymes. GPx converts H_2O_2 into H_2O by using GSH and converts GSH into GSSG (Ulusu and Turan 2005, Can et al. 2005, Turan et al. 2001, Ulusu et al. 2003b, Zhong and Holmgren 2000, Ulusu et al. 2003a).

On the other hand, sulfation is a posttranslational modification of cells and has critical roles in the biodegradation, metabolization, and elimination of xenobiotics processes. Sulfotransferase enzymes catalyze the sulfate conjugation EDCs to eliminate them from their toxic effects (Schmidt et al. 2017, Harris et al. 2007). These enzymes catalyze a reaction between a substrate and 3'-phosphoadenosine 5'-phosphosulfate and 3'-phosphoa-denosine 5'-phosphosulfate is accepted as a universal sulfate donor (James 2021, Klaassen and Boles 1997). Glucuronic acid is also an important small molecule that plays an essential role in biotransformation and eliminating xenobiotics. The UDP-glucuronosyltransferase enzyme reacts with glucuronic acid and the substrate xenobiotics to make them much more water-soluble. Glucuronic acid molecule is synthesized via the glucuronic acid pathway, directly connected with glycolysis and the pentose phosphate pathway (Lock 2010, Oesch-Bartlomowicz and Oesch 2007). Bisphenol A and genistein are detoxified via glucuronic acid, sulfate and phthalate plasticizers, polybrominated diphenyl ether, isononyl cyclohexane-1,2-dicarboxylate and DEHP are metabolized via glucuronic acid (Engel et al. 2018, Engel et al. 2017, Bursztyka et al. 2008).

Additionally, mitochondria are the primary source of oxidative stress because of oxidative phosphorylation. ROS are produced in mitochondria and cytoplasm and cleared by antioxidant enzymes including GR, superoxide dismutase (SOD), catalase (CAT), and GPx. Phthalates such as DEHP, BPA, DBP, MEHP, and DiBP can bind and activate peroxisome proliferator activating receptors (PPAR), especially PPAR-α leading to the enlargement of mitochondria and impair mitochondrial metabolism (Aydemir et al. 2019a-c).

PPARs comprise three subtypes (PPARα, δ, and γ) are the primary regulators of antioxidant defense, lipid, and mitochondria metabolism (Kim 2013). Since PPAR-α is responsible for regulating glucose and lipid metabolism, upregulation of PPAR-α causes liver dysfunction, altered lipid metabolism, impaired glucose transport, enhanced oxidative stress, and triggered inflammatory response leading to cancer, metabolic syndrome, diabetes, and CVDs (Chou et al. 2018).

Role of the Phthalates-Induced Oxidative Stress in the Disease Pathogenesis

Infertility

According to the World Health Organization (WHO) data, infertility is described as a couple's failure to conceive and accounts for 8-12% of the world population according to the World Health Organization (WHO) data (Pigini et al. 2022). Oxidative stress is directly correlated with decreased quality of gametes and infertility, also, the role of the phthalates-induced oxidative stress in male and female infertility has been reported previously (Adeoye et al. 2017, Pigini et al. 2022). Long-chain phthalates are used as a plasticizer.

Short-chain ones are added in the solvents in almost all industrial products such as cosmetics, food wrappings, pharmaceuticals, toys, and households. Therefore, humans are exposed to phthalates daily, tightly associated with infertility. DEHP, DBP, DINP, DMP, and DEP are the most used phthalates in industrial products, and since they are not covalently bound, they leach from the products to the air, soil, water, and dust (Katsikantami et al. 2016, Panagiotou et al. 2021a). Phthalates have been found in the lungs, liver, serum, urine, follicular fluid, amniotic fluid, and adipose tissue of humans as indicators of life-long exposure to the phthalates that start during fetal life (Hannon and Flaws 2015). Phthalates and their metabolized molecules cause ovarian toxicity by targeting follicles at different stages during folliculogenesis, leading to infertility in humans because of the depletion of ovarian reserve. On the other hand, phthalates cause testicular defects, diminished sperm count, shorter anogenital distance, impairment in the steroid hormone synthesis, and reduced androgen levels in male individuals (Panagiotou et al. 2021b).

According to the literature, impaired oxidative stress metabolism is directly correlated with male and female infertility. In male individuals, elevated levels of oxidative stress can damage the sperm membrane causing decreased motility and altering sperm DNA. Urine phthalate and phthalate metabolite levels are associated with high levels of oxidative stress in individuals. Several studies have indicated that DEHP, MEHP, MEHHP, and MEOHP are found in infertile male and female individuals (Wang et al. 2016, Guo et al. 2014). On the other hand, impaired G6PD, 6-PGD, GR, and GST enzyme activities indicating altered PPP and oxidative stress metabolism correlated with tissue damage have been reported in testis tissue of DEHP-treated rats (Aydemir et al. 2019a-c). Additionally, higher MCNP levels in the urine are associated with higher mitochondrial DNA copy number (mtDNAcn) and deletions in the mtDNA (Huffman et al. 2018). ROS increases upon elevated levels of oxidative stress resulting in the attacking of ROS to the proteins, lipids, and nucleic acid. The 8-oxo-dGuo (8-oxo-7,8-dihydro-2-deoxyguanosine) is produced because of oxidative damage of DNA and associated with aging, hypertension, diabetes, cancer, and epigenetic alterations. 8-oxo-dGuo is one of the most used oxidative stress markers and increased in the urine of male and female individuals upon DEHP, DEP, DnBP, MEP, MBzP, MEHP BzBP, and MnBP administration (Pigini et al. 2022). Since follicular fluid (FF) is vital for oocyte development and fertilization, FF is controlled during *in vitro* fertilization (IVF) process. Elevated levels of 8-hydroxy-2′-deoxyguanosine (8-OHdG), malondialdehyde (MDA), and reduced total-antioxidant capacity (TAC) have been detected in FF upon phthalate exposure (Yuan et al. 2020).

Metabolic Syndrome

Metabolic syndrome (MetS) is considered a public health problem affecting both men and women in all age groups worldwide and characterized by insulin resistance, dyslipidemia, chronic inflammation, diabetes, and impaired oxidative stress metabolism (Haverinen et al. 2021) MetS are three times more common than diabetes mellitus (DM) in many populations (Saklayen, 2018). Body mass index (BMI) measurement is one of the significant criteria for defining obesity and metabolic syndrome. According to the literature, individuals with equal or greater than 30 kg/m2 can be accepted as obese, whereas people with BMI greater than 27 may have metabolic syndrome (Chamorro-Garcia and Veiga-Lopez, 2021, Kobo et al. 2019). Since BMI is not only criteria for defining metabolic syndrome, additional key features should be evaluated besides BMI, for instance, waist circumstances over 35 inches for women and 40 inches for men, blood pressure over 130/85 mmHg, fasting triglyceride level higher than 150 mg/dl, high-density lipoprotein (HDL) less than 40 mg/dl for men and 50mg/dl for women (P. L. Huang, 2009).

EDCs play a crucial role in endocrine-related adverse effects on the metabolism by mimicking hormones and causing metabolic syndrome, obesity, diabetes, and causing weight gain (Fénichel & Chevalier, 2017). Phthalates are accepted as 'environmental obesogen' molecules that can affect lipid metabolism normal endocrine regulation and interfere with the action of hormones, increase fatty acid synthesis, accumulate adipose tissue, cause weight gain, and promote obesity and metabolic syndrome (Darbre 2017, Gupta et al. 2020). Higher exposure to various phthalates is associated with insulin resistance and metabolic syndrome. Phthalates are generally used in industrial products, food containers, and food packing (Huang et al. 2021, Ko et al. 2019). The risk of exposure to phthalates is closely related to various health problems such as insulin resistance, metabolic syndrome, high blood sugar, type-2 diabetes mellitus. The metabolic syndrome is not a disease but a common metabolic disorder that results in an increased risk of essential conditions such as high blood pressure (hypertension), stroke, cardiovascular disease, high blood sugar, high serum triglycerides, type-2 diabetes mellitus, excess body fat around the waist (abdominal, visceral obesity) and obesity (Grundy 2006, Eckel et al. 2005, Huang et al. 2021).

Phthalates have several adverse health effects on the pregnant woman causing epigenetic and hormonal changes, lipid accumulation, circulating lipid concentration, dyslipidemia, and insulin resistance. Prenatal exposure to phthalate metabolites increases BMI in boys and girls (Ashrap et al. 2022, Philips et al. 2017). Exposure to the phthalates, including MBP, MBzP, MEHP, MMP, MEOHP, and MEHHP, is tightly associated with obesity, blood pressure, BMI and adiposity markers, lipid profile (Xia et al. 2018, Amin et al. 2018). DEHP exposure can increase the G6PD and 6PGD enzyme activities involved in the fatty acid synthesis metabolism (Aydemir and Ulusu 2020a, Tandogan et al. 2011c). PPAR-γ is upregulated upon phthalate administration and increases the risk of obesity and insulin resistance, contributing to the MetS pathogenesis. PPAR-γ induces adipocyte production, excessive calorie intake, hyperglycemia, inflammatory response, and insulin resistance (Du et al. 2021). Elevated levels of oxidative stress during MetS progression dysregulate the production of adipocytokines, including adiponectin, irisin, monocyte chemoattractant protein-1 (MCP-1), TNF-α, leptin, and interleukin-6 (IL-6), contributing to an inflammatory state in the body, also induces oxidative stress as well. On the other hand, inflammatory markers such as TNF-α, IL-1, and IL-6 are elevated because of impaired adipose function that contributes to the tissue's impairment redox status (Monserrat-Mesquida et al. 2020). In the light of this information, phthalates induce oxidative stress and impair lipid and glucose metabolism contributing to the MetS pathogenesis (Aydemir et al. 2019a-d).

Diabetes Mellitus

Diabetes mellitus (DM) is an important life-long chronic disease and considered a major public health problem worldwide. The prevalence of DM increases every year worldwide, and numbers of type 1 and type 2 diabetic people account for 463 million in 2019. All statistical analyses show the number of patients with diabetes is rising with in alarming rate that is predicted that 578 million people in 2030 and 700 million people in 2045 will have DM (Saeedi et al. 2019). Insulin hormone is secreted dependent on the blood glucose level. In DM pathogenesis, glucose-induced insulin secretion is dysregulated so that insulin hormone concentration would be deficient or there is a problem in the receptors insulin binds. Still, the sending to the signal and the cells cannot take glucose inside the cells, which causes elevation of glucose in the blood. Phthalate exposure is tightly associated with DM pathogenesis via inducing epigenetic changes, attacking pancreas beta cells and immune cells (Patel et al. 2022; Predieri et al. 2020).

Exposure to phthalates, such as MMP, MnBP, MiBP, MCPP, and DEHP metabolites, are associated with an increased risk factor for DM (Liang et al. 2022, Zhang et al. 2022). The effects of phthalates on gestational diabetes were examined according to the pregnant women's trimesters and reported that in the first-trimester MBP, MCNP, and MCPP were negatively associated with gestational diabetes but then in the 2nd trimester, MCNP and MCPP also showed negative correlation to the impaired glucose tolerance test but in high concentrations of MiBP and MHBP were associated with elevated glucose levels (James-Todd et al. 2022). Administration of DEHP, DBP, and bisphenol A (BPA) induces type-2 diabetes mellitus development in laboratory animals via dysregulation of pancreas tissue (Baralić et al. 2021). Karabulut and Barlas (2021) reported that oxidative stress is a toxigenic mechanism of MEHP and MBP toxicity on INS-1 cells. Their results showed that phthalate metabolites caused changes in gene expression at the molecular level by increasing oxidative stress in pancreatic beta cells, resulting in a decrease in insulin synthesis. Therefore, it is assumed that MEHP and MBP-mediated beta cell dysfunctions are an important factor in insulin resistance or type 2 diabetes.

Elevated levels of oxidative stress, dysregulation of adipose function, and enhanced inflammatory cytokines are observed during phthalate administration and directly correlated with DM pathogenesis. Adiponectin is secreted from adipose tissue and responsible for insulin sensitivity and anti-inflammatory status; however, adiponectin secretion is dysregulated during DM pathogenesis. Moreover, according to the literature, decreased adiponectin levels, enhanced oxidative stress, and inflammatory status has been reported upon phthalate administration. Serum biomarkers correlated with oxidative stress such as c-reactive protein (CRP), alkaline phosphatase (ALP), absolute neutrophil count (ANC), and ferritin levels elevated upon MMP, MnBP, MiBP, MCPP MBzP, MEHHP, MEOHP, MCPP, MECPP, and MEHP levels in the patients with diabetes (Duan et al. 2017). Since DEHP treatment impaired glucose tolerance and transport, glucose metabolism in liver and muscle, glycogen synthesis, phthalate-induced oxidative stress is suggested to contribute to the pathogenesis of type 2 DM in humans(Duan et al. 2017). Several studies have shown that phthalate exposure, including DEHP, increases body weight, serum glucose levels, body fat mass, and food intake via higher estrogen receptor (ER1) expression in adipose tissue (LEE,

HWANG, and CHOI 2014). Estrogens are the primary energy and glucose homeostasis regulators regulating insulin resistance, adipose tissue function, and glucose tolerance in humans. Phthalates bind to the ERs, causing reduced estrogen levels in the organism, leading to increased fat mass and altered insulin resistance in laboratory animals (Klöting et al. 2015).

DEHP reduces the expression of insulin receptor and glucose transporter 4 (GLUT4) genes involved in glucose uptake, circulation, and oxidation according to the *in vitro* and *in vivo* studies. In vivo studies have revealed that DEHP decreased blood glucose utilization, hepatic glycogenesis, serum insulin, and testosterone levels; on the other hand, it increased serum blood glucose and estradiol levels. DEHP administration also caused impaired glucose uptake and oxidation in the adipose tissue leading to the DM and MetS pathogenesis. DEHP, MEHP, and dicyclohexyl phthalate (DCHP) have let the activation of PPAR-α and PPAR-γ cause fatty acid oxidation, adipocyte differentiation, enhanced lipid accumulation, and expression of adipocytic proteins (Rengarajan et al. 2007). Additionally, thyroid hormone function has a vital role in the metabolic processes and energy metabolism; thus, phthalate administration resulted in impaired thyroid hormone function, causing obesity and impaired glucose metabolism, according to the literature. Pdx-1 and Ucp-2 genes have a key role in the β-cell function, pancreatic homeostasis, and development; however, gene expression has been impaired upon DEHP administration in the rats (Stojanoska et al. 2017, Güven et al. 2016). We have previously reported that DEHP impaired blood glucose levels, serum biochemistry parameters, G6PD and 6PGD activities in the detoxification organs liver and kidney supporting impaired glucose metabolism and enhanced oxidative stress metabolism in the rats that can be a possible contributor to the DM pathogenesis (Aydemir et al. 2018).

Cardiovascular Diseases

According to the world health organization (WHO), cardiovascular diseases (CVDs) are the major cause of death (Mariana and Cairrao 2020). Smoking, a diet with high calories, lifestyle, low physical activity, and genetic susceptibility correlates with a higher risk of having CVDs in humans. According to the literature, higher blood pressure, atherosclerosis, obesity, metabolic syndrome, and cardiometabolic risk contribute to the pathogenesis of CVDs and are correlated with phthalate exposure such as DEHP, benzyl butyl phthalate (BBzP), DMP, and DBP (Mariana and Cairrao 2020). Adipose tissue function is impaired during CVDs pathogenesis because of the impaired oxidative stress, energy, and inflammation metabolisms.

DEHP induces tumor necrosis factor α (TNF-α), resulting in adipose tissue lipolysis, reduced insulin sensitivity, impaired glucose transporter metabolism, and insulin signaling (Callaghan et al. 2021). For instance, BPA induces NOD-like receptor protein 3 (NLRP3) inflammasome via elevated levels of ROS in adipose cells, and ROS-induced immune cells are recruited to the adipose tissue, which triggers both inflammation and oxidative stress. Additionally, BPA can directly inhibit the activity of antioxidant enzymes such as GR, GPx, catalase (CAT), and SOD in the adipose tissue (Meli et al. 2020). Mitochondrial metabolism of heart tissue is impaired upon BPA and DEHP administration, for instance, ATP depletion, cytochrome-c release, loss of mitochondrial membrane potential, and mass leading to cardiac dysfunction (J.-S. Schmidt et al. 2012). On the other hand, phthalates are potent agonists of the pregnane X receptor (PXR), which can be activated by steroids, hormones, and numerous xenobiotic chemicals. According to the literature, hypercholesterolemia is induced via PXR activation upon phthalate exposure in laboratory animals, proving phthalate-induced impairment of lipid metabolism (Sui et al. 2021).

According to the literature, hypertension is considered one of the significant contributors to CVDs and increases upon phthalate administration. Phthalates and their metabolites cause high blood pressure, elevated levels of malondialdehyde (MDA) as lipid peroxidation marker, reduced GPx and SOD1 activity that is directly associated with endothelial dysfunction leading to hypertension and CVDs (Lu et al. 2018). On the other hand, phthalates and their metabolized products impair inflammatory response by increasing interleukin-6 (IL-6), IL-10, C-reactive protein (CRP) L-1β, IL-8, CXCL2, CXCL3, CXCL6, CCL3, MMP10, and CSF2 levels, causing the phthalate-mediated inflammatory response causing hypertension (Adrogué and Madias 2016, Lu et al. 2018). Angiotensin-converting enzyme (ACE) and endothelin-1 are upregulated in the cardiac tissue of the laboratory animals upon phthalate treatment. Since ACE is responsible for the conversion of angiotensin I to angiotensin II involved in vasoconstrictor activity, same as endothelin-1, upregulation of ACE and endothelin-1 vasoconstriction increase vascular resistance. Moreover, according to the literature, heart failure, myocardial infarction, kidney dysfunction, and hypertension are correlated with elevated endothelin-1 levels (Jaimes et al. 2017).

Several studies have reported that phthalate levels and their metabolites in urine are tightly correlated with elevated levels of oxidative stress and biomarker of various diseases such as diabetes, CVDs, metabolic syndrome, and infertility. CRP, fibrinogen, and D-dimer levels elevated phthalate-administered individuals having CVDs (Pigini et al. 2022, Kim 2013, Monserrat-Mesquida et al. 2020, Duan et al. 2017). MnBP, DEHP, and DnBP administration are associated with the serum's oxidative stress and inflammation biomarkers, such as bilirubin, fibrinogen, alkaline phosphatase, endothelial, and platelet microparticles (EMPs and PMPs). EMPs such as CD31+/CD42a and PMPs including CD31+/CD42a+ are considered biomarkers of endothelial dysfunction and CVDs because of apoptotic endothelial cells and cardiotoxicity. Moreover, impaired antioxidant defense and elevated ROS levels contribute significantly to endothelial dysfunction, arterial stiffness, and damage during CVDs progression (Chu, Wu, and Su 2021). Besides, phthalates contribute to the pathogenesis of diabetes and metabolic syndrome associated with CVDs risk as well; thus, exposure to phthalates contribute to CVDs pathogenesis in different aspects, including oxidative stress, inflammation, endothelial dysfunction, obesity, insulin resistance, obesity, and metabolic syndrome (Aydemir et al. 2018).

Cancer

Cancer is a multi-step and complex disease that arises from four steps: initiation, promotion, progression, and metastasis. Impaired antioxidant defense and elevated levels of ROS cause DNA mutations and damage during cancer progression, invasion, angiogenesis, and metastasis. On the other hand, high levels of oxidative stress lead to inflammation contributing to cancer progression and metastasis (Reuter et al. 2010). Phthalates can induce carcinogenesis directly by binding to the nuclear receptors such as androgen receptors (AR), ERs, PPAR, and vitamin D receptors (VDR) or indirectly by enhanced oxidative stress and inflammatory responses. Phthalates can induce steroid and hormone-dependent cancers such as breast cancer, testicular cancer, and non-small lung cell cancer (NSCLC) by activating nuclear receptors, including ER and AR. Additionally, nuclear receptors play a vital role in the extracellular matrix (ECM) regulation, and upregulation of nuclear receptors is associated with metastasis and tumor microenvironment because of the dysregulation of ECM (Du et al. 2021). Moreover, enhanced oxidative stress and inflammatory response are significant contributors to the ECM dysregulation during various diseases such as cancer and neurological disorders (Aydemir et al. 2022).

PXR receptor, also known as NR1I2, is activated via xenobiotics, hormones, and drugs, upregulating transcription factor ETS-1 involved in the cell invasion via activating matrix metalloproteinases (MMPs) the primary site of tumor cells leading to the invasive cancer cell growth and metastasis. Phthalate-induced PXR activation leads to the ETS-1 mediated *in vitro* and *in vivo* invasion of hepatocellular carcinoma (HCC) cells, according to the literature (Du et al. 2021). On the other hand, phthalates such as DEHP upregulate PPAR-α leading to impaired lipid metabolism, enhanced oxidative stress metabolism, and enhanced peroxisomal β-oxidation. Hydrogen peroxide (H_2O_2) is produced mainly in the liver via peroxisomal β-oxidation, and H_2O_2 is converted into H_2O via CAT and GPx enzymes. Phthalate administration reduces antioxidant enzyme activity, including CAT, GR, and GPx, where increases ROS levels such as H_2O_2 via PPAR-α activation, thus impaired redox homeostasis can induce carcinogenesis, tumor invasion, and metastasis (Chou et al. 2018, Aydemir et al. 2019c-e).

According to the literature, long-term or lifetime exposure to phthalates such as DEHP contributes to the liver, breast, prostate, and testicular cancer pathogenesis. Prostate cancer is an androgen-dependent tumor; age, ethnicity, obesity, and family history are associated with an increased risk factor for prostate cancer. Reduced levels of testosterone and increased body weight lead to more aggressive tumor progression for prostate cancer. AR and ER are expressed in human prostate glands activated upon phthalate administration, leading to prostate cancer cell growth, advancement, and metastasis (Chuang et al. 2020). *In vitro* studies showed that DEHP, BBP, and DBP induce prostate cancer cell proliferation via ERK5 and p38 pathways. Also, AR activation-induced cell growth in prostate cancer cell lines, including LnCap and PC-3 (Zhu et al. 2018). Phthalate-induced oxidative stress has been detected in patients with prostate cancer; for instance, elevated levels of 8-OH-dG and DNA strand breakages have been measured in those patients (Chang et al. 2018).

DEHP exposure is associated with an increased risk of testicular dysregulation and cancer via elevated levels of oxidative stress. We have previously reported administration of EDCs, including DEHP and butylparaben, impaired oxidative stress metabolism in testis tissue correlated with tissue damage in rats (Aydemir et al. 2019a-c. Nuclear factor-erythroid 2 related factor (Nrf2) is vital for protecting cells against chemically-induced oxidative stress and controlling the expression of various antioxidant enzymes, including SOD, GPx, and GR. Nrf2 is abundant in Leydig cells responsible for testosterone production, and their function is impaired upon DEHP treatment via Nrf-2 mediated Notch1 pathway that may lead to impaired testis function and cancer (Tang et al. 2018). Also, DBP induces testicular toxicity via elevated levels of oxidative stress, apoptosis of spermatogenic cells, and membrane damage of testicular cells, where Leydig cells are the most vulnerable cell type against phthalate-induced oxidative stress in testis tissue. Enhanced oxidative stress causes lipid peroxidation (LPO) attacking cell membrane and mitochondrial membrane that leads to impaired tissue function and reduced levels of testosterone hormone (Erkekoglu et al. 2010).

Hepatocellular cancer (HCC) is the sixth most common cancer globally, while smoking, obesity, hepatitis, and alcohol are associated with higher risk with HCC in humans (Du et al. 2021). Phthalate administration is tightly correlated with enlargement, impaired glucose metabolism, enhanced oxidative stress, and carcinogenesis in the liver. DEHP and BBP administration induced DNA damage, tumor growth, impaired apoptosis, and impaired energy metabolism in HCC cells. Aryl hydrocarbon receptor (AhR) is associated with angiogenesis and metastasis, where phthalate-induced ER activation resulted in the activation of the MEK, p38 kinase, and PI3K pathways leading to the cancer initiation and progression. (Rusyn et al. 2006, Tsai et al. 2014). Interestingly phthalates exposure such as DEHP, BBP contributes to the drug resistance in various types of cancers, including breast and colon (Jadhao et al. 2021, Hsieh et al. 2022). The correlation of breast cancer, prostate, and thyroid cancer with exposure to phthalates has been reported in the literature (Liu et al. 2021). ERs are found in the breast, and thyroid tissue is stimulated upon phthalate administration leading to tumorigenesis (Lee et al. 2014).

In conclusion, phthalates and their metabolized products contribute to the cancer pathogenesis via activating ERs and ARs, altering hormone metabolism and impaired oxidative stress metabolism. There are several studies indicating correlation between urinary phthalates levels and cancer pathogenesis, however role of the mechanisms of phthalate-induced oxidative stress should be further investigated.

Conclusion

EDCs can be derived from organic or inorganic sources and impair hormone metabolism of humans and wildlife. They are found in almost all types of industrial products such as toys, pharmaceuticals, cosmetics, food wrappings, furniture, paints, solvents, plasticizer, and households. Phthalates have different mechanisms to alter hormone metabolism, including mimicking or antagonizing hormones, altering hormone synthesis, dysregulation of hormone transport, and activation/repression of hormone receptors. Since EDCs are xenobiotics, they metabolized by the detoxification enzymes in the liver, gut, skin and kidney. During metabolization process, EDCs and their harmful metabolized metabolites exert harmful effects via different metabolism including impaired oxidative stress metabolism, inflammation, impaired hormone homeostasis and altered detoxification. Impaired oxidative stress is involved in the various disease pathogenesis such as diabetes, cancer, obesity, metabolic syndrome, infertility, neurological disorders and cardiovascular diseases. Phthalate-induced oxidative stress is impaired via alteration of the anti-oxidant enzymes activities and activating peroxisome proliferator activating receptors (PPAR), especially PPAR-α leading to the enlargement of mitochondria and impair mitochondrial metabolism. In conclusion, phthalates and their harmful metabolites lead to the enhanced oxidative stress contributing to the pathogenesis of various diseases including cancer, cardiovascular diseases, infertility, neurological disorders, cardiovascular diseases, obesity, metabolic syndrome and diabetes.

References

Adeoye, O., Olawumi, J., Opeyemi, A., Christiania, O. 2017. "Review on the Role of Glutathione on Oxidative Stress and Infertility." *JBRA Assisted Reproduction* Mar 1;22(1):61-66. doi:10.5935/1518-0557.20180003.

Adrogué, Horacio J., and Nicolaos E. Madias. 2016. "Sodium and Potassium in the Pathogenesis of Hypertension." *Current Opinion in Nephrology and Hypertension*, December, 1. doi:10.1097/MNH.0000000000000301.

Amin, M. M., Ebrahimpour, K., Parastar, S., Shoshtari-Yeganeh, B., Hashemi, M., Mansourian, M., Poursafa, P., Fallah, Z., Rafiei, N., Kelishadi, R. 2018. "Association of Urinary Concentrations of Phthalate Metabolites with Cardiometabolic Risk Factors and Obesity in Children and Adolescents." *Chemosphere* 211 (November): 547–56. doi:10.1016/j.chemosphere.2018.07.172.

Ashrap, P., Aung, M. T., Watkins, D. J., Mukherjee, B., Rosario-Pabón, Z., Vélez-Vega, C. M., Alshawabkeh, A., Cordero, J. F., Meeker, J. D. 2022. "Maternal Urinary Phthalate Metabolites are Associated with Lipidomic Signatures Among Pregnant Women in Puerto Rico." *J Expo Sci Environ Epidemiol* Jan 24. doi: 10.1038/s41370-022-00410-3. Epub ahead of print. PMID: 35075242.

Aydemir, D., Karabulut, G., Şimşek, G., Gok, M., Barlas, N., Ulusu, N. N. 2018. "Impact of the Di(2-Ethylhexyl) Phthalate Administration on Trace Element and Mineral

Levels in Relation of Kidney and Liver Damage in Rats." *Biological Trace Element Research* 186 (2). doi:10.1007/s12011-018-1331-0.

Aydemir, D., Karabulut, G., Şimşek, G., Gok, M., Barlas, N., Ulusu, N. N. 2019a. "Data the DEHP Induced Changes on the Trace Element and Mineral Levels in the Brain and Testis Tissues of Rats." *Data in Brief* Sep 17;26:104526. doi:10.1016/j.dib.2019.104526.

Aydemir, D., Hashemkhani, M., Acar, H. Y., Ulusu N. N. 2019b. "In Vitro Interaction of Glutathione S-Transferase-Pi Enzyme with Glutathione-Coated Silver Sulfide Quantum Dots: A Novel Method for Biodetection of Glutathione S-Transferase Enzyme." *Chemical Biology and Drug Design* Dec;94(6):2094-2102. doi:10.1111/ cbdd.13614.

Aydemir, D., Hashemkhani, M., Durmusoglu, E. G., Yagci-Acar, H., Ulusu, N. N. 2019c. "A New Substrate for Glutathione Reductase: Glutathione Coated Ag_2S Quantum Dots." *Talanta* 194 (March): 501–6. doi:10.1016/j.talanta.2018.10.049.

Aydemir, D., Sarayloo, E., Ulusu, N. N. 2019d. "Rosiglitazone-Induced Changes in the Oxidative Stress Metabolism and Fatty Acid Composition in Relation with Trace Element Status in the Primary Adipocytes." *Journal of Medical Biochemistry* Sep 2;39(3):267-275. doi:10.2478/jomb-2019-0041.

Aydemir, D., Oztasci, B., Barlas, N., Ulusu, N. N. 2019e. "Effects of butylparaben on antioxidant enzyme activities and histopathological changes in rat tissues." *Arh Hig Rada Toksikol* Dec 1;70(4):315-324. doi: 10.2478/aiht-2019-70-3342. PMID: 32623865.

Aydemir, D., Oztasci, B., Barlas, N., Ulusu, N. N. 2020a. "Influence of the Butylparaben Administration on the Oxidative Stress Metabolism of Liver, Kidney and Spleen." *Turkish Journal of Biochemistry* 45 (6): 689–94. doi:10.1515/tjb-2020-0048.

Aydemir, D., Ulusu, N. N. 2020b. "The Possible Role of The Glucose-6-Phosphate Dehydrogenase Enzyme Deficiency in The Polyneuropathies." *The Journal of Basic and Clinical Health Sciences* 4 (3): 212-217. doi:10.30621/jbachs.2020.1151.

Aydemir, D., Malik, A. N., Kulac, I., Basak, A. N., Lazoglu, I., Ulusu, N. N. 2022. "Impact of the ALS Disease on the Biomechanical Properties and Oxidative Stress Metabolism of the Lung Tissue Correlated with the Human Mutant SOD1^{G93A} Protein Accumulation." *Frontiers in Bioengineering and Biotechnology*, https://doi.org/10.3389/fbioe.2022.810243.

Baralić, K., Živančević, K., Jorgovanović, D., Javorac, D., Radovanović, J., Gojković, T., Buha Djordjevic, A., Ćurčić, M., Mandinić, Z., Bulat, Z., Antonijević, B., and Đukić-Ćosić, D. 2021. "Probiotic reduced the impact of phthalates and bisphenol A mixture on type 2 diabetes mellitus development: Merging bioinformatics with in vivo analysis." *Food and Chemical Toxicology*, 154, 112325. https://doi.org/10.1016/j.fct.2021.112325.

Braun, J., M. 2017. "Early-Life Exposure to EDCs: Role in Childhood Obesity and Neurodevelopment." *Nature Reviews Endocrinology* 13 (3): 161–73. doi:10.1038/nrendo.2016.186.

Bursztyka, J., E. Perdu, K. Pettersson, I. Pongratz, M. Fernández-Cabrera, N. Olea, L. Debrauwer, D. Zalko, and J.P. Cravedi. 2008. "Biotransformation of Genistein and Bisphenol A in Cell Lines Used for Screening Endocrine Disruptors." *Toxicology in Vitro* 22 (6): 1595–1604. doi:10.1016/j.tiv.2008.06.013.

Cai, X., Young, G. M., and Xie, W. 2021. "The xenobiotic receptors PXR and CAR in liver physiology, an update". *Biochimica et Biophysica Acta (BBA) - Molecular Basis of Disease*, 1867(6), 166101. https://doi.org/10.1016/j.bbadis.2021.166101.

Callaghan, M. A., Alatorre-Hinojosa, S., Connors, L. T., Singh, R. D., Thompson, J. A. 2021. "Plasticizers and Cardiovascular Health: Role of Adipose Tissue Dysfunction." *Frontiers in Pharmacology,* 11. https://doi.org/10.3389/fphar.2020.626448.

Can, B., Ulusu, N. N., Kilinç, K., Leyla Acan, N., Saran, Y., and Turan, B. 2005. "Selenium Treatment Protects Diabetes-Induced Biochemical and Ultrastructural Alterations in Liver Tissue." *Biological Trace Element Research*, 105(1–3), 135–150. https://doi.org/10.1385/BTER:105:1-3:135.

Chamorro-Garcia, R., Veiga-Lopez, A. 2021. "The New Kids on the Block: Emerging Obesogens." *Advances in Pharmacology*, 29, 457–84. doi:10.1016/bs.apha.2021. 05. 003.

Chang, W.-H., Lee, C.-C., Yen, Y.-H., and Chen, H.-L. 2018. "Oxidative damage in patients with benign prostatic hyperplasia and prostate cancer co-exposed to phthalates and to trace elements." *Environment International*, *121*, 1179–1184. https://doi.org/10.1016/j.envint.2018.10.034.

Chou, C.-K., Yang, Y.-T., Yang, H.-C., Liang, S.-S., Wang, T.-N., Kuo, P.-L., Wang, H.-M. D., Tsai, E.-M., and Chiu, C.-C. 2018. "The Impact of Di(2-ethylhexyl)phthalate on Cancer Progression." *Archivum Immunologiae et Therapiae Experimentalis*, *66*(3), 183–197. https://doi.org/10.1007/s00005-017-0494-2.

Chu, P.-C., Wu, C., and Su, T.-C. 2021. "Association between Urinary Phthalate Metabolites and Markers of Endothelial Dysfunction in Adolescents and Young Adults." *Toxics*, *9*(2), 33. https://doi.org/10.3390/toxics9020033.

Cooper, A.J.L., and M.H. Hanigan. 2018. "Metabolism of Glutathione S-Conjugates: Multiple Pathways." *In Comprehensive Toxicology*, 363–406. Elsevier. doi:10.1016/B978-0-12-801238-3.01973-5.

Darbre, P. D. 2017. "Endocrine Disruptors and Obesity." *Current Obesity Reports* 6 (1): 18–27. doi:10.1007/s13679-017-0240-4.

Diamanti-Kandarakis, E., Bourguignon, J.-P., Giudice, L. C., Hauser, R., Prins, G. S., Soto, A. M., Zoeller, R. T., and Gore, A. C. 2009. "Endocrine-Disrupting Chemicals: An Endocrine Society Scientific Statement." *Endocrine Reviews*, *30*(4), 293–342. https://doi.org/10.1210/er.2009-0002.

Duan, Y., Wang, L., Han, L., Wang, B., Sun, H., Chen, L., Zhu, L., and Luo, Y. 2017. "Exposure to phthalates in patients with diabetes and its association with oxidative stress, adiponectin, and inflammatory cytokines." *Environment International*, *109*, 53–63. https://doi.org/10.1016/j.envint.2017.09.002.

Dutta, S., Haggerty, D. K., Rappolee, D. A., Ruden, D. M. 2020. "Phthalate Exposure and Long-Term Epigenomic Consequences: A Review." *Frontiers in Genetics* 11 (May). doi:10.3389/fgene.2020.00405.

Du, Y., Shi, X., Ma, W., Wen, P., Yu, P., Wang, X., Fang, P., Chen, A., Gao, Z., and Cui, K. 2021. "Phthalates promote the invasion of hepatocellular carcinoma cells by enhancing the interaction between Pregnane X receptor and E26 transformation specific sequence 1." *Pharmacological Research*, *169*, 105648. https://doi.org/10.1016/j.phrs.2021.105648.

Eckel, R. H., Grundy, S. M., Zimmet, P.Z. 2005. "The Metabolic Syndrome." *The Lancet* 365 (9468): 1415–28. doi:10.1016/S0140-6736(05)66378-7.

Engel, A., Buhrke, T., Imber, F., Jessel, S., Seidel, A., Völkel, W., and Lampen, A. 2017. "Agonistic and Antagonistic Effects of Phthalates and Their Urinary Metabolites on the Steroid Hormone Receptors ERα, ERβ, and AR." *Toxicology Letters*, *277*, 54–63. https://doi.org/10.1016/j.toxlet.2017.05.028.

Engel, A., Buhrke, T., Kasper, S., Behr, A.-C., Braeuning, A., Jessel, S., Seidel, A., Völkel, W., and Lampen, A. 2018. "The Urinary Metabolites of DINCH ® Have an İmpact on the Activities of the Human Nuclear Receptors ERα, ERβ, AR, PPARα and PPARγ." *Toxicology Letters*, *287*, 83–91. https://doi.org/10.1016/j.toxlet.2018. 02.006.

Erkekoglu, P., Rachidi, W., Yuzugullu, O. G., Giray, B., Favier, A., Ozturk, M., and Hincal, F. 2010. "Evaluation of Cytotoxicity and Oxidative DNA Damaging Effects of di(2-ethylhexyl)-phthalate (DEHP) and mono(2-ethylhexyl)-phthalate (MEHP) on MA-10 Leydig Cells and Protection by Selenium." *Toxicology and Applied Pharmacology*, *248*(1), 52–62. https://doi.org/10.1016/j.taap.2010.07.016.

Fénichel, P., and Chevalier, N. 2017. "Environmental Endocrine Disruptors: New Diabetogens?" *Comptes Rendus Biologies* 340 (9–10): 446–52. doi:10.1016/j.crvi. 2017.07.003.

Fernandez-Marcos, P. J., and Nóbrega-Pereira, S. 2016. "NADPH: New Oxygen for the ROS Theory of Aging." *Oncotarget* 7 (32): 50814–15. doi:10.18632/oncotarget.107 44.

Forman, H. J., Zhang, H., Rinna, A. 2009a. "Glutathione: Overview of Its Protective Roles, Measurement, and Biosynthesis." *Molecular Aspects of Medicine* 30 (1–2): 1–12. doi:10.1016/j.mam.2008.08.006.

Gök, M., Ulusu, N. N., Tarhan, N., Tufan, C., Ozansoy, G., Arı, N., and Karasu, Ç. 2016. "Flaxseed Protects Against Diabetes-Induced Glucotoxicity by Modulating Pentose Phosphate Pathway and Glutathione-Dependent Enzyme Activities in Rats." *Journal of Dietary Supplements*, *13*(3), 339–351. https://doi.org/10.3109/19390211.2015. 1036188.

Gore, A. C., V. A. Chappell, S. E. Fenton, J. A. Flaws, A. Nadal, G. S. Prins, J. Toppari, and R. T. Zoeller. 2015. "EDC-2: The Endocrine Society's Second Scientific Statement on Endocrine-Disrupting Chemicals." *Endocrine Reviews* 36 (6): E1–150. doi:10.1210/er.2015-1010.

Grundy, S. M. 2006. "Metabolic Syndrome: Connecting and Reconciling Cardiovascular and Diabetes Worlds." *Journal of the American College of Cardiology* 47 (6): 1093–1100. doi:10.1016/j.jacc.2005.11.046.

Guo, Y., Weck, J., Sundaram, R., Goldstone, A. E., Buck Louis, G., and Kannan, K. 2014. "Urinary Concentrations of Phthalates in Couples Planning Pregnancy and Its Association with 8-Hydroxy-2′-deoxyguanosine, a Biomarker of Oxidative Stress: Longitudinal Investigation of Fertility and the Environment Study." *Environmental Science & Technology*, *48*(16), 9804–9811. https://doi.org/10.1021/es5024898.

Güven, C., Dal, F., Aydoğan Ahbab, M., Taskin, E., Ahbab, S., Adin Çinar, S., Sırma Ekmekçi, S., Güleç, Ç., Abacı, N., Akçakaya, H. 2016. "Low dose monoethyl phthalate (MEP) exposure triggers proliferation by activating PDX-1 at 1.1B4 human pancreatic beta cells." *Food and Chemical Toxicology*, *93*, 41–50. https://doi.org/10.1016/j.fct.2016.04.023.

Hannon, P. R., Flaws, J.A. 2015. "The Effects of Phthalates on the Ovary." *Frontiers in Endocrinology 6* (February). doi:10.3389/fendo.2015.00008.

Harris, R., Turan, N., Kirk, C., Ramsden, D., and Waring, R. 2007. "Effects of Endocrine Disruptors on Dehydroepiandrosterone Sulfotransferase and Enzymes Involved in PAPS Synthesis: Genomic and Nongenomic Pathways." *Environmental Health Perspectives*, *115*(Suppl 1), 51–54. https://doi.org/10.1289/ehp.9365.

Haverinen, E., Paalanen, L., Palmieri, L., Padron-Monedero, A., Noguer-Zambrano, I., Sarmiento Suárez, R., and Tolonen, H. 2021. "Comparison of Metabolic Syndrome Prevalence Using Four Different Definitions – A Population-Based Study in Finland." *Archives of Public Health*, *79*(1), 231. https://doi.org/10.1186/s13690-021-00749-3.

Hsieh, T.-H., Hsu, C.-Y., Yang, P.-J., Chiu, C.-C., Liang, S.-S., Ou-Yang, F., Kan, J.-Y., Hou, M.-F., Wang, T.-N., and Tsai, E.-M. 2022. "DEHP Mediates Drug Resistance by Directly Targeting AhR in Human Breast Cancer." *Biomedicine & Pharmacotherapy*, *145*, 112400. https://doi.org/10.1016/j.biopha.2021.112400.

Huang, P. L. 2009. "A Comprehensive Definition for Metabolic Syndrome." *Disease Models & Mechanisms* 2 (5–6): 231–37. doi:10.1242/dmm.001180.

Huang, Y.-C., Huang, P.-R., Lo, Y.-T. C., Sun, C.-W., Pan, W.-H., Wang, S.-L., and Huang, H.-B. 2021. "Food Processing and Phthalate Exposure: The Nutrition and Health Survey in Taiwan (1993–1996 and 2005–2008)." *Frontiers in Nutrition*, *8*. https://doi.org/10.3389/fnut.2021.766992.

Huffman, A. M., Wu, H., Rosati, A., Rahil, T., Sites, C. K., Whitcomb, B. W., and Richard Pilsner, J. 2018. "Associations of urinary phthalate metabolites and lipid peroxidation with sperm mitochondrial DNA copy number and deletions." *Environmental Research*, *163*, 10–15. https://doi.org/10.1016/j.envres.2018.01.023.

Jadhao, M., Tsai, E.-M., Yang, H.-C., Chen, Y.-F., Liang, S.-S., Wang, T.-N., Teng, Y.-N., Huang, H.-W., Wang, L.-F., and Chiu, C.-C. 2021. "The Long-Term DEHP Exposure Confers Multidrug Resistance of Triple-Negative Breast Cancer Cells through ABC Transporters and Intracellular ROS." *Antioxidants*, *10*(6), 949. https://doi.org/10.3390/antiox10060949.

Jaimes, R., Swiercz, A., Sherman, M., Muselimyan, N., Marvar, P. J., and Posnack, N. G. 2017. "Plastics and Cardiovascular Health: Phthalates May Disrupt Heart Rate Variability and Cardiovascular Reactivity." *American Journal of Physiology-Heart and Circu-latory Physiology*, *313*(5), H1044–H1053. https://doi.org/10.1152/ajpheart.00364.2017.

James, M. O. 2021. "Drug Metabolism: Phase II Enzymes." *In Reference Module in Biomedical Sciences*. Elsevier. doi:10.1016/B978-0-12-820472-6.00123-7.

James-Todd, T., Ponzano, M., Bellavia, A., Williams, P. L., Cantonwine, D. E., Calafat, A. M., Hauser, R., Quinn, M. R., Seely, E. W., and McElrath, T. F. 2022. "Urinary Phthalate and DINCH Metabolite Concentrations and Gradations of Maternal Glucose İntolerance." *Environment International*, *161*, 107099. https://doi.org/10.1016/j.envint.2022.107099.

Katsikantami, I., Sifakis, S., Tzatzarakis, M. N., Vakonaki, E., Kalantzi, O.-I., Tsatsakis, A. M., and Rizos, A. K. 2016. "A Global Assessment of Phthalates Burden and Related

Links to Health Effects." *Environment International*, *97*, 212–236. https://doi.org/10.1016/j.envint.2016.09.013.

Kim, T. 2013. "Peroxisome-Proliferator-Activated Receptors Regulate Redox Signaling in the Cardiovascular System." *World Journal of Cardiology* 5 (6): 164. doi:10.4330/wjc.v5.i6.164.

Klaassen, C. D., Boles, J. W. 1997. "The Importance of 3'-phosphoadenosine 5'-phosphosulfate (PAPS) in the Regulation of Sulfation." *The FASEB Journal* 11 (6): 404–18. doi:10.1096/fasebj.11.6.9194521.

Klöting, N., Hesselbarth, N., Gericke, M., Kunath, A., Biemann, R., Chakaroun, R., Kosacka, J., Kovacs, P., Kern, M., Stumvoll, M., Fischer, B., Rolle-Kampczyk, U., Feltens, R., Otto, W., Wissenbach, D. K., von Bergen, M., and Blüher, M. 2015. "Di-(2-Ethylhexyl)-Phthalate (DEHP) Causes Impaired Adipocyte Function and Alters Serum Metabolites." *Plos One 10*(12), e0143190. https://doi.org/10.1371/journal.pone.0143190.

Ko, N.-Y., Lo, Y.-T. C., Huang, P.-C., Huang, Y.-C., Chang, J.-L., and Huang, H.-B. 2019. "Changes in İnsulin Resistance Mediate the Associations between Phthalate Exposure and Metabolic Syndrome." *Environmental Research*, *175*, 434–441. https://doi.org/10.1016/j.envres.2019.04.022.

Kobo, O., Leiba, R., Avizohar, O., and Karban, A. 2019. "Normal Body Mass İndex (BMI) Can Rule Out Metabolic Syndrome." *Medicine*, *98*(9), e14712. https://doi.org/10.1097/MD.0000000000014712.

Kondolot, M., Ozmert, E. N., Ascı, A., Erkekoglu, P., Oztop, D. B., Gumus, H., Kocer-Gumusel, B., and Yurdakok, K. 2016. "Plasma Phthalate and Bisphenol A Levels and Oxidant-Antioxidant Status in Autistic Children." *Environmental Toxicology and Pharmacology*, *43*, 149–158. https://doi.org/10.1016/j.etap.2016.03.006.

Küblbeck, J., Niskanen, J., Honkakoski, P. 2020. "Metabolism-Disrupting Chemicals and the Constitutive Androstane Receptor CAR." *Cells* 9 (10): 2306. doi:10.3390/cells9102306.

Lee, H.-R., Hwang, K.-A., and Choı, K.-C. 2014. "The Estrogen Receptor Signaling Pathway Activated by Phthalates is Linked with Transforming Growth Factor-B in the Progression of LNCaP Prostate Cancer Models." *International Journal of Oncology*, *45*(2), 595–602. https://doi.org/10.3892/ijo.2014.2460.

Liang, Q.-X., Lin, Y., Fang, X.-M., Gao, Y.-H., and Li, F. 2022. "Association Between Phthalate Exposure in Pregnancy and Gestational Diabetes: A Chinese Cross-Sectional Study." *International Journal of General Medicine*, *Volume 15*, 179–189. https://doi.org/10.2147/IJGM.S335895.

Liu, G., Cai, W., Liu, H., Jiang, H., Bi, Y., and Wang, H. 2021. "The Association of Bisphenol A and Phthalates with Risk of Breast Cancer: A Meta-Analysis." *International Journal of Environmental Research and Public Health*, *18*(5), 2375. https://doi.org/10.3390/ijerph18052375.

Lock, E.A. 2010. "Renal Xenobiotic Metabolism." *In Comprehensive Toxicology*, 55–79. Elsevier. doi:10.1016/B978-0-08-046884-6.00803-4.

Lu, X., Xu, X., Lin, Y., Zhang, Y., and Huo, X. 2018. "Phthalate Exposure as a Risk Factor for Hypertension." *Environmental Science and Pollution Research*, *25*(21), 20550–20561. https://doi.org/10.1007/s11356-018-2367-6.

Mariana, M., and Cairrao, E. 2020. "Phthalates Implications in the Cardiovascular System." *Journal of Cardiovascular Development and Disease*, *7*(3), 26. https://doi.org/10.3390/jcdd7030026.

Meli, R., Monnolo, A., Annunziata, C., Pirozzi, C., and Ferrante, M. C. 2020. "Oxidative Stress and BPA Toxicity: An Antioxidant Approach for Male and Female Reproductive Dysfunction." *Antioxidants*, *9*(5), 405. https://doi.org/10.3390/antiox9050405.

Monserrat-Mesquida, M., Quetglas-Llabrés, M., Capó, X., Bouzas, C., Mateos, D., Pons, A., Tur, J. A., and Sureda, A. 2020. "Metabolic Syndrome is Associated with Oxidative Stress and Proinflammatory State." *Antioxidants*, *9*(3), 236. https://doi.org/10.3390/antiox9030236.

Moolna, A., Bowsher, C. G. 2010. "The Physiological Importance of Photosynthetic Ferredoxin NADP+ Oxidoreductase (FNR) Isoforms in Wheat." *Journal of Experimental Botany* 61 (10): 2669–81. doi:10.1093/jxb/erq101.

Oesch-Bartlomowicz, B., Oesch, F. 2007. "Mechanisms of Toxification and Detoxification Which Challenge Drug Candidates and Drugs." *In Comprehensive Medicinal Chemistry II*, 193–214. Elsevier. doi:10.1016/B0-08-045044-X/00124-3.

Ozcan, M., Aydemir, D., Bacanlı, M., Anlar, H. G., Ulusu, N. N., and Aksoy, Y. 2021. "Protective Effects of Antioxidant Chlorophyllin in Chemically Induced Breast Cancer Model In vivo." *Biological Trace Element Research*, *199*(12), 4475–4488. https://doi.org/10.1007/s12011-021-02585-6.

Panagiotou, E. M., Ojasalo, V., Damdimopoulou, P. 2021. "Phthalates, Ovarian Function and Fertility in Adulthood." *Best Practice & Research Clinical Endocrinology & Metabolism*, *35*(5), 101552. https://doi.org/10.1016/j.beem.2021.101552.

Patel, R., Parmar, N., Pramanik Palit, S., Rathwa, N., Ramachandran, A. V., and Begum, R. 2022. "Diabetes Mellitus and Melatonin: Where Are We?" *Biochimie*. https://doi.org/10.1016/j.biochi.2022.01.001.

Philips, Elise M., Vincent W.V. Jaddoe, and Leonardo Trasande. 2017. "Effects of Early Exposure to Phthalates and Bisphenols on Cardiometabolic Outcomes in Pregnancy and Childhood." *Reproductive Toxicology* 68 (March): 105–18. doi:10.1016/j.reprotox.2016.08.015.

Pigini, D., Caporossi, L., Paci, E., Capanna, S., Viganò, P., Alteri, A., Rabellotti, E., Buonaurio, F., Papaleo, B., and Tranfo, G. 2022. "Phthalate Exposure and Biomarkers of Oxidation of Nucleic Acids: Results on Couples Attending a Fertility Center." *Toxics*, *10*(2), 61. https://doi.org/10.3390/toxics10020061.

Predieri, B., Bruzzi, P., Bigi, E., Ciancia, S., Madeo, S. F., Lucaccioni, L., and Iughetti, L. 2020. "Endocrine Disrupting Chemicals and Type 1 Diabetes." *International Journal of Molecular Sciences*, *21*(8), 2937. https://doi.org/10.3390/ijms21082937.

Rengarajan, S., Parthasarathy, C., Anitha, M., Balasubramanian, K. 2007. "Diethylhexyl Phthalate İmpairs İnsulin Binding and Glucose Oxidation in Chang Liver Cells." *Toxicology in Vitro*, *21*(1), 99–102. https://doi.org/10.1016/j.tiv.2006.07.005.

Reuter, S., Gupta, S. C., Chaturvedi, M. M., and Aggarwal, B. B. 2010. "Oxidative Stress, İnflammation, and Cancer: How Are They Linked?" *Free Radical Biology and Medicine*, *49*(11), 1603–1616. https://doi.org/10.1016/j.freeradbiomed.2010.09.006.

Rusyn, I., Peters, J. M., and Cunningham, M. L. 2006. "Modes of Action and Species-Specific Effects of Di-(2-ethylhexyl)Phthalate in the Liver." *Critical Reviews in Toxicology*, *36*(5), 459–479. https://doi.org/10.1080/10408440600779065.

Saccoccia, F., Angelucci, F., Boumis, G., Carotti, D., Desiato, G., Miele, A., and Bellelli, A. 2014. "Thioredoxin Reductase and Its Inhibitors." *Current Protein & Peptide Science*, *15*(6), 621–646. https://doi.org/10.2174/1389203715666140530091910.

Saeedi, P., Petersohn, I., Salpea, P., Malanda, B., Karuranga, S., Unwin, N., Colagiuri, S., Guariguata, L., Motala, A. A., Ogurtsova, K., Shaw, J. E., Bright, D., and Williams, R. 2019. "Global and Regional Diabetes Prevalence Estimates for 2019 and Projections for 2030 and 2045: Results from the International Diabetes Federation Diabetes Atlas, 9th edition." *Diabetes Research and Clinical Practice*, *157*, 107843. https://doi.org/ 10.1016/j.diabres.2019.107843.

Saklayen, M. G. 2018. "The Global Epidemic of the Metabolic Syndrome." *Current Hypertension Reports* 20 (2): 12. doi:10.1007/s11906-018-0812-z.

Schmidt, J.-S., Schaedlich, K., Fiandanese, N., Pocar, P., and Fischer, B. 2012. "Effects of Di(2-ethylhexyl) Phthalate (DEHP) on Female Fertility and Adipogenesis in C3H/N Mice." *Environmental Health Perspectives*, *120*(8), 1123–1129. https://doi.org/10.1289/ehp.1104016.

Schmidt, N., Page, D., Tiehm, A. 2017. "Biodegradation of Pharmaceuticals and Endocrine Disruptors with Oxygen, Nitrate, Manganese (IV), Iron (III) and Sulfate as Electron Acceptors." *Journal of Contaminant Hydrology* 203 (August): 62–69. doi:10.1016/j.jconhyd.2017.06.007.

Serrano, S. E., Braun, J., Trasande, L., Dills, R., and Sathyanarayana, S. 2014. "Phthalates and Diet: A Review of the Food Monitoring and Epidemiology Data." *Environmental Health*, *13*(1), 43. https://doi.org/10.1186/1476-069X-13-43.

Stojanoska, M. M., Milosevic, N., Milic, N., and Abenavoli, L. 2017. "The İnfluence of Phthalates and Bisphenol A on the Obesity Development and Glucose Metabolism Disorders." *Endocrine*, *55*(3), 666–681. https://doi.org/10.1007/s12020-016-1158-4.

Sui, Y., Meng, Z., Chen, J., Liu, J., Hernandez, R., Gonzales, M. B., Gwag, T., Morris, A. J., and Zhou, C. 2021. "Effects of Dicyclohexyl Phthalate Exposure on PXR Activation and Lipid Homeostasis in Mice." *Environmental Health Perspectives*, *129*(12). https://doi.org/10.1289/EHP9262.

Tandoğan, B., Kuruüzüm-Uz, A., Sengezer, C., Güvenalp, Z., Demirezer, L. Ö., and Nuray Ulusu, N. 2011. "*In vitro* Effects of Rosmarinic Acid on Glutathione Reductase and Glucose 6-Phosphate Dehydrogenase." *Pharmaceutical Biology*, *49*(6), 587–594. https://doi.org/10.3109/13880209.2010.533187.

Tandoğan, B., Ulusu, N. N. 2007. "The Inhibition Kinetics of Yeast Glutathione Reductase by Some Metal Ions." *Journal of Enzyme Inhibition and Medicinal Chemistry* 22 (4): 489–95. doi:10.1080/14756360601162147.

Tandoğan, B., Ulusu, N. N. 2010. "Purification and Kinetics of Bovine Kidney Cortex Glutathione Reductase." *Protein & Peptide Letters* 17 (5): 667–74. doi:10.2174/092986610791112684.

Tang, X., Wu, S., Shen, L., Wei, Y., Cao, X., Wang, Y., Long, C., Zhou, Y., Li, D., Huang, F., Liu, B., and Wei, G. 2018. "Di-(2-ethylhexyl) Phthalate (DEHP)-İnduced Testicular Toxicity through Nrf2-Mediated Notch1 Signaling Pathway in Sprague-

Dawley Rats." *Environmental Toxicology*, *33*(7), 720–728. https://doi.org/10.1002/tox.22559.

Tsai, C.-F., Hsieh, T.-H., Lee, J.-N., Hsu, C.-Y., Wang, Y.-C., Lai, F.-J., Kuo, K.-K., Wu, H.-L., Tsai, E.-M., and Kuo, P.-L. 2014. "Benzyl Butyl Phthalate İnduces Migration, İnvasion, and Angiogenesis of Huh7 Hepatocellular Carcinoma Cells through Nongenomic AhR/G-Protein Signaling." *BMC Cancer*, *14*(1), 556. https://doi.org/10.1186/1471-2407-14-556.

Turan, B., Acan, N. L., Ulusu, N. N., and Tezcan, E. F. 2001. "A Comparative Study on Effect of Dietary Selenium and Vitamin E on Some Antioxidant Enzyme Activities of Liver and Brain Tissues." *Biological Trace Element Research*, *81*(2), 141–152. https://doi.org/10.1385/BTER:81:2:141.

Ulusu, N. N., Acan, N. L., Turan, B., and Tezcan, E. F. 2003. "Inhibition of Glutathione Reductase by Cadmium Ion in Some Rabbit Tissues and the Protective Role of Dietary Selenium." *Biological Trace Element Research*, *91*(2), 151–156. https://doi.org/10.1385/BTER:91:2:151.

Ulusu, N. N., Turan, B. 2005. "Beneficial Effects of Selenium on Some Enzymes of Diabetic Rat Heart." *Biological Trace Element Research* 103 (3): 207–16. doi:10.1385/BTER:103:3:207.

Wallner, P., Kundi, M., Hohenblum, P., Scharf, S., and Hutter, H.-P. 2016. "Phthalate Metabolites, Consumer Habits and Health Effects." *International Journal of Environmental Research and Public Health*, *13*(7), 717. https://doi.org/10.3390/ijerph13070717.

Wang, Y.-X., Zeng, Q., Sun, Y., You, L., Wang, P., Li, M., Yang, P., Li, J., Huang, Z., Wang, C., Li, S., Dan, Y., Li, Y.-F., and Lu, W.-Q. 2016. "Phthalate Exposure in Association with Serum Hormone Levels, Sperm DNA Damage and Spermatozoa Apoptosis: A Cross-Sectional Study in China." *Environmental Research*, *150*, 557–565. https://doi.org/10.1016/j.envres.2015.11.023.

Xia, B., Zhu, Q., Zhao, Y., Ge, W., Zhao, Y., Song, Q., Zhou, Y., Shi, H., and Zhang, Y. 2018. "Phthalate Exposure and Childhood Overweight and Obesity: Urinary Metabolomic Evidence." *Environment International*, *121*, 159–168. https://doi.org/10.1016/j.envint.2018.09.001.

Yuan, X.-Q., Du, Y.-Y., Liu, C., Guo, N., Teng, X.-M., Hua, X., Yao, Y.-C., Deng, Y.-L., Zeng, Q., Deng, T.-R., and Li, Y.-F. 2020. "Phthalate Metabolites and Biomarkers of Oxidative Stress in the Follicular Fluid of Women Undergoing İn vitro Fertilization." *Science of The Total Environment*, *738*, 139834. https://doi.org/10.1016/j.scitotenv.2020.139834.

Zhang, H., Ben, Y., Han, Y., Zhang, Y., Li, Y., Chen, X. 2022. "Phthalate Exposure and Risk of Diabetes Mellitus: Implications from a Systematic Review and Meta-Analysis." *Environmental Research*, *204*, 112109. https://doi.org/10.1016/j.envres.2021.112109.

Zhong, L., Holmgren, A. 2000. "Essential Role of Selenium in the Catalytic Activities of Mammalian Thioredoxin Reductase Revealed by Characterization of Recombinant Enzymes with Selenocysteine Mutations." *Journal of Biological Chemistry*, *275*(24), 18121–18128. https://doi.org/10.1074/jbc.M000690200.

Zhu, M., Huang, C., Ma, X., Wu, R., Zhu, W., Li, X., Liang, Z., Deng, F., Wu, J., Geng, S., Xie, C., and Zhong, C. 2018. "Phthalates Promote Prostate Cancer Cell Proliferation through Activation of ERK5 and p38." *Environmental Toxicology and Pharmacology*, *63*, 29–33. https://doi.org/10.1016/j.etap.2018.08.007.

Chapter 8

Epigenetic Effects of Phthalates

Unzile Yaman[1] and Belma Kocer-Gumusel[2,*]
[1]Katip Celebi University, Faculty of Pharmacy,
Department of Toxicology, İzmir, Turkey
[2]Lokman Hekim University, Faculty of Pharmacy,
Department of Toxicology, Ankara, Turkey

Abstract

Phthalates are plasticizers that are used as an additive in many customer products and the production of polyvinyl chloride (PVC) plastics. Due to their abundant use, they are ubiquitously present in the environment and can easily enter the human body by dermal absorption, ingestion, or inhalation. It is also possible to be exposed to those chemicals throughout life, especially in critical developmental periods such as pregnancy, lactation, and puberty. It is well-known that phthalates may act as an endocrine disruptor and cause toxicity primarily in the reproductive and neuroendocrine systems. Multiple *in vitro*, *in vivo*, and human studies showed a certain relation with conditions such as infertility, obesity, cancer, and diabetes. Epigenetics are important mechanisms in the ability of phthalates to modify health and disease, and this group of chemicals is epigenetically toxic. Over the last decade, research on the mechanisms underlying phthalate toxicity has expanded. Increasing evidence suggests that the epigenetic mechanisms including DNA methylation, histone modifications, and miRNAs play an important role in pathologies as a result of estrogenic, anti-estrogenic, and anti-androgenic effects of phthalates. These mechanisms are also involved in developmental programming and epigenetic alterations in early life may cause serious adverse effects on both exposed and future generations. This chapter will

* Corresponding Author's Email: belma.gumusel@lokmanhekim.edu.tr.

In: Phthalates: Environmental and Health Effects
Editors: Müfide Aydoğan Ahbab and Nurhayat Barlas
ISBN: 978-1-68507-970-3

focus on epigenetic modifications caused by phthalates and the outcomes of these possible toxic effects.

Keywords: Phthalates, epigenetic, endocrine disruptor, DNA methylation, histone modifications, miRNAs

Introduction

Phthalates are commonly used plasticizers and are produced abundantly. They are mainly used in consumer products for their ability to increase material flexibility. It is known that di-(2ethylhexyl) phthalate (DEHP) is produced by over 2 million tons annually worldwide. Different phthalates have different molecular weights, and their usage is decided according to their molecular weight. Phthalates with high molecular weight such as DEHP and diisononyl phthalate (DiNP) are more likely to be used in the production of raincoats, shoes, food packaging, toys and medical equipment. However, low molecular weight phthalates such as dimethyl phthalate (DMP), diethyl phthalate (DEP) and dibutyl phthalate (DBP) are preferred for the production of personal care products, insecticides and covering (Schettler 2006). The molecular weight of phthalates is also important for their route of exposure and metabolism. While oral exposure is the main route of high molecular weight phthalates, low molecular weight phthalates enter the body dermally or by inhalation. The elimination half-life of these plasticizers may change between hours and days and they generally show no tendency to accumulate in the body. However, in the studies, it has been shown that different phthalates exist at different levels in the urine of participants of the studies due to their abundant usage (Kavlock et al. 1996, Diamanti-Kandarakis et al. 2009, Schug et al. 2011, Latini, Verrotti, and De Felice 2004). Such worldwide production and exposure to phthalates raised concerns about health concerns both for human and environment.

Over the last decades, studies have shown that phthalate exposure is associated with various disorders. Although reproductive disorders are the main concern, it is well known that exposure to these chemicals is also associated with the case of hormone-dependent cancers, obesity, neurotoxicity and even autoimmunity. Given that people are frequently exposed to these chemicals throughout their life, it is important to understand their mechanism of toxicity. Evidence has shown that phthalates and their metabolites may cause oxidative stress since they generally undergo oxidation reactions (van't

Erve et al. 2019). It is also known that phthalates are also epigenetically toxic chemicals. Thus, exposure to plasticizers may change gene expressions by altering DNA methylation, histone modifications (acetylation, methylation, phosphorylation, ubiquitination, sumoylation and ADP ribosylation) and/or miRNA levels and these changes may cause adverse health effects (Dolinoy, Huang, and Jirtle 2007). Alterations in gene expressions that are caused by up and down regulations in epigenetic marks may persist throughout life and they may be inherited transgenerationally. These permanent differences may cause neural, immune and endocrine disorders and late-onset diseases such as cancers and diabetes. Underlying mechanisms of these long-lasting effects of endocrine disruptors such as phthalates continue to be enlightened and it is known that they tend to involve in epigenetic programming of gene expressions during the early stages of life. It is also strongly evidenced that cumulative adverse effects of these chemicals could be mediated through epigenetic mechanisms (Kundakovic and Champagne 2011).

In this chapter, we described the relationship between phthalates and different states of pathologies and the role of epigenetic modifications as an underlying mechanism of phthalate toxicity.

Epigenetic Mechanisms

Epigenetics is the science of gene expression and stability changes caused by modifications in chromatin without the changes in DNA sequence. In other words, epigenetics defines the changes in phenotype in the absence of genotypic changes. All molecular changes that occur on DNA or on histones that are closely related to DNA without any change in the nucleotide sequence are considered epigenetic modifications. Epigenetic modifications can determine which gene is transcribed, worked or silenced. For example, skin cells and liver, brain, lung or muscle cells contain the same genome, however, they all have quite different metabolisms and phenotypes that are entirely due to the fact that the same gene is transcribed in different ways (some genes are silenced and some are turned on) through epigenetic modifications. DNA methylation-mediated epigenetic silencing is one way to silence genes, resulting in transcriptional differences. This silencing mechanism also explains why identical twins carry the same genome but do not have the same phenotype (Portela and Esteller 2010, Talbert and Henikoff 2006).

Most of the epigenetic modifications occur in sperm and oocytes. All epigenetic markers such as methylated or acetylated locations are deleted and rewritten during meiosis, called "reprogramming." Reprogramming allows the fertilized cells to start "from scratch" and create their own epigenetic changes (Kanherkar, Bhatia-Dey, and Csoka 2014, Teperek and Miyamoto 2013). However, some epigenetic modifications in the reproductive cells can sometimes escape this reprogramming process and be transferred to the next generation. The state of epigenetic traces (e.g., DNA methylation, histone acetylation) occurring in the chromatin and being transmitted stably through gametes is called transgenerational epigenetic inheritance.

The aim of epigenetic mechanisms is to regulate gene expressions by creating reversible modifications on DNA, histones and miRNAs. These modifications cause alterations in the packaging of the genome and the interpretation of the genes which plays a vital role in the persistence of physiological, biochemical and molecular reactions.

DNA Methylation

Transcription begins in promoter regions that are rich in CG sequences. These cytosine and guanine bases are linked by phosphate, are called as CpG region and the regions on DNA that are rich in CpG are called as CpG islands. DNA methylation is the attachment of a methyl (-CH_3) group to DNA bases. Although DNA methylation could be seen on other bases, it generally occurs by a methyl group binding to the fifth carbon of cytosine (5-mC). The majority of methylation reactions are located in the promoter region of DNA due to the density of CpG regions. A gene becomes silent when is methylated (Gibney and Nolan 2010, Teperek and Miyamoto 2013).

DNA methyl transferase (DNMT) enzyme family transfers a methyl group from S-adenosylmethionine (SAM) to the cytosine in DNA. There are 4 major enzymes (DNMT1, DNMT3A, DNMT3B, DNMT3C) and a cofactor (DNMT3L) to maintain methylation, de novo methylation (reprogramming) and protect the cell from retrotransposon activity (Jin, Li, and Robertson 2011).

DNMT1 is the main enzyme of the DNMT family. It primarily ensures that both strands in DNA are fully methylated and thus DNA methylation profile continues during the replication. DNMT3A and DNMT3B are involved in the methylation of new CpG sites which are mainly responsible for de novo methylation. DNMT3C is responsible for silencing the promoter regions of new retrotransposons formed in male germ cells by methylation. DNMT3L is expressed in oocytes during the preservation of hereditary characteristics from the mother. There is also DNMT2 which is responsible for RNA methylation in embryonic stem cells. In addition to the DNMT family, enzymes containing methyl binding sites such as methyl CpG binding protein 2 (MeCP2), methyl-CpG binding domain protein 1 (MBD1), methyl-CpG binding domain protein 2 (MBD2) and methyl-CpG binding domain protein 4 (MBD4) may be attached to the methylated DNA, preventing the binding of transcription factors, thereby silencing the gene (Raddatz et al. 2013, Bogdanović and Veenstra 2009).

Histone Modifications

Nuclear DNA does not appear free and linear state. It is highly condensed and wrapped around histones. This structure consisting of histones and wrapped DNA is called as nucleosome or histone octamer. The N-terminal of the outer surface of the nucleosome is positively charged and this structure contains 15-38 amino acids known as histone tail. Each nucleosome contains two of each of the H2A, H2B, H3 and H4 histones and 147 DNA base pairs which are folded 1.7 times in an octamer structure (Mariño-Ramírez et al. 2005). Amino acids in the N-terminal tails of these four significant histones are subjected to enzyme-catalyzed post-translational modifications to regulate gene expression and DNA-histone interactions (Morales and Richard-Foy 2000). These modifications are methylation, phosphorylation, acetylation, deamination, ADP ribosylation, tail cutting, proline isomerization, ubiquitination and sumoylation. In many species, histone H3 acetylation occurs at lysine (K) 9, 14, 18, 23 and 56; methylation occurs at arginine (R) 2 and K 4, 9, 27, 36 and 79; phosphorylation occurs at serine (S) positions 10, 28, threonine (T) 3 and 11. In addition, it is known that H4 acetylation occurs at K 5, 8, 12 and 16; methylation occurs at R3 and K20; phosphorylation occurs at S1 (Wood et al. 2009).

Modifications in histone proteins are vital since they are important for forming heterochromatin (compressed) and euchromatin (open) forms of the chromatin structure, thus regulating gene expression, DNA replication, recombination and genome stability (Bannister and Kouzarides 2011). In the case of hyperacetylation of histones such as H3K4, H3K36, H3K79 trimethylation and H3K9 acetylation histone modifications are added to or removed from the structure by regulatory enzymes called writers and erasers (Kouzarides 2007). These enzymes regulate transcription by recognizing specific amino acids containing certain groups. Histone modifications allow the regulation of chromatin structure by changing the electrostatic charge, and thus the formation of the substituent group is recognized by different adapter proteins (Sadakierska-Chudy and Filip 2015). In other words, histone modifications regulate access of transcription factors to promoter regions and interactions between DNA and octamer. Therefore, quantitative measurement of different histone modifications may provide important information about epigenetic regulation in pathophysiological conditions and may contribute to the development of therapies targeting histone-regulating enzymes (Deb et al. 2016).

Non-Coding RNAs

Non-coding RNAs play a key role in gene expression and ensuring genomic stability. Regulatory roles of short non-coding RNAs such as tRNAs, rRNAs, small nuclear RNAs (snRNAs) and small nucleolar RNAs (snoRNAs) are well known. snRNAs generally are derived from larger RNA precursors and microRNAs (miRNAs), short interfering RNAs (siRNAs), PIWI-interacting RNAs (piRNAs) and repeat-associated RNAs (rasiRNAs) are included in this group.

In recent years, the most studied non-coding RNAs are miRNAs due to their recent discovery as post-transcriptional regulators. These short (19-22 nucleotides), endogenous, single-stranded, non-coding RNAs regulate approximately 30% of the genes (Lewis et al. 2003). miRNAs are non-coding RNA molecules regulating the expression of many genes by suppressing translation in the post-translational stage or by directly inducing mRNA degradation with the RNA interfering silencing junction. In addition, miRNAs regulate the translational efficiency or stability of the targeted mRNA in gene silencing. The effect of miRNA on the target sequence depends on the ratio of base pairing between miRNA and mRNA. In the case of no match, miRNA suppresses the translation of mRNA; when the opposite, miRNA cleaves and degrades the mRNA.

siRNAs have similar nucleotide lengths but differ from miRNAs since they are double-stranded RNAs. miRNAs have a maturation pathway in which their biogenesis begins in the nucleus by RNA polymerase II. Transcription products in the nucleus form the hairpin structured pri-miRNAs. These pri-miRNAs are converted to pre-miRNAs with a length of 70-120 bases by RNAse III enzyme. pre-miRNAs are transported to the cytoplasm by exportin

5 and transformed into mature miRNAs by interacting with an endonuclease named Dicer.

Recent studies showed that miRNAs may be associated with various pathology because of the abnormal expressions of specific miRNAs in some cases. For example, miR-223-3p upregulation was shown in the patient having prostate cancer (Wei et al. 2014). Since miRNAs can also be detectable in circulation, they may be used as biomarker in some diseases such as cancer, autoimmune diseases and neuropathologies.

Phthalates and Epigenetic Effects

As mentioned above epigenetic mechanisms are vital for developmental activities and diseases. Environmental chemicals such as phthalates may affect the expression of genes and such genes may be inherited to the next generation by the mechanism of epigenetic modifications. Especially in the last decade, researchers have been stated that the changes caused by phthalates on the epigenetic fingerprints may cause different states of pathologies such as reproductive diseases, obesity, cancer, neurotoxicity and autoimmunity (Singh and Li 2012).

Reproductive Toxicity of Phthalates and Epigenetic Mechanisms

In mammalian cells, while DNA methylation patterns in somatic cells are fixed, embryos in the preimplantation process are broadly reprogrammed. Mammalian sperms and oocytes have high methylation status until fertilization. Both paternal and maternal genome undergoes passive demethylation during fertilization. Subsequently, de-novo methylation begins throughout the whole genome. Exposure to phthalates at any stage of this delicate process may disturb the methylation and cause abnormal epigenetic changes In gametes, embryos or early germ cells (Jin, Li, and Robertson 2011).

The main metabolite of DEHP, monoethyl hexyl phthalate (MEHP), is shown that it may change genome-wide and gene-specific methylation during *in vitro* maturation of oocytes which resulted in hypomethylation both in DNA and the expression of H3K4me2 (Zhang et al. 2018). Exposure to DEHP in the gestational period may result in hypermethylation in F1 female mice while it causes hypomethylation in F3 generation (Rattan et al. 2019). It is also important to state that DEHP exposure during early embryonic development may lead to abnormal methylation patterns gene specifically, especially in Stra8 and Lhx8 which are responsible for the retinoic acid synthesis and is a transcription factor for the establishment of newborn mouse ovary, respectively, thus perturbing early folliculogenesis (Zhang et al. 2015, Zhang et al. 2014). Although the mechanism of these changes is still not clear, according to a study conducted in adult female rats exposed to DBP, phthalates may change methylation profiles by downregulating the expression of DNMT1 in the ovary (Liu and Craig 2019).

Expression of only the maternal or paternal allele in the offspring is called gene imprinting. Methylation patterns directly affect imprinting by activating or silencing the parental alleles. Sometimes, differentially methylated regions (DMRs) on the genes may resist demethylation during fertilization and may be inherited to the next generation instead of elimination or production of own imprinting. This resistance may affect the transfer of nutrients through placenta which is an important mechanism for fetal intrauterine growth, postnatal behavior and brain development (Reik and Walter 2001). It is known that DEHP exposure during the intrauterine period may cause lower methylation of maternal insulin-like growth factor 2 receptor (Igf2r) and paternally expressed gene 3 (Peg3) in mice which are related to the lower expression of Dnmt3b and Dnmt3 (Li et al. 2014a). Similarly, a miRNAseq analysis of the effect of DEHP on the expression profile of miRNA in mouse ovary found that differentially expressed miRNAs could regulate ovarian development by targeting the MAPK, mTOR, FoxO signaling pathways (Zhang et al. 2019). It is also important to state that phthalate exposure presents a nonmonotonic dose-response relationship which means low-dose exposure may cause obvious epigenetic changes than higher doses (Liu et al. 2018).

During spermatogenesis, DNA in the sperm head goes through an extensive remodeling process and this change causes changes in the whole nuclear structure and epigenetic profile. In normal spermatogenesis, spermatid genome conformation is changed by acetylation of histones and DNA helix structure begins to open with the help of topoisomerases. Subsequently, the transition proteins (TNP1 and TNP2) and the protamines bind to DNA. When spermatogenesis ends, protamine heterochromatin in the sperm genome are formed 6-20 times more tightly than histone heterochromatin. For this reason, sperm DNA is transcriptionally inactive and thus becomes more resistant to nuclease attacks or factors such as radiation or toxic chemicals (Casas and Vavouri 2014).

Most epigenetic regulation occurs during spermatogenesis and conception. Therefore, any intervention at this stage may cause serious problems resulting in male infertility. Apart from DNA packaging in the spermatid nucleus, epigenetic reprogramming occurs at nearly every step of spermatogenesis. These rearrangements are closely related to many processes such as chromosome structure and XY sex chromosome formation. In gene silencing studies, it has been determined that sex-specific genes are expressed in different ways during sperm formation. Many epigenetic regulators such as DNA methyltransferases, histone-modifying enzymes and regulatory enzymes play an active role in these processes. However, it has been understood that DNA methylation profiles in sperm differ between individuals as well as in sperm belonging to the same person, thus providing the emergence of phenotypic characters that will completely distinguish the next generation from each other (Sasaki and Matsui 2008). Epigenetic modifications in sperm are made mainly by DNA methylation. It has been understood that DNA methylation errors are associated with genetic diseases such as immunodeficiency, centromere instability and facial anomalies syndrome (ICF), Rett syndrome[1], X-linked dominant or non-specific mental retardation, and alpha thalassemia. These diseases caused by epigenetic changes may be associated with gene errors (eg LIT1, H19, IGF2, UBE3A), deletions (15q-13) or uniparental disomy.

Oligoasthenoteratospermia and oligospermia phenotypes mostly occur due to gene expression disorders, which in turn caused by DNA methylation. However, in a study, it was determined that sperm DNA methylation profiles were significantly and consistently different in fertile and infertile men (Hazzouri et al. 2000). In addition, it has been reported in the same study that the quality of embryos formed during *in vitro* fertilization is determined by sperm DNA, and accordingly, embryo quality can be predicted by looking at sperm DNA methylations in normospermic men. Therefore, by considering the role of epigenetic modifications in sperm formation and maturation, some disorders in the epigenetic profiles of infertile men may be the answer to unexpected complications observed during infertility treatment (Marques et al. 2008).

---

[1] Rett syndrome is a rare genetic disorder that affects brain development, resulting in severe mental and physical disability. Mutations of the methyl-CpG binding protein 2 (MECP2) gene are the most prevalent cause of classical Rett cases.

On the other hand, post-translational histone modifications play an active role in the maintenance of sperm cell functions. The structure of chromatin must become loose, which is accomplished by histone acetylation for transcription factors to attach to DNA. Likewise, the gene is silenced as a result of deacetylation. Testis-specific bromodomain (Brdt) recognizes acetylated lysines at the N-terminus of the histone tail, resulting in a healthy or diseased phenotype. Changes in H3K9 acetylation and H3K27 trimethylation reduce Brdt expression and thus prevent healthy sperm formation. Lack of demethylation in H3K9 reduces TNP1 and P1 expressions. Thus, during sperm production, histones cannot be fully located and DNA damage occurs (Steilmann et al. 2010). A decrease in H4 acetylation in spermatids results in abnormal spermatogenesis and infertility. In addition, the disruption of acetylation of important genes, especially in histone H4K12ac, during spermatogenesis disrupts the structure of sperm chromatins, causing this disorder to continue in the zygote, thus transferring it to the next generation (Paradowska et al. 2012).

Histone methyltransferase or histone demethylase plays an important role in gene activation and silencing by providing methylation and demethylation of lysines in H3 and H4. H3K4 methylation ensures gene expression, while H3K9 and H3K27 trimethylation are responsible for gene silencing and the formation of heterochromatin. During meiosis, many mono, di, or trimethylations occur in H3K4, H3K9 and H3K27, but especially H3K9 must be demethylated at the end of meiosis (Kouzarides 2007).

The JMDA1 gene is the most important epigenetic regulator expressed in testicles, responsible for the demethylation of monomethyl and trimethyl H3K9. It has no activity on trimethyl H3K9. It shows its transcriptional activity by decreasing histone methylation and increasing histone acetylation. Its deficiency causes infertility by causing apoptosis and inhibition of spermatid elongation. The deficiency of this gene changes not only the methylation but also the acetylation profile. Expressions of vital genes for chromatin condensation, such as TNP1, TNP2, P1 and P2, are dependent on acetylation, and therefore their rates in spermatids are significantly reduced in JMDA1 deficiency (Shi et al. 2004).

Phthalates, Lipid Metabolism and Epigenetic Mechanisms

Phthalates may dysregulate lipid metabolism by several pathways and this may lead to obesity which has become an epidemic with over 4 million people dying each year as a result of being overweight according to the World Health Organization. Over the last decade, studies have shown the most important mechanism leading to the impairment of lipid metabolism is the stimulation of peroxisome proliferator-activated receptors (PPARs) by a peroxisome proliferator such as phthalates. PPARs are a novel subfamily of nuclear receptors dimerizing with retinoid X receptor (RXR) and they bind to PPAR-responsive DNA regulatory elements controlling the expression of genes involved in adipogenesis, glucose, lipid, and cholesterol metabolism. The activation of RXR-PPAR dimer stimulates oxidation reactions, hereby, this results in different levels of expression of several genes regulating fat cell development (Thomas et al. 2011).

Recent studies showed that these changes in PPAR metabolism may also be epigenetically inherited. To mention transgenerational inheritance, the expression patterns should persist at least two generations after the first exposure. Recent literature highlighted that the obesogenic effects of phthalates are based on their ability to bind nuclear receptors. These receptors are responsible for methyl and acetyltransferases which regulate gene expression and alter the epigenetic profile (Ozgyin et al. 2015). As the main target of obesogens and the key element of adipogenesis, PPARs are prone to be affected by environmental exposure. However, studies focusing on the epigenetic effects of phthalates from the point of view of lipid metabolism are limited.

In a gestational exposure study, it is shown that DBP exposure may cause obesity significantly in F3 generation and these changes are epigenetically inherited by the change of sperm epimutations in F1 generation (Manikkam et al. 2013). This is a great example of male obesity that may be transmitted through the female germline. In a study, it is shown that urinary monocarboxy-isononyl phthalate (MCNP) concentrations were positively associated with sperm mitochondria DNA copy number which is an epigenetic biomarker for cellular oxidative stress, lipid metabolism and environmental exposure (Huffman et al. 2018). According to another study investigating benzyl butyl phthalate (BBP) to regulate the mesenchymal stem cell epigenome to drive adipogenesis, BBP exposure enhanced lipid accumulation and adipogenesis in a dose-dependent manner. In addition to this, it enhances H3K9 acetylation while decreasing H3K9 dimethylation and its mechanism is through PPARγ, as PPARγ knockdown led to decreased H3K9ac and rescued H3K9me2 during BBP exposure (Sonkar, Powell, and Choudhury 2016). Similarly in another study investigating gestational and lactational exposure to phthalates, it is found that gene expression of lipid metabolism pathways was altered in testis and adipose tissue of male offsprings and DNA methylation was increased at two loci of lipid metabolism genes. Differentially methylated CpGs were also identified in a tissue-specific manner (Moody et al. 2019). miR-34a-5p is a key miRNA involved in obesity and regulates the downstream pathway. Sirtuin is also a significant epigenetic modulator for lipid metabolism. It is found that BBP exposure resulted in increased expression levels of miR-34a-5p with an associated increase in adipogenesis. BBP was also significantly decreased the sirtuins in gene expression levels which means BBP exposure demonstrated the involvement of epigenetic regulation by altering the expression patterns of miR-34a-5p and perturbing the energy homeostasis of the differentiating adipocytes by altering sirtuin activity, resulting in increased adipogenesis, subsequently, obesity.

In utero DEHP exposure may also induce fat accumulation and alter lipid metabolism and adipogenesis in F1 generation by changing mRNA expression levels of T-box 15 and Gpc4 which are developmental genes which are important in obesity and body fat distribution (Gu et al. 2016). Human studies also show similar results. In a study conducted with children of pregnant women, it has been shown that perinatal exposure to phthalates (monobutyl phthalate (MBP), mono-isobutyl phthalate (MiBP), monobenzyl phthalate (MBzP)) changes skin thickness and BMI (please add open name)-for age in girls and those changes are positively associated with H19 methylation (Bowman et al. 2019).

There are also studies aiming to investigate the ability of phthalates to bind estrogenic receptors and the relation of epigenetic mechanisms. However, this connection still remains unclear and mechanistic studies are needed.

Phthalates and Epigenetic Mechanisms in Other Pathologies

In recent years, studies about epigenetic pathways in various pathologies such as reproductive diseases, cancer, developmental and behavioral dysfunctions, obesity, diabetes and even immune diseases have been conducted for the purpose of understanding the underlying mechanism and finding specific gene regulations having a role in the transgenerational inheritance of these states. Although gene-specific epigenetic regulations are gradually being understood in some specific cancer types, more detailed and mechanistic data are needed to clarify these mechanisms for other common diseases.

Phthalates lead to various types of cancer because of their xenoestrogenic properties. In the case of phthalate exposure, (abundant production and usage), the exposure starts prenatally and continues during the whole life. It is known that early-life exposure to environmental chemicals such as phthalates is considered for the increasing prevalence of not only reproductive diseases but also other pathologies such as cancer. DEHP has been known as an estrogen receptor agonist which may promote the cell proliferation of estrogen receptor α-positive (ERα-positive) breast cancer cells. In a recent study, researchers found that DEHP exposure may cause alterations in genome-wide DNA methylation in breast cancer cell line MCF-7 cells. According to this study, DEHP affects the ERs in the cells by hypermethylation of 700 genes and hypomethylation of 221 genes through the Wnt/β-catenin signaling pathway (Chou et al. 2019). Similarly, phthalates and their metabolites may increase methylation levels to elevate ADAM33 gene expression which is a transmembrane glycoprotein that mediates changes in cell adhesion and plays an important role in cancer progression (Yang et al. 2018). In addition, it was shown that DEHP exposure may induce global DNA hypermethylation with selective upregulation of DNMT1 which means it may potentially induce the epigenetic alterations that might increase the risk of breast cancer (Ghosh et al. 2022). As mentioned above DEHP has reproductive toxicity, especially for male reproductive organs, therefore, it may induce pathological changes in the prostate as well. In a study, it was found that DEHP exposure changed the DNA methylation of six prostate carcinogenesis-related genes (ESR2/GSTP1/NKX3.1/PSCA/PTGS2/Rassf1a), increased methylation levels of the promoter CpG site and PSCA mRNA expression which is an important biomarker of prostate cancer (Xia et al. 2018).

High molecular weight phthalates such as DEHP, BBP and their monoesters are known to be related to allergies, asthma, wheezing, hay fever, itchy rashes, and eczema. Phthalates are presumed to cause oxidative stress and induce inflammatory cytokines by changing the expression of specific genes. Especially DEHP and BBP are associated with alterations of the response of T helper type 2 (Th2) by suppressing IFN-α/IFN-β expressions via epigenetic regulation (Kuo et al. 2013). In a study about phthalate exposure and DNA hypomethylation of TNFα which is an inflammatory cytokine that may increase asthma risk in children, differential methylation patterns have been observed in three genes-androgen receptors, TNFα, and IL-4 causing asthma in children by inducing allergic inflammation (Wang et al. 2015). Similarly, another study involving a transgenerational asthma model in mice showed that maternal exposure to BBP may cause allergic airway inflammation in the F2 generations by inducing global DNA hypermethylation in CD4+ T cells (Jahreis et al. 2018).

Phthalate-induced epigenetic modifications play a crucial role in behavioral pathologies through gene expression regulation. Especially prenatal/postnatal exposure to phthalates may cause behavioral dysregulation by inducing peripheral or neuronal inflammation via global hypomethylation in DNA and decreasing DNMT1 expressions. Those changes may aggravate autism-like symptoms and inflammation in adulthood through epigenetic regulation (Nadeem et al. 2021). The most commonly used phthalate DEHP is metabolized into MEHP, and it represents the toxic effects of DEHP. In an *in vitro* study, MEHP exposure upregulated the expression of mRNA of choline acetyl transferase, a marker for cholinergic neurons, and downregulated tyrosine hydroxylase, a marker for dopaminergic neurons, suggesting that exposure to MEHP may affect neuron differentiation (Chen et al. 2011). A low molecular weight phthalate, DBP exposure affects neuroprotection by upregulating the aromatase and reducing the expression of phosphate CREB and BDNF which are the important neuroprotective proteins in the hippocampus (Li et al. 2014b). It is also important to state that, these epigenetic modifications in the brain may be transgenerationally inherited. It was shown that prenatal and postnatal DEHP exposure may modify nonsocial behaviors in F3 generation (Quinnies et al. 2015, Quinnies et al. 2017). In a similar study, researchers found that these transgenerational effects of DEHP exposure may be related to the changes in expression of both nuclear estrogen receptor genes (Esr1 and Esr2), that were either up-or down-regulated in the amygdala in a dose- and sex-specific manner (Goldsby, Wolstenholme, and Rissman 2017).

Conclusion

Phthalates, as the most abundant endocrine disruptors with exposure across all life stages, are a key concern for transgenerational effects. Emerging evidence indicates that epigenetic mechanisms have the potential for understanding the toxicity and developing biomarkers to predict risk and susceptibility to possible developing diseases. It is still important to note that epigenetic fingerprints vary across individuals. Thus, more detailed and mechanistic studies are urgently needed in order to better understand the phthalate exposure to these disease-associated epigenetic alterations. Forming an in-depth understanding and knowledge base for such processes will enable more precise predictions of the harmful potential of phthalates, as well as more targeted and effective disease prevention initiatives.

References

Bannister, A. J. and Tony, K. 2011. "Regulation of chromatin by histone modifications." *Cell Research* 21 (3):381-395.

Bogdanović, O. and Veenstra, G. J. C. 2009. "DNA methylation and methyl-CpG binding proteins: developmental requirements and function." *Chromosoma* 118 (5):549-565.

Bowman, A., Peterson, K. E., Dolinoy, D. C., Meeker, J. D., Sánchez, B. N., Mercado-Garcia, A., Téllez-Rojo, M. M., and Goodrich, J. M. 2019. "Phthalate exposures, DNA methylation and adiposity in Mexican children through adolescence." *Frontiers in Public Health*:162.

Casas, E. and Vavouri, T. 2014. "Sperm epigenomics: challenges and opportunities." *Frontiers in Genetics* 5:330.

Chen, T., Yang, W., Li, Y., Chen, X., and Xu, S. 2011. "Mono-(2-ethylhexyl) phthalate impairs neurodevelopment: inhibition of proliferation and promotion of differentiation in PC12 cells." *Toxicology Letters* 201 (1):34-41.

Chou, C. K., Huang, H. W., Yang, C. F., Dahms, H. U., Liang, S. S., Wang, T. N., Kuo, P. L., Hsi, E., Tsai, E. M., and Chiu, C. C. 2019. "Reduced camptothecin sensitivity of estrogen receptor-positive human breast cancer cells following exposure to di (2-ethylhexyl) phthalate (DEHP) is associated with DNA methylation changes." *Environmental Toxicology* 34 (4):401-414.

Deb, M., Sengupta, D., Kar, S., Rath, S. K., Roy, S., Das, G., and Patra, S. K. 2016. "Epigenetic drift towards histone modifications regulates CAV1 gene expression in colon cancer." *Gene* 581 (1):75-84.

Diamanti-Kandarakis, E., Bourguignon, J. P., Giudice, L. C., Hauser, R., Prins, G. S., Soto, A. M., Zoeller, R. T., and Gore, A. C. 2009. "Endocrine-disrupting chemicals: an Endocrine Society scientific statement." *Endocrine Reviews* 30 (4):293-342.

Dolinoy, D. C., Huang, D., and Jirtle, R. L. 2007. "Maternal nutrient supplementation counteracts bisphenol A-induced DNA hypomethylation in early development." *Proceedings of the National Academy of Sciences* 104 (32):13056-13061.

Ghosh, K., Chatterjee, B., Nalla, K., Behera, B., Mukherjee, A., and Kanade, S. R. 2022. "Di-(2-ethylhexyl) phthalate triggers DNA methyltransferase 1 expression resulting in elevated CpG-methylation and enrichment of MECP2 in the p21 promoter *in vitro*." *Chemosphere*:133569.

Gibney, E. R. and Nolan, C. M. 2010. "Epigenetics and gene expression." *Heredity* 105 (1):4-13.

Goldsby, J. A., Wolstenholme, J. T., and Rissman, E. F. 2017. "Multi-and transgenerational consequences of bisphenol A on sexually dimorphic cell populations in mouse brain." *Endocrinology* 158 (1):21-30.

Gu, H., Liu, Y., Wang, W., Ding, L., Teng, W., and Liu, L. 2016. "In utero exposure to di-(2-ethylhexyl) phthalate induces metabolic disorder and increases fat accumulation in visceral depots of C57BL/6J mice offspring." *Experimental and Therapeutic Medicine* 12 (6):3806-3812.

Hazzouri, M., Pivot-Pajot, C., Faure, A. K., Usson, Y., Pelletier, R., Sèle, B., Khochbin, S., and Rousseaux, S. 2000. "Regulated hyperacetylation of core histones during mouse spermatogenesis: involvement of histone-deacetylases." *European Journal of Cell Biology* 79 (12):950-960. doi: https://doi.org/10.1078/0171-9335-00123.

Huffman, A. M., Wu, H., Rosati, A., Rahil, T., Sites, C. K., Whitcomb, B. W., and Richard Pilsner, J. 2018. "Associations of urinary phthalate metabolites and lipid peroxidation with sperm mitochondrial DNA copy number and deletions." *Environmental Research* 163:10-15.

Jahreis, S., Trump, S., Bauer, M., Bauer, T., Thürmann, L., Feltens, R., Wang, Q., Gu, L., Grützmann, K., Röder, S., Averbeck, M., Weichenhan, D., Plass, C., Sack, U., Borte, M., Dubourg, V., Schüürmann, G., Simon, J. C., von Bergen, M., Hackermüller, J., Eils, R., Lehmann, I., and Polte, T. 2018. "Maternal phthalate exposure promotes allergic airway inflammation over 2 generations through epigenetic modifications." *Journal of Allergy and Clinical Immunology* 141 (2):741-753.

Jin, B., Li, Y., and Robertson, K. D. 2011. "DNA methylation: superior or subordinate in the epigenetic hierarchy?" *Genes & cancer* 2 (6):607-617.

Kanherkar, R. R., Bhatia-Dey, N., and Csoka, A. B. 2014. "Epigenetics across the human lifespan." *Frontiers in cell and developmental biology* 2:49.

Kavlock, R. J., Daston, G. P., DeRosa, C., Fenner-Crisp, P., Gray, L. E., Kaattari, S., Lucier, G., Luster, M., Mac, M. J., Maczka, C., Miller, R., Moore, J., Rolland, R., Scott, G., Sheehan, D. M., Sinks, T., and Tilson, H. A. 1996. "Research needs for the risk assessment of health and environmental effects of endocrine disruptors: a report of the US EPA-sponsored workshop." *Environmental Health Perspectives* 104 (suppl 4): 715-740.

Kouzarides, T. 2007. "Chromatin modifications and their function." *Cell* 128 (4):693-705.

Kundakovic, M., and Champagne, F. A. 2011. "Epigenetic perspective on the developmental effects of bisphenol A." *Brain, Behavior, and Immunity* 25 (6):1084-1093.

Kuo, C. H., Hsieh, C. C., Kuo, H. F., Huang, M. Y., Yang, S. N., Chen, L. C., Huang, S. K., and Hung, C. H. 2013. "Phthalates suppress type I interferon in human plasmacytoid dendritic cells via epigenetic regulation." *Allergy* 68 (7):870-879.

Latini, G., Verrotti, A., and De Felice, C. 2004. "Di-2-ethylhexyl phthalate and endocrine disruption: a review." *Current Drug Targets-Immune, Endocrine & Metabolic Disorders* 4 (1):37-40.

Lewis, B. P., Shih, I. H., Jones-Rhoades, M. W., Bartel, D. P., and Burge, C. B. 2003. "Prediction of mammalian microRNA targets." *Cell* 115 (7):787-798.

Li, L., Zhang, T., Qin, X. S., Ge, W., Ma, H. G., Sun, L. L., Hou, Z. M., Chen, H., Chen, P., Qin, G. Q., Shen, W., and Zhang, X. F. 2014a. "Exposure to diethylhexyl phthalate (DEHP) results in a heritable modification of imprint genes DNA methylation in mouse oocytes." *Molecular Biology Reports* 41 (3):1227-1235.

Li, X., Jiang, L., Cheng, L., and Chen, H. 2014b. "Dibutyl phthalate-induced neurotoxicity in the brain of immature and mature rat offspring." *Brain and Development* 36 (8):653-660.

Liu, J., Wang, W., Zhu, J., Li, Y., Luo, L., Huang, Y., and Zhang, W. 2018. "Di (2-ethylhexyl) phthalate (DEHP) influences follicular development in mice between the weaning period and maturity by interfering with ovarian development factors and microRNAs." *Environmental Toxicology* 33 (5):535-544.

Liu, X., and Craig, Z. R. 2019. "Environmentally relevant exposure to dibutyl phthalate disrupts DNA damage repair gene expression in the mouse ovary." *Biology of Reproduction* 101 (4):854-867.

Manikkam, M., Tracey, R., Guerrero-Bosagna, C., and Skinner, M. K. 2013. "Plastics derived endocrine disruptors (BPA, DEHP and DBP) induce epigenetic transgenerational inheritance of obesity, reproductive disease and sperm epimutations." *PloS one* 8 (1):e55387.

Mariño-Ramírez, L., Kann, M. G., Shoemaker, B. A., and Landsman, D. 2005. "Histone structure and nucleosome stability." *Expert Review of Proteomics* 2 (5):719-729.

Marques, C. J., Costa, P., Vaz, B., Carvalho, F., Fernandes, S., Barros, A., and Sousa, M. 2008. "Abnormal methylation of imprinted genes in human sperm is associated with oligozoospermia." *Molecular Human Reproduction* 14 (2):67-74. doi: 10.1093/molehr/gam093.

Moody, L., Hernández-Saavedra, D., Kougias, D. G., Chen, H., Juraska, J. M., and Pan, Y. X. 2019. "Tissue-specific changes in Srebf1 and Srebf2 expression and DNA methylation with perinatal phthalate exposure." *Environmental Epigenetics* 5 (2):dvz009.

Morales, V., and Richard-Foy, H. 2000. "Role of histone N-terminal tails and their acetylation in nucleosome dynamics." *Molecular and Cellular Biology* 20 (19):7230-7237.

Nadeem, A., Al-Harbi, N. O., Ahmad, S. F., Alhazzani, K., Attia, S. M., Alsanea, S., Alhoshani, A., Mahmood, H. M., Alfardan, A. S., and Bakheet, S. A. 2021. "Exposure to the plasticizer, Di-(2-ethylhexyl) phthalate during juvenile period exacerbates autism-like behavior in adult BTBR T+ tf/J mice due to DNA hypomethylation and enhanced inflammation in brain and systemic immune cells." *Progress in Neuro-Psychopharmacology and Biological Psychiatry* 109:110249.

Ozgyin, L., Erdős, E., Bojcsuk, D., and Balint, B. L. 2015. "Nuclear receptors in transgenerational epigenetic inheritance." *Progress in Biophysics and Molecular Biology* 118 (1-2):34-43.

Paradowska, A. S., Miller, D., Spiess, A. N., Vieweg, M., Cerna, M., Dvorakova-Hortova, K., Bartkuhn, M., Schuppe, H. C., Weidner, W., and Steger, K. 2012. "Genome wide identification of promoter binding sites for H4K12ac in human sperm and its relevance for early embryonic development." *Epigenetics* 7 (9):1057-1070. doi: 10.4161/epi.21556.

Portela, A., and Esteller, M. 2010. "Epigenetic modifications and human disease." *Nature Biotechnology* 28 (10):1057-1068.

Quinnies, K. M., Doyle, T. J., Kim, K. H., and Rissman, E. F. 2015. "Transgenerational effects of di-(2-ethylhexyl) phthalate (DEHP) on stress hormones and behavior." *Endocrinology* 156 (9):3077-3083.

Quinnies, K. M., Harris, E. P., Snyder, R. W., Sumner, S. S., and Rissman, E. F. 2017. "Direct and transgenerational effects of low doses of perinatal di-(2-ethylhexyl) phthalate (DEHP) on social behaviors in mice." *PLoS One* 12 (2):e0171977.

Raddatz, G., Guzzardo, P. M., Olova, N., Fantappié, M. R., Rampp, M., Schaefer, M., Reik, W., Hannon, G. J., and Lyko, F. 2013. "Dnmt2-dependent methylomes lack defined DNA methylation patterns." *Proceedings of the National Academy of Sciences* 110 (21):8627-8631.

Rattan, S., Beers, H. K., Kannan, A., Ramakrishnan, A., Brehm, E., Bagchi, I., Irudayaraj, J., and Flaws, J. A. 2019. "Prenatal and ancestral exposure to di (2-ethylhexyl) phthalate alters gene expression and DNA methylation in mouse ovaries." *Toxicology and Applied Pharmacology* 379:114629.

Reik, W., and Walter, J. 2001. "Genomic imprinting: parental influence on the genome." *Nature Reviews Genetics* 2 (1):21-32.

Sadakierska-Chudy, A., and Filip, M. 2015. "A comprehensive view of the epigenetic landscape. Part II: Histone post-translational modification, nucleosome level, and chromatin regulation by ncRNAs." *Neurotoxicity Research* 27 (2):172-197.

Sasaki, H., and Matsui, Y. 2008. "Epigenetic events in mammalian germ-cell development: reprogramming and beyond." *Nature Reviews Genetics* 9 (2):129-140. doi: 10.1038/nrg2295.

Schettler, T. 2006. "Human exposure to phthalates via consumer products." *International Journal of Andrology* 29 (1):134-139.

Schug, T. T., Janesick, A., Blumberg, B., and Heindel, J. J. 2011. "Endocrine disrupting chemicals and disease susceptibility." *The Journal of Steroid Biochemistry and Molecular Biology* 127 (3-5):204-215.

Shi, Y., Lan, F., Matson, C., Mulligan, P., Whetstine, J. R., Cole, P. A., Casero, R. A., and Shi, Y. 2004. "Histone demethylation mediated by the nuclear amine oxidase homolog LSD1." *Cell* 119 (7):941-953.

Singh, S., and Li, S. S. 2012. "Epigenetic effects of environmental chemicals bisphenol A and phthalates." *International Journal of Molecular Sciences* 13 (8):10143-10153.

Sonkar, R., Powell, C. A., and Choudhury, M. 2016. "Benzyl butyl phthalate induces epigenetic stress to enhance adipogenesis in mesenchymal stem cells." *Molecular and Cellular Endocrinology* 431:109-122.

Steilmann, C., Cavalcanti, M. C., Bartkuhn, M., Weidner, W., Steger, K., and Paradowska, A. 2010. "1887 The interaction of modified histones with the bromodomain testis-specific (BRDT) gene and its mRNA level in sperm of fertile and infertile men." *Journal of Urology* 183 (4S):e733-e733. doi: doi:10.1016/j.juro.2010.02.1840.

Talbert, P. B., and Henikoff, S. 2006. "Spreading of silent chromatin: inaction at a distance." *Nature Reviews Genetics* 7 (10):793-803.

Teperek, M., and Miyamoto, K. 2013. "Nuclear reprogramming of sperm and somatic nuclei in eggs and oocytes." *Reproductive Medicine and Biology* 12 (4):133-149.

Thomas, K., Sung, D. Y., Chen, X., Thompson, W., Chen, Y. E., McCarrey, J., Walker, W., and Griswold, M. 2011. "Developmental patterns of PPAR and RXR gene expression during spermatogenesis." *Front Biosci (Elite Ed)* 3:1209-20.

Van T Erve, T. J., Rosen, E. M., Barrett, E. S., Nguyen, R., Sathyanarayana, S., Milne, G. L., Calafat, A. M., Swan, S. H., and Ferguson, K. K. 2019. "Phthalates and phthalate alternatives have diverse associations with oxidative stress and inflammation in pregnant women." *Environmental Science & Technology* 53 (6):3258-3267.

Wang, I. J., Karmaus, W. J., Chen, S. L., Holloway, J. W., and Ewart, S. 2015. "Effects of phthalate exposure on asthma may be mediated through alterations in DNA methylation." *Clinical Epigenetics* 7 (1):1-9.

Wei, Y., Yang, J., Yi, L., Wang, Y., Dong, Z., Liu, Z., Ou-yang, S., Wu, H., Zhong, Z., Yin, Z., Zhou, K., Gao, Y., Yan, B., and Wang, Z. 2014. "MiR-223-3p targeting SEPT6 promotes the biological behavior of prostate cancer." *Scientific Reports* 4 (1):1-8.

Wood, C., Snijders, A., Williamson, J., Reynolds, C., Baldwin, J., and Dickman, M. 2009. "Post-translational modifications of the linker histone variants and their association with cell mechanisms." *The FEBS Journal* 276 (14):3685-3697.

Xia, B., Wang, Y., Wang, X., Wu, J., Song, Q., Sun, Z., and Zhang, Y. 2018. "In utero and lactational exposure of DEHP increases the susceptibility of prostate carcinogenesis in male offspring through PSCA hypomethylation." *Toxicology Letters* 292:78-84.

Yang, P. J., Hou, M. F., Tsai, E. M., Liang, S. S., Chiu, C. C., Ou-Yang, F., Kan, J. Y., Peng, C. Y., and Wang, T. N. 2018. "Breast cancer is associated with methylation and expression of the a disintegrin and metalloproteinase domain 33 (ADAM33) gene affected by endocrine-disrupting chemicals." *Oncology Reports* 40 (5):2766-2777.

Zhang, J. N., Zhang, R. Q., Liu, J. C., Li, L., Shen, W., and Sun, X. F. 2019. "Di (2-ethylhexyl) phthalate exposure impairs the microRNAs expression profile during primordial follicle assembly." *Frontiers in Endocrinology* 10:877.

Zhang, T., Li, L., Qin, X. S., Zhou, Y., Zhang, X. F., Wang, L. Q., De Felici, M., Chen, H., Qin, G. Q., and Shen, W. 2014. "Di(2-ethylhexyl) phthalate and bisphenol A exposure impairs mouse primordial follicle assembly *in vitro*." *Environmental and Molecular Mutagenesis* 55 (4):343-353.

Zhang, X. F., Zhang, T., Han, Z., Liu, J. C., Liu, Y. P., Ma, J. Y., Li, L., and Shen, W. 2015. "Transgenerational inheritance of ovarian development deficiency induced by maternal diethylhexyl phthalate exposure." *Reproduction, Fertility and Development* 27 (8):1213-1221.

Zhang, Y., Wang, T., Lan, M., Zang, X. W., Li, Y. L., Cui, X. S., Kim, N. H., and Sun, S. C. 2018. "Melatonin protects oocytes from MEHP exposure-induced meiosis defects in porcine." *Biology of Reproduction* 98 (3):286-298.

Chapter 9

Recent Advances in Biosensor Based Phthalate Analysis

Erkut Yılmaz[1], Müfide Aydoğan Ahbab[2], Fatma Gülruy Aydın[3] and Emir Alper Türkoğlu[4,*]

[1]Department of Biotechnology, Faculty of Science and Letters, Aksaray University, Aksaray, Turkey
[2]Hamidiye Vocational School of Health Services, University of Health Sciences Turkey, İstanbul, Turkey
[3]Department of Pharmacognosy, Faculty of Pharmacy, University of Health Sciences Turkey, İstanbul, Turkey
[4]Department of Pharmaceutical Biotechnology, Faculty of Pharmacy, University of Health Sciences Turkey, İstanbul, Turkey

Abstract

Phthalates are found in dye solvents, glues, cosmetics, personal care products, detergents and a variety of other products in addition to their use as plasticizers. For this reason, phthalates are called as "the everywhere chemical." Despite their wide usage, people are becoming more concerned about phthalates with the better understanding of their effects on organisms and the environment. Many regulatory agencies classify phthalates as priority pollutants and restrict or prohibit their use. This situation has increased the importance of monitoring and detection of phthalates in various environmental and biological matrices including drinking and surface water, soil, sediment, indoor and/or outdoor air, food, milk, blood, saliva and urine. Conventional phthalate detection methods are usually laboratory-based and have significant drawbacks such as the requirement for appropriate laboratory settings and skilled

* Corresponding Author's Email: alper.turkoglu@sbu.edu.tr.

In: Phthalates: Environmental and Health Effects
Editors: Müfide Aydoğan Ahbab and Nurhayat Barlas
ISBN: 978-1-68507-970-3

workers as well as long test periods, expensive and complex processes. As a result, there is a growing interest on novel analytical techniques for detecting phthalates from a variety of media in a cost-effective, fast, selective and sensitive manner. Biosensor-based methods present alternatives to conventional detection approaches for the determination of phthalate from complicated matrixes. This chapter focuses on the recent approaches for biosensor-based phthalate analysis including biological/biomimetic recognition elements and novel sensor materials such as nanomaterials, metal-organic frameworks and micro or nano electromechanical systems.

Keywords: phthalate, biosensor, biorecognition, nanomaterial

Introduction

Plasticizers are used as additives in the plastic industry, primarily in polyvinyl chloride (PVC) products. The most common plasticizers used in the manufacture of plastic materials are phthalate acid esters (PAEs), which have a common chemical structure, dialkyl or alkyl/aryl esters of 1,2-benzene-dicarboxylic acid. The alkyl groups can vary in length and structure (linear, branched or cyclic ring). The differences of alkyl groups enable PAEs to have their unique physical and chemical properties (National Research Council 2009). Although more than 25 PAEs are used in commercial applications, the most common PAEs used in consumer products are dimethyl phthalate (DMP), diethyl phthalate (DEP), dibutyl phthalate (DBP), diisobutyl phthalate (DIBP), benzylbutyl phthalate (BzBP), dicyclohexyl phthalate (DCHP), di(2-ethylhexyl) phthalate (DEHP), di-n-octyl phthalate (DnOP), di-isononyl phthalate (DINP) and di-isodecyl phthalate (DIDP) (Wang et al. 2019).

PAEs are divided into two classes based on their molecular weight. Low-molecular-weight PAEs with one to four carbons in alkyl groups, such as DMP, DEP, DBP, and DIBP, are primarily utilized as solvents for finishing products in cosmetics, pharmaceuticals, waxes, inks, and insecticides. High-molecular-weight PAEs contain five or more carbons in alkyl groups such as DEHP, DOP, and DINP (Schettler 2006). PAEs are produced in high volumes and primarily used in construction and buildings, polyethylene terephthalate (PET) bottles, plastic tubing, food packaging and processing materials, automobiles, containers, vinyl toys, vinyl floor coverings and building products (Zhang et al. 2021).

Production of PAEs has increased since the 1930s due to their ubiquitous usage. The annual global production of phthalate was 4.7 million tons in 2006 and has reached approximately 6-8 million tons (Net et al. 2015, Baloyi et al. 2021, Seyoum and Pradhan 2019). Since PAEs are not covalently bound to the molecular structure of the plastic polymer, they can leach, migrate and evaporate into the environment. Several studies have revealed that PAEs have contaminated air, terrestrial, and aquatic environments, including seas, rivers, lakes, and sediments (Lee et al. 2019, Peijnenburg and Struijs 2006, Adeniyi et al. 2011, Cho et al. 2014, Paluselli et al. 2018, Fromme et al. 2002, Yang et al. 2014), as well as the biota (Wofford et al. 1981, Staples et al. 1997, Munshi et al. 2013).

For the past two decades, phthalates have been to the focus of public attention due to their possible harmful effects on both wildlife and human health. Many of the phthalates or PAEs and their metabolites are classified as endocrine disrupting chemicals (EDCs), which can interfere with the normal hormonal activities of organisms (La Merrill et al. 2020). The PAEs enter the body through the gastrointestinal tract, dermal absorption, inhalation and prenatal administration. PAEs exhibit toxic, carcinogenic, mutagenic and teratogenic effects on animals and humans even at low concentrations (Chang et al. 2021). Initially, human and animal studies have focused on the adverse effects of PAEs on the reproductive system and endocrine-disrupting activities (Parks et al. 2000, Gray Jr et al. 2000, Akingbemi et al. 2001, Duty et al. 2003, Latini et al. 2003, Mylchreest et al. 2002, Jarfelt et al. 2005, Moore et al. 2001, Sun and Liu 2017). Subsequently, human exposure to PAEs has been associated to cardiovascular disease, neurological disorders, thyroid disease, and respiratory system diseases (Trasande et al. 2013, Muscogiuri and Colao 2017, Zhao et al. 2016, Morgenstern et al. 2017, Weng et al. 2017, Ku et al. 2015, Hoppin et al. 2013, Chopra et al. 2014).

Certain PAEs have been subject to regulation, restriction and prohibition by the governments due to relevance to the risks they pose to human health, especially to children. BBP, DBP, DEHP, DINP, DIDP, DNOP and DIBP are restricted to a maximum content of 0.1% by weight of the plasticized material (individually or in combination) by The Registration, Evaluation, Authorisation and Restriction of Chemicals (REACH) regulation for all consumer products placed in the EU market (ECHA 2018). In Europe, DEHP was the first PAE restricted in toys and other childcare articles, which can directly contact to the mouths of children in 1999, and then five PAEs (DBP, BBP, DINP, DIDP and DNOP) in these articles that are available above 0.1% concentration were banned (Eureach_Annex_Xvii 2007). The Consumer

Product Safety Commission (CPSC) also banned the products that contain more than 0.1% by weight of certain phthalates used in toys for children and childcare articles in the US (CPSC 2017).

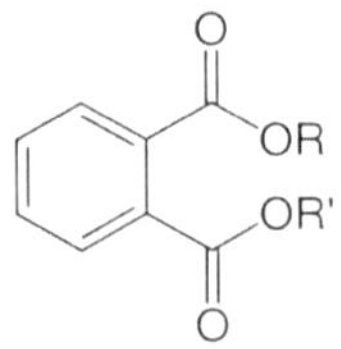

Figure 1. General structure of phthalates.

Phthalates are also found in paint solvents, adhesives, cosmetics, personal care products, detergents and many other products in addition to their use as plasticizers. Therefore, phthalates are also called as "the everywhere chemical." Figure 1 depicts their general chemical structure. Here R and R' are generally 4-15 carbon length alkyl groups.

Phthalates are not chemically bound to materials they are added to, so they migrate to contacted matrix (Wormuth et al. 2006). The melting and boiling points of phthalate esters range from roughly -25°C to 5°C and 230°C to 486°C, respectively. Most phthalates are liquid at room temperature and are low-vapor-pressure compounds (Staples et al. 1997).

Methods and Techniques for Phthalate Analysis

Phthalates are classified as priority pollutants and are restricted/prohibited by many regulatory agencies (the United States Consumer Product Safety Commission 2008, (EU) 2018/2005 2018) due to their possible carcinogenic, endocrine-disrupting, and mutagenic effects (De Jong et al. 2020). Therefore, detecting phthalate levels in cosmetics, food, textiles and a variety of other products is critical.

Phthalates have been commonly analyzed by several techniques such as (i) gas chromatography (GC) in combination with mass spectrometry detector (MS) and/or GC/MS (capillary) (Otezo et al. 2015, Berset and Etter-Holzer 2001), electron capture detector (ECD) (Jaworek et al. 2013) and photo-ionization detection (FID) (Net et al. 2015), (ii) liquid chromatography using UV (Salazar-Beltrán et al. 2017), DAD (Shen et al. 2007, Xie et al. 2016) and mass spectrometric detection (Sendón et al. 2012). GC-MS ensures higher resolution and effective separation of phthalates from several environmental matrices. LC-UV is a cost-effective technique that provides satisfactory performance and comparable limits of detection (LODs) than those analyzed by LC-MS and GC-MS methods (Otezo et al. 2015, Zaater et al. 2014).

Conventional analysis methods for phthalate determination can be divided into two categories: spectrometric methods and chromatographic methods.

Spectrometric Methods

UV-visible spectrophotometry and fluorescence spectroscopy are commonly used spectrometric approaches for phthalate analysis (Qureshi et al. 2016). The presence of phthalate esters can also be detected using FT-Raman spectroscopy. With the use of appropriate reference samples, quantitative determination of the phthalate ester content is also possible (Nørbygaard and Berg 2004). Even though spectroscopic methods can provide relatively faster and less expensive measurements, they are not commonly used due to selectivity and sensitivity issues. Even so, in some cases, they can provide promising results. DiScenza et al. (2019) reported a cyclodextrin-promoted fluorescence modulation method to detect phthalate esters from human saliva with a promising selectivity and sensitivity with 89 nM LOD value. Even though there have been some promising results, the lack of separation and preconcentration steps limits the use of direct spectroscopic methods for phthalate analysis.

Chromatographic Methods

Gas chromatography and high-performance liquid chromatography are the most commonly used chromatographic methods for phthalate analysis. These methods are highly selective and sensitive owing to the use of various solid phase extraction techniques and extremely sensitive mass detectors. As a result, they are primarily used as gold standards for the analysis of phthalates. Although phthalate detection is generally a laboratory-based process, this procedure possesses some disadvantages due to the need for special laboratory conditions and trained personnel, long test times, as well as expensive and complex processes (Zia et al. 2013). Therefore, some analytical techniques for detecting phthalates in various environments in a cost-effective, rapid, selective, and sensitive manner are required (Zhou et al. 2017). Besides traditional methods, there are rapidly developing novel methods to detect phthalates from various media, such as bioassays, arrays, and biosensors.

Bioassays and Arrays

The most common immunoassay strategies for quantifying PAEs are enzyme-linked immunoassay (ELISA), biotin-streptavidin enzyme-linked immunoassay (BA-ELISA), fluorescence immunoassay (FIA), chemiluminescence immunoassay (CL-ELISA) and time-resolved immunoassay (TRFIA) (Li and Zhang 2020). By the use of novel nanoparticles with enzymes and antibodies, these relatively new bioanalytical tools offer promising expectations.

Biosensors

Biosensors are basic analytical tools that mimic the functional, structural, and compositional characteristics of nature. The recognition part of the biosensor reacts the with analyte, and this interaction is readily converted to a signal by a transducer for signal production (Guo 2012). These devices have provided valuable solutions because of their rapid, cost-effective, and user-friendly nature. Biosensors exhibit many advantages over conventional methods due to their sensitive, simple and label-free analysis potentials, even in complicated matrices (Türkoğlu 2021). Sensor-based analysis systems can contain a wide range of materials, including biological materials, organic/inorganic chemicals, membranes, nanoparticles, microfluidics, semiconductors, and fluorescent materials. Therefore, these studies necessitate a highly multidisciplinary approach (Hu and Niemeyer 2019).

A biosensor platform is composed of two main parts: a recognition system and a physicochemical transducer. The recognition system provides the selectivity needed for the measurements while the transducer translates the physico-chemical changes that occur during the recognition event to an optical, electrical, thermal or magnetism-based read-outs. The design of the recognition part is a crucial step in the preparation of biosensors. Some biomolecules, including antibodies, proteins, enzymes and nucleic acids, act as recognition elements for biosensor (Türkoğlu 2021). These structures are known for their selectivity toward a variety of target molecules. Even though they all have unique recognition capabilities, they are also easily degraded (Palchetti and Mascini 2010).

Aptamers are known as synthetic antibodies and these biostructures can be used for the preparation of biological recognition elements. Aptamers are single-stranded oligonucleotides that fold into certain structures and bind to specific targets. They are generally produced via a multistep enrichment process from a library of thousands of DNA, RNA, or synthetic XNA (Eremeeva et al. 2019).

Molecularly imprinted polymers (MIPs) are artificial receptors that mimic natural biorecognition mechanisms for target structures such as ions, molecules, supramolecules, and even whole cells (Yilmaz et al. 2017). In general, MIPs are used for phthalate analysis in two different ways, as a preconcentrator via solid-phase extraction, or as a direct recognition element on a variety of sensor surfaces (Bolat et al. 2019, Zhang et al. 2013).

New generation systems and materials have been combined with biosensor systems and/or transducers to increase functionality, sensitivity and selectivity. A variety of nanomaterials has been used as sensor materials due to their unique properties. Their usage as sensor material applies to all transducer types. Their optical properties enhance plasmons and provide flourescent emissions. Quantum dots and metallic nanoparticles like gold and silver have been extensively used for the unique optical properties. Additionally, carbon nanotubes, graphene, and nanowires are commonly used, especially for electrochemical sensors due to their unique electrical properties (Wang 2005).

Metal-organic frameworks (MOFs) are commonly used in optical sensors. MOFs provide an ordered large porous structure with a high metal loading capacity for the sensor systems to which they are attached. MOF-based sensor systems operate by the releasing metal ions from the framework. The released metal ions may cause a color change, affect enzyme activity or change the electrochemical properties of the media to increase the sensor sensitivity (Du et al. 2021).

Micro or nano electromechanical systems (MEMs/NEMs) combine mechanic and electrochemical functionality to the sensor systems to which they are attached. Their use in sensor systems aims miniaturization and enhanced electrical properties. So, they are generally used in electrochemical systems (Zhu et al. 2020).

Biosensors have been largely categorized due to their transducers such as optical, electrochemical, mass-based and calorimetric (Türkoğlu 2021). Therefore, biosensor-based phthalate analysis described below has been evaluated within this framework. It can clearly be said that literature seems to focus on the phthalate derivatives illustrated in Figure 2 for the biosensor-based studies. These derivatives are also the most common and widely used phthalate derivatives in various industries. In human-beings, their exposure routes are known as ingestion, inhalation and dermal exposure (Rastogi et al. 2006). Due to these exposure routes, it is important to detect phthalates even in gaseous media. The COVID-19 pandemic appears to have an indirect effect on phthalate exposure. Some recent studies have linked PAE in face masks to the risk of inhalation exposure (Xie et al. 2022, Wang et al. 2022).

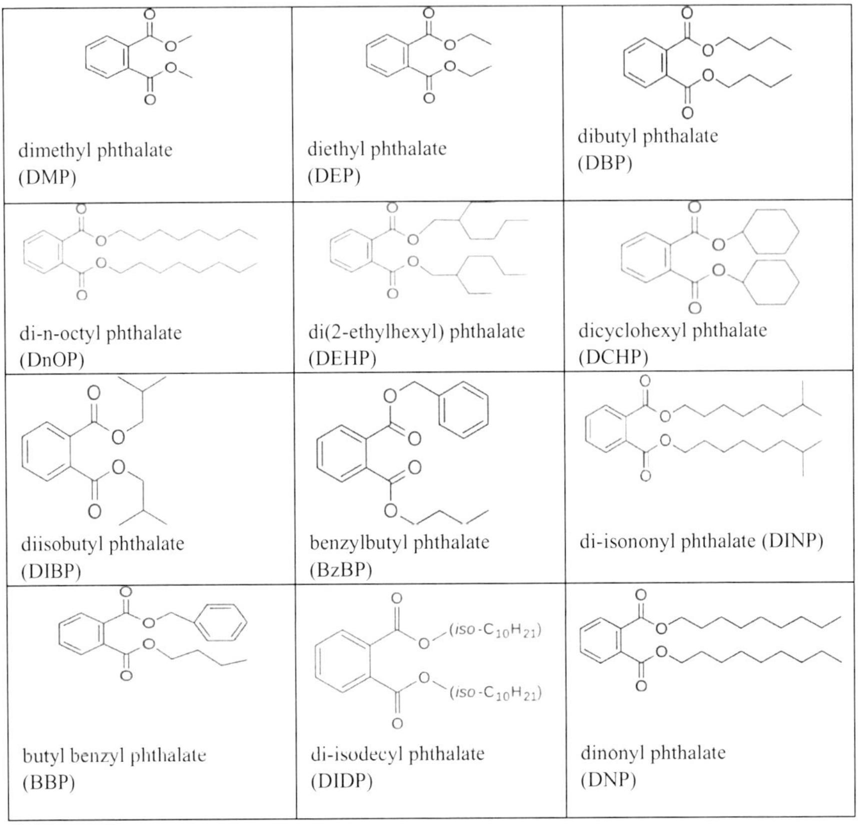

Figure 2. Most common PAEs in biosensor based studies.

Phthalate Analysis via Biosensors

Mass Sensitive Biosensors

The piezoelectric effect was first investigated in the 19th century by Pierre and Jacques Curie (Xu et al. 2021) and it has been applied since the 20th century (Tichý et al. 2010). The piezoelectric effect can be introduced as the ability of voltage or current generation in response to applied mechanical stress. Piezoelectric-based materials function as oscillators that operate according to the piezoelectric effect principles and can detect interactions occurring on their surfaces. Therefore, this type of material is quite suitable for biosensor-based applications. The piezoelectric biosensors are widely used devices that measure the bio-interaction between the target molecule and the ligand in an easy, cost-effective, and label-free manner (Pohanka 2017). Quartz crystal microbalance (QCM) is an extensively applied piezoelectric transducer (Du et al. 2013) that converts mass change into an electrical signal (Ngo et al. 2014). QCM biosensors are used in medical diagnosis, environmental monitoring, food science, quantification and interaction of biomolecules because of their cost-effective, portable, selective (Sener et al. 2010, Özgür et al. 2013), sensitive, rapid, and reliable features (Park and Lee 2018). In addition to their widespread use, QCM biosensors are also commonly preferred for the effective detection of phthalates (Habuka et al. 2005, Habuka and Yamaha 2007).

There are some investigations about the QCM-based phthalate detection in the literature (Wang et al. 2013, Zhang et al. 2015, Chen et al. 2017). Being liquid at room temperature, DBP is also present as a low concentration vapor. It is urgent need to detect DBP due to its potent estrogenic effect. In order to obtain easy, rapid and sensitive DBP detection, Au decorated porous ZnO microspheres were produced for the recognition part of the QCM sensor. Crystalline structures of the Au decorated ZnO microspheres were analyzed by X-ray diffraction (XRD) analysis, and structural and morphological investigations were characterized by scanning electron microscopy (SEM). Fabricated sensor detected DBP with a high sensitivity of 38.1 Hz/ppb in the range from 2 to 30 ppb with theoretically calculated detection limit below 1 ppb. According to ZnO based and Au decorated ZnO based QCM studies for DBP detection, Au contributed high sensitivity and selectivity to target compound. After the long-term stability test, the sensor also showed acceptable long term stability features (Zhang et al. 2015).

Chen et al. (2017) examined the wireless-electrodeless QCM with dissipation (QCM-D) as a sensing system to monitor DBP vapor concentration in the air. Nickel hydroxide based nanofilm was constructed as sensing element for QCM system. Structure and morphology of nano-$Ni(OH)_2$ were investigated by SEM. According to SEM results, morphology of $Ni(OH)_2$ was sheet like. Optimization of film thickness was performed to obtain more recognition sites and higher sensitivity. Thickness of the nanofilm analysis indicated that optimal nanofilm thickness was preferred as 3.46 $\mu g/mm^2$. The wireless-electrodeless QCM-D biosensor detected DBP in the range of 0.4-40 ppb with the detection limit of 0.4 ppb. The sensor also demonstrated a sensitivity of 7.3 Hz/ppb for DBP.

A QCM based gas sensor with the polyaniline nanofibers as sensing element was developed to detect DBP in the air. Polyaniline nanofiber was synthesized and coated on the surface of QCM. Characterization of the polyaniline nanofiber-based film was performed by SEM and Brunauer-Emmett-Teller (BET) analysis. SEM result showed that polyaniline nanofiber-based film included nanowires with a diameter of about 60 nm. The surface area and pore size of the nanofilm were obtained from BET results as 14.18 m^2/g and 60.25 nm, respectively. The polyaniline nanofiber based QCM sensor detected DBP in the range from 0.02 to 0.4 ppm. LOD of the sensor was calculated as 0.02 ppm. Sensing response and selectivity characteristics of the QCM sensor were studied with the use of 0.8 ppm DBP, 8 ppm ethanol, 8 ppm acetone and 8 ppm acetaldehyde. The sensor possessed a very high selectivity to DBP despite the 10 times higher concentration of ethanol, acetone and acetaldehyde. Moreover, the response of the sensor was almost same during 60-day long-term stability studies (Wang et al. 2013).

Electrochemical Biosensors

Electrochemical biosensors are the most commonly used and widely available types in the biosensor market (Zhao and Jiang 2010) due to their desired detection limits, high sensitivity, cost effective, user-friendly, simple instrumentation and portable features (Srivastava et al. 2020). Electrochemical biosensors are simple devices that detect electrical changes of electrochemical processes on an electrode surface (Jain et al. 2022). Antibodies and/or antibody fragments, proteins, nucleotide and carbohydrate-based bio-molecules, phages and artificial cells have been examined in the design of recognition element for electrochemical biosensors (Kuralay et al. 2013,

Cesewski and Johnson 2020). Different transducers have been proposed for electrochemical biosensor. Amperometric, potentiometric, conductometric, field effect and/or ion change transducers have been used according to type of analyte (Matter et al. 2021). Amperometric and potentiometric transducers have been commonly used types of electrochemical biosensors (Narlawar et al. 2022). Electrochemical biosensors have been extensively employed in molecular and medical diagnosis (Hua et al. 2022, Sadique et al. 2021, Hasan et al. 2021), fermentation process (Villalonga et al. 2022), water quality monitoring (Tsopela et al. 2016), detection of drugs (Kurbanoglu et al. 2020), military operations (Colozza et al. 2019) and environmental monitoring (Chung et al. 2021). Combining the advantages of electrode modification with sensitive electroanalytical techniques, the detection of phthalates has become a popular topic in recent years (El-Sharif et al. 2022).

Noh et al. (2015) produced a microfluidic device with preconcentration channels and micellar electrokinetic separation combined to glassy carbon electrode. Proposed biomimetic sensor probe successfully preconcentrated, separated and detected trace amounts of the phthalates such as DEP, DBP, BBP, DEHP and DCHP. The detection limits for all analytes were determined to be between 12.5 and 35.2 pM. The proposed method was successfully applied to the analysis of real samples such as manicure, PVC plastics and mammalian cells, paving the way for the development of sex-related disorder analysis strategies.

Bolat et al. (2019) presented a impedimetric MIP-based sensor for DBP recognition and they achieved a low detection limit as 4.5 nM with a imprinting factor of 4.85 via DBP imprinted polypyrrole film on hand-made pencil graphite electrode.

In another study, Zia et al. (2015) reported MEMS based interdigital planar sensor for phthalate detection from aqueous solution. They produced repeated parallel patterns to strength the signal to noise ratio. A self-assembled monolayer of 3-aminopropyltrietoxysilane (APTES) with embedded molecular imprinted polymer (N,N-methlene-bis-acrylamide, methacry-lamide, ammonium persulfate based) was used for selective recognition of DEHP in the range of 1 to 50 ppm.

Annamalai and Vasudevan (2020) reported an enzyme and nanocomposite material based voltametric method with the LOD values in the range of 0.03 to 0.08 nM for DEHP, DEP, DMP, DBP and BBP. Their nanocomposite material consisted of immobilized esterase enzyme, multi-walled carbon nanotubes (MWCNTs), cupper nanoparticles and nafion. The esterase enzyme, that already has the ability to hydrolyze phthalate esters, used in the study was purified from bacteria. The use of modified enzyme on sensor surface provided the required selectivity for the system when the other parts of the composite nano material enhanced sensor response.

Han et al. (2017) proposed an DNA aptamer and electrochemical sensor based total phthalate analysis platform for group-specific to the basic PAE skeleton with a LOD value of 10 pM via voltametric determination on gold electrode. The results showed that SELEX (systematic evolution of ligands by exponential enrichment) enriched DNA aptamers can be used as highly selective affinity material even for highly hydrophobic phthalate molecules.

Optical Sensors

Optical biosensors are a powerful alternative to traditional analytical techniques because of their high precision, sensitivity and small size. Optical based sensors rely on measurement of the change of optical characteristics like polarization and refraction due to the interaction of target molecules with sensing structures. Optic-based biosensors have been performed in the detection of biomarkers, drugs, toxic materials, even viruses and whole cells (Yilmaz et al. 2017, Özgür et al. 2020).

Surface Plasmon Resonance (SPR), imaging SPR (SPRi), localized surface plasmon resonance (LSPR), evanescent wave fluorescence biosensors, bioluminescent optical fibre biosensors, optical waveguide interferometric biosensors, reflectometric interference spectroscopy biosensors, surface-enhanced raman scattering biosensors (SERS) and ellipsometric biosensors are the most common optical biosensors (Pirzada and Altintas 2020).

Optic based sensory systems have been used in the detection of phthalates in recent years. Tang et al. (2018) developed an optical fiber based immunosensing platform for PAEs. Optical fiber was coated with antigens instead of antibodies contrary to their widespread use in the literature. This provided a better protection to fluorescent-labeled antibodies. Fluorescent-labeled antibodies and PAEs solution were mixed thoroughly and pre-reacted at 37°C for 5 minutes. The coated antigen modified probe was inserted in the sample cell and the developed immunosensor was used to detect several PAEs in greenhouse soils with great success.

Moon et al. (2016) offered a very different approach for endocrine disrupting chemicals including phthalic anhydride. Their M13-bacteriophage arrays changed color with exposure to the gaseous phase chemicals. Consequently, all selected EDCs gave a different color due to exposure.

In a study by Lim et al. (2018), a DEHP-specific aptamer was identified, and a quantum dot based aptasensor accompanying portable analyzer was developed. The sensor achieved the detection of DEHP in the range from 0.0005 to 100 ng/mL with a limit of quantitation (LOQ) of 0.5 pg/mL.

Other Sensors

Zhu et al. (2018) produced a colorimetric immunosensor based on horseradish peroxidase and copper-based metal-organic frameworks (Cu-MOFs). For the detection of trace DBP, Cu-MOFs were first applied to the colorimetric immunosensor for signal amplification to improve the sensitivity of method. First, a 96-well plate was coated with phthalate antigen, then DBP and the polyclonal antibody (Ab_1) were added sequently into each well. Then Cu-MOFs labelled second antibody (Cu-MOFs@Ab2) was used as signal amplification for the detection of trace DBP and measured the absorbance change. The established method had LOD of 1 μg/L for DBP. They conducted experiments on river samples, liqueur, red wine, and milk samples and showed that the produced sensor can be used to detect trace contaminations in a variety of samples.

Geng et al. (2012) proposed a fish cell-based biosensor system to detect genotoxicity. The system was particularly useful in detecting the genotoxicity of DEHP. Neverthless the fish cell-based sensor had a serious drawback. It could produce false positive results in response to sodium butyrate and other agents. This situation affected the usability of the system.

Conclusion and Recommendation

All the transduction methods mentioned above have advantages and disadvantages over each other. Furthermore, issues such as non-specific adsorption, low mass transfer rate, insufficient signal/noise ratio, reproducibility and reusability are also essential for sensor-based methods (Morales and Halpern 2018). Fortunately, using highly selective biological and biomimetic materials on transducers can effectively overcome these issues.

Phthalate industry has a tendency to replace lower molecular weighted PAEs with the guidance of the relevant regulations due to lower migration capabilities of higher molecular weighted phthalates (more than 6 carbon backbone). According to reviewed literature, the focus of researchers on low molecular weighted phthalates is quite obvious due to their higher solubility and possibility of greater accumulation on organism and environment. Therefore, increasing attention on analysis of higher molecular weight phthalates seems to be a necessity. Moreover, for biosensing methods, the less water soluble phthalates are challenging due to sensitivity requirements. Phthalates possess a high solubility in lipids and alcohol but a low solubility in water. However, studies on the detection of phthalates with sensors have focused on aqueous media (Bolat et al. 2019).

Phthalate detection from air samples is another area that needs attention in terms of public health. There are only few studies on biosensor-based phthalate determination in air samples. These studies are based on QCM based detections. Although the volatility of phthalates is low, analysis should be performed from air samples, especially in hazardous environments such as plastic production facilities.

Personal protective equipments like face masks are seems to novel target media due to COVID-19 pandemia. Regular and long-term uses of face mask in the pandemia have increased the potantial phthalate exposure risk for human-beings. In this regard, biosensors may be essential analytical tools for rapid, real-time and on-site detection for phthalates in the future.

Lee et al. (2022) evaluated risk assesment of phthalate migration from daily plastic products with gold nanoflower decorated aptasensor for DEHP. Biosensors, which are suitable for online monitoring, can be used as a migration monitoring tool to produce safer materials and evaluate health risk assesment.

The use of nanomaterials for phthalate biosensing is expected to increase in the future. Due to increased sensitivity with the help of nanomaterials, an increased usage of pseudo natural/biomimetic/semi synthetic recognition elements (aptamers, molecular imprinted materials etc.) have been also expected. Although there has been no example yet according to trends in biosensing investigations, Miniaturized Total Analysis System (μTAS) based devices will be the frontier target for multi-analysis of phthalates.

References

Adeniyi, A. A., Okedeyi, O. O. and Yusuf, K. A. 2010. "Flame ionization gas chromatographic determination of phthalate esters in water, surface sediments and fish species in the Ogun river catchments, Ketu, Lagos, Nigeria." *Environmental Monitoring and Assessment* 172 (1-4): 561-569.

Akingbemi, B. T., Youker, R. T., Sottas, C. M., Ge, R., Katz, E., Klinefelter, G. R., Zirkin, B. R. and Hardy, M. P. 2001. "Modulation of rat leydig cell steroidogenic. function by Di(2-Ethylhexyl)Phthalate." *Biology of Reproduction* 65 (4): 1252-1259.

Annamalai, J. and Vasudevan, N. 2020. "Detection of phthalate esters in PET bottled drinks and lake water using esterase/PANI/CNT/CuNP based electrochemical biosensor." *Analytica Chimica Acta* 1135: 175-186.

Baloyi, N. D., Tekere, M., Maphangwa, K. W. and Masindi, V. 2021. "Insights into the prevalence and impacts of phthalate esters in aquatic ecosystems." *Frontiers in Environmental Science* 9: 263.

Berset, J-D. and Etter-Holzer, R. 2001. "determination of phthalates in crude extracts of sewage sludges by high-resolution capillary gas chromatography with mass spectrometric detection." *Journal of AOAC International* 84(2): 383-391.

Bolat, G., Yaman, Y. T. and Abaci, S. 2019. "Molecularly imprinted electrochemical impedance sensor for sensitive dibutyl phthalate (DBP) determination." *Sensors and Actuators B: Chemical,* 299: 127000.

Cesewski, E. and Johnson, B. N. 2020. "Electrochemical biosensors for pathogen detection." *Biosensors and Bioelectronics* 159: 112214.

Chang, W. H., Herianto, S., Lee, C. C., Hung, H. and Chen, H. L. 2021. "The effects of phthalate ester exposure on human health: A review." *Science of The Total Environment,* 786: 147371.

Chen, D., Sun, X., Zhang, K., Fan, G., Wang, Y., Li, G. and Hu, R. 2017. "A Noncontact Dibutyl Phthalate Sensor Based on a Wireless-Electrodeless QCM-D Modified with Nano-Structured Nickel Hydroxide." *Sensors* 17: 1681.

Cho, E., Khim, J., Chung, S., Seo, D. and Son, Y. 2014. "Occurrence of micropollutants in four major rivers in Korea." *Science of The Total Environment* 491-492: 138-147.

Chopra, V., Harley, K., Lahiff, M. and Eskenazi, B. 2014. "Association between phthalates and attention deficit disorder and learning disability in U.S. children, 6-15 years." *Environmental Research* 128: 64-69.

Chung, T. H., Meshref, M. N. A. and Dhar, B. R. 2021. "A review and roadmap for developing microbial electrochemical cell-based biosensors for recalcitrant environmental contaminants, emphasis on aromatic compounds." *Chemical Engineering Journal* 424: 130245.

Colozza, N., Kehe, K., Dionisi, G., Popp, T., Tsoutsoulopoulos, A., Steinrits, D., Moscone, D. and Arduini, F. 2019. "A wearable origami-like paper-based electrochemical biosensor for sulfur mustard detection." *Biosensors and Bioelectronics* 419: 15-23.

Consumer Product Safety Commision. 2017. *Consumer Product Safety Commision: Prohibition of Children's Toys and Child Care Articles Containing Specified Phthalates: Determinations Regarding Certain Plastics.* In Vol. 82, No. 167, edited by U.S. Consumer Product Safety Commission: Federal Register.

De Jong, W. H., T. Borges, R. M. Ion, D. Panagiotakos, E. Testai, T. Vermeire, U. Bernauer, C. Rousselle, Sté Bégué, H. M. Kopperud, M. R. Milana, T. Schmidt, F. Pignatti, E. Stoyanova, K. Volk, R. Bertollini, P. De Voogt, R. Duarte-Davidson, P. Hoet, R. Kraetke, A. Proykova, T. Samaras, M. Scott, R. Slama, M. Vighi, and S.

Zacharo. 2020. "Guidelines on the benefit-risk assessment of the presence of phthalates in certain medical devices covering phthalates which are carcinogenic, mutagenic, toxic to reproduction (CMR) or have endocrine-disrupting (ED) properties." *Regulatory Toxicology and Pharmacology* 111:104546. doi: https://doi.org/10.1016/j.yrtph.2019.104546.

DiScenza, D. J., Smith, M. A., Intravaia, L. E. and Levine, M. 2018. "Efficient Detection of Phthalate Esters in Human Saliva via Fluorescence Spectroscopy." *Analytical Letters* 52: 1-17.

Du, L., Chen, W., Zhu, P., Tian, Y., Chen, Y. and Wu, C. 2021. "Applications of functional metal-organic frameworks in biosensors." *Biotechnology Journal* 16 (2): 1900424.

Du, L., Wu, C., Peng, H., Zou, L., Zhao, L., Huang, L. and Wang, P. 2013. "Piezoelectric olfactory receptor biosensor prepared by aptamer-assisted immobilization." *Sensors and Actuators B: Chemical* 187: 481-487.

Duty, S. M., Singh, N. P., Silva, M. J., Barr, D. B., Brock, J. W., Ryan, L., Herrick, R. F., Christiani, D. C. and Hauser, R. 2002. "The relationship between environmental exposures to phthalates and DNA damage in human sperm using the neutral comet assay." *Environmental Health Perspectives* 111 (9): 1164-1169.

El-Sharif, H. F., Patel, S., Ndunda, E. N. and Reddy, S. M. 2022. "Electrochemical detection of dioctyl phthalate using molecularly imprinted polymer modified screen-printed electrodes." *Analytica Chimica Acta* 1196: 339547.

Eremeeva, E., Fikatas, A., Margamuljana, L., Abramov, M., Schols, D., Groaz, E. and Herdewijn, P. 2019. "Highly stable hexitol based XNA aptamers targeting the vascular endothelial growth factor." *Nucleic Acids Research* 47(10): 4927-4939.

Eureach_Annex_Xvii. 2007. "EUREACH entry 51 and 52 of Annex XVII of the REACH regulation." *O. J. Eur. Commun.* 49 (L396):1-849.

European Union. 2018/2005. 2018. "Commission Regulation (EU) 2018/2005 of 17 December 2018 Amending Annex XVII to Regulation (EC) No 1907/2006 of the European Parliament and of the Council Concerning the Registration, Evaluation, Authorisation and Restriction of Chemicals (REACH) as regards Bis(2-Ethylhexyl) Phthalate (DEHP), Dibutyl Phthalate (DBP), Benzyl Butyl Phthalate (BBP) and Diisobutyl Phthalate (DIBP)."

Fromme, H., Küchler, T., Otto, T., Pilz, K., Müller, J. and Wenzel, A. 2002. "Occurrence of phthalates and bisphenol A and F in the environment." *Water Research* 36(6): 1429-1438.

Geng, D., Zhang, Z. and Guo, H. 2012. "Development of a fish cell biosensor system for genotoxicity detection based on DNA damage-induced trans-activation of p21 gene expression." *Biosensors* 2(3): 318-340.

Gray, L. E. 2000. "Perinatal exposure to the phthalates DEHP, BBP, and DINP, but not DEP, DMP, or DOTP, alters sexual differentiation of the male rat." *Toxicological Sciences* 58(2): 350-365.

Guo, X. 2012. "Surface plasmon resonance based biosensor technique: A review." *Journal of Biophotonics* 5(7): 483-501.

Habuka, H., Tawada, M., Takeuchi, T. and Aihara, M. 2005. "Gas velocity influence on silicon surface organic contamination evaluated using quartz crystal microbalance." *Journal of the Electrochemical Society* 152(11): G862-G866.

Habuka, H. and Yamaha, D. 2007. "Physisorption and Desorption of Diethyl Phthalate and Isopropanol on a Silicon Surface." *Journal of the Electrochemical Society* 154(12): H1031-H1035.

Han, Y., Diao, D., Lu, Z., Li, X., Guo, Q., Huo, Y., Xu, Q., Li, Y., Cao, S., Wang, J., Wang, Y., Zhao, J., Li, Z., He, M., Luo, Z. and Lou, X. 2017. "Selection of group-specific phthalic acid esters binding DNA aptamers via rationally designed target immobilization and applications for ultrasensitive and highly selective detection of phthalic acid esters." *Analytical Chemistry* 89(10): 5270-5277.

Hasan, M. R., Ahommed, M. S., Daizy, M., Bacchu, M. S., Ali, M. R., Al-Mamun, M. R., Aly Saad Aly, M., Khan, M. Z. H. and Hossain, S. I. 2021. "Recent development in electrochemical biosensors for cancer biomarkers detection." *Biosensors and Bioelectronics: X* 8: 100075.

Hoppin, J. A., Jaramillo, R., London, S. J., Bertelsen, R. J., Salo, P. M., Sandler, D. P. and Zeldin, D. C. 2013. "Phthalate exposure and allergy in the U.S. population: Results from NHANES 2005-2006." *Environmental Health Perspectives* 121(10): 1129–1134.

Hu, Y. and Niemeyeri C. M. 2019. "From DNA nanotechnology to material systems engineering." *Advanced Materials* 31(26): 1806294.

Hua, X., Fan, J., Yang, L., Wang, J., Wen, Y., Su, L. and Zhang, X. 2022. "Rapid detection of miRNA via development of consecutive adenines (polyA)-based electrochemical biosensors." *Biosensors and Bioelectronics* 198: 113830.

Jain, U., Saxena, K., Hooda, V., Balayan, S., Singh, A. P., Tikadar, M. and Chauhan, N. 2022. "Emerging vistas on pesticides detection based on electrochemical biosensors - An update." *Food Chemistry* 371: 131126.

Jarfelt, K., Dalgaard, M., Hass, U., Borch, J., Jacobsen, H. and Ladefoged, O. 2005. "Antiandrogenic effects in male rats perinatally exposed to a mixture of di(2-ethylhexyl) phthalate and di(2-ethylhexyl) adipate." *Reproductive Toxicology* 19(4): 505-515.

Jaworek K. and Czaplicka, M. 2013. "Determination of Phthalates in Polymer Materials-Comparison of GC/MS and GC/ECD Methods." *Polímeros: Ciência e Tecnologia* 23(6): 718-724.

Ku, H. Y., Su, P. H., Wen, H. J., Sun, H. L., Wang, C. J., Chen, H. Y., Jaakkola, J. J. K., Wang, S. L. and TMICS Group. 2015. "Prenatal and postnatal exposure to phthalate esters and asthma: a 9-year follow-up study of a taiwanese birth cohort." *PLOS ONE,* 10(4): e0123309.

Kuralay, F., Yılmaz, E., Uzun, L. and Denizli, A. 2013. "Cibacron Blue F3GA modified disposable pencil graphite electrode for the investigation of affinity binding to bovine serum albumin." *Colloids and Surfaces B: Biointerfaces* 110: 270-274.

Kurbanoglu, S., Erkmen, C. and Uslu, B. 2020. "Frontiers in electrochemical enzyme based biosensors for food and drug analysis." *TrAC Trends in Analytical Chemistry*, 124: 115809.

La Merrill, M. A., Vandenberg, L. N., Smith, M. T., Goodson, W., Browne, P., Patisaul, H. B., Guyton, K. Z., Kortenkamp, A., Cogliano, V. J., Woodruff, T. J., Rieswijk, L., Sone, H., Korach, K. S., Gore, A. C., Zeise, L. and Zoeller, R. T. 2020. "Consensus on the key characteristics of endocrine-disrupting chemicals as a basis for hazard identification." *Nature Reviews Endocrinology* 16: 45-57.

Latini, G., De Felice, C., Presta, G., Del Vecchio, A., Paris, I., Ruggieri, F. and Mazzeo, P. 2003. "Exposure to Di(2-ethylhexyl)phthalate in humans during pregnancy: A preliminary report." *Biology of the Neonate* 83(1): 22-24.

Lee, K., Gurudatt, N. G., Heo, W., Hyun, K. A. and Jung, H. I. 2022. "Ultrasensitive detection and risk assessment of di (2-ethylhexyl) phthalate migrated from daily-use plastic products using a nanostructured electrochemical aptasensor." *Sensors and Actuators B: Chemical* 357: 131381.

Lee, Y. M., Lee, J. E., Choe, W., Kim, T., Lee, J. Y., Kho, Y., Kyungho, C. and Zoh, K. D. 2019. "Distribution of phthalate esters in air, water, sediments, and fish in the Asan Lake of Korea." *Environment International* 126: 635-643.

Li, L., and Zhang, M. 2020. "Development of immunoassays for the determination of phthalates." *Food and Agricultural Immunology* 31(1): 303-316.

Lim, H. J., Kim, A. R., Yoon, M. Y., You, Y., Chua, B. and Son, A. 2018. "Development of quantum dot aptasensor and its portable analyzer for the detection of di-2-ethylhexyl phthalate." *Biosensors and Bioelectronics*, 121: 1-9.

Matter, I. A., Darwesh, O. M. and Matter, H. A. B. 2021. "Nanosensors for herbicides monitoring in soil." In A. Amrane, D. Mohan, T. A. Nguyen, A. A. Assadi, & G. Yasin (Eds.), *Nanomaterials for Soil Remediation* (pp. 221–237). Elsevier.

Moon, J. S., Lee, Y., Shin, D. M., Kim, C., Kim, W. G., Park, M., Han, J., Song, H., Kim, K. and Oh, J. W. 2016. "Identification of Endocrine Disrupting Chemicals using a Virus-Based Colorimetric Sensor." *Chemistry-An Asian Journal* 11(21): 3097-3101.

Moore, R. W., Rudy, T. A., Lin, T. M., Ko, K. and Peterson, R. E. 2001. "Abnormalities of sexual development in male rats with in utero and lactational exposure to the antiandrogenic plasticizer di(2-ethylhexyl) phthalate." *Environmental Health Perspectives* 109(3): 229-237.

Morales, M. A. and Halpern, J. M. 2018. "Guide to Selecting a Biorecognition Element for Biosensors." *Bioconjugate Chemistry* 29(10): 3231-3239.

Morgenstern, R., Whyatt, R. M., Insel, B. J., Calafat, A. M., Liu, X., Rauh, V. A., Herbstmanb, J., Bradwin, G. and Factor-Litvak, P. 2017. "Phthalates and thyroid function in preschool age children: Sex specific associations." *Environment International* 106: 11-18.

Munshi, A. B., Karim, N., Shaukat, S., Hashmi, D., Boardman, G. D. and Flick, G. J. 2013. "Toxicity of phthalate esters in fish and shellfish from virginia beach using Matrix Solid Phase Dispersion (MSPD) and GC-MS." *Journal of the Chemical Society of Pakistan* 35(6): 1463-1471.

Muscogiuri, G. and Colao, A. 2017. "Phthalates: new cardiovascular health disruptors?" *Archives of Toxicology* 91(3): 1513-1517.

Mylchreest, E., Sar, M., Wallace, D. G. and Foster, P. M. D. 2002. "Fetal testosterone insufficiency and abnormal proliferation of Leydig cells and gonocytes in rats exposed to di(n-butyl) phthalate." *Reproductive Toxicology* 16(1): 19-28.

Narlawar, S., Coudhury, S. and Gandhi, S. 2022. "Magnetic properties-based biosensors for early detection of cancer." In R. Khan, A. Parihar & S.K. Sanghi (Eds.), *Biosensor Based Advanced Cancer Diagnostics From Lab to Clinics* (pp. 165-178). Elsevier.

National Research Council. 2009. "Phthalates and cumulative risk assessment: the tasks ahead." *National Research Council (US) Committee on the Health Risks of Phthalates*. Washington (DC): National Academies Press (US).

Net, S., Delmont, A., Sempéré, R., Paluselli, A. and Ouddane, B. 2015. "Reliable quantification of phthalates in environmental matrices (air, water, sludge, sediment and soil): A review." *Science of the Total Environment* 515-516: 162-180.

Net, S, Sempéré, R., Delmont, A., Paluselli, A. and Ouddane, B. 2015. "Occurrence, fate, behavior and ecotoxicological state of phthalates in different environmental matrices." *Environmental Science & Technology* 49(7): 4019-4035.

Ngo, V. K. T., Nguyen, D. G., Nguyen, H. P. U., Tran, V. M., Nguyen, T. K. M., Huynh, T. P., Lam, Q. V., Huynh, T. D. and Truong, T. N. L. 2014. "Quartz crystal microbalance (QCM) as biosensor for the detecting of Escherichia coli O157:H7." *Advances in Natural Sciences: Nanoscience and Nanotechnology* 5(4): 045004.

Noh, H. B., Gurudatt, N. G., Won, M. S. and Shim, Y. B. 2015. "Analysis of phthalate esters in mammalian cell culture using a microfluidic channel coupled with an electrochemical sensor." *Analytical Chemistry* 87(14): 7069-7077.

Nørbygaard, T. and Berg, R. W. 2004. "Analysis of phthalate ester content in poly (vinyl chloride) plastics by means of fourier transform raman spectroscopy." *Applied Spectroscopy*. 58(4): 410-413.

Otezo, P., Saha, S. K., Moane, S., Barron, J., Clancy, G. and Murray, P. 2015. "Improved method for rapid detection of phthalates in bottled water by gas chromatography–mass spectrometry." *Journal of Chromatography B* 997: 229-235.

Özgür, E., Topçu, A. A., Yılmaz, E. and Denizli, A. 2020. "Surface plasmon resonance based biomimetic sensor for urinary tract infections." *Talanta* 212: 120778.

Özgür, E., Yılmaz, E., Şener, G., Uzun, L., Say, R. and Denizli, A. 2013. "A new molecular imprinting-based mass-sensitive sensor for real-time detection of 17β-estradiol from aqueous solution." *Environmental Progress & Sustainable Energy* 32(4): 1164-1169.

Palchetti I. and Mascini M. 2010. "Biosensor technology: a brief history." In: P., Malcovati, A., Baschirotto, A., d'Amico, C., Natale. (eds) *Sensors and Microsystems. Lecture Notes in Electrical Engineering* (pp 15-23), Springer, Dordrecht.

Paluselli, A., Aminot, Y., Galgani, F., Net, S. and Sempéré, R. 2018. "Occurrence of phthalate acid esters (PAEs) in the northwestern Mediterranean Sea and the Rhone River." *Progress in Oceanography* 163: 221-231.

Park, H. J. and Lee, S. S. 2018. "A quartz crystal microbalance-based biosensor for enzymatic detection of hemoglobin A1c in whole blood." *Sensors and Actuators B* 258: 836-840.

Parks, L. G., Ostby, J. S., Lambright, C. R., Abbott, B. D., Klinefelter, G. R., Barlow, N. J. and L. E. Gray Jr., L. E. 2000. "The plasticizer diethylhexyl phthalate induces malformations by decreasing fetal testosterone synthesis during sexual differentiation in the male rat." *Toxicological Sciences* 58(2): 339-349.

Peijnenburg, W. J. G. M., and Struijs, J. 2006. "Occurrence of phthalate esters in the environment of the Netherlands." *Ecotoxicology and Environmental Safety* 63(2): 204-215.

Pirzada, M. and Altintas, Z. 2020. "Recent progress in optical sensors for biomedical diagnostics." *Micromachines*. 11(4): 356.

Pohanka, M. 2017. "The piezoelectric biosensors: principles and applications, a review." *International Journal of Electrochemical Science* 12: 496-506.

Qureshi, M. S., Yusoff, A. R., Wirzal, M. D., Barek, J., Afridi, H. I. and Üstündag, Z. 2015. "Methods for the determination of endocrine-disrupting phthalate esters." *Critical Reviews in Analytical Chemistry* 46(2): 146-159.

Rastogi, S. K., Kesavachandran, C., Mahdi, F. and Pandey, A. 2006. "Phthalate exposure and health outcomes." *Indian Journal of Occupational and Environmental Medicine* 10: 111-115.

Sadique, M. A., Yadav, S., Ranjan, P., Khan, M. A., Kumar, A. and Khan, R. 2021. "Rapid detection of SARS-CoV-2 using graphene-based IoT integrated advanced electrochemical biosensor." *Materials Letters* 305: 130824.

Salazar-Beltrán, D., Hinojosa-Reyes, L., Ruiz-Ruiz, E., Hernández-Ramírez, A. and Guzmán-Mar, J. L. 2017. "Determination of phthalates in bottled water by automated on-line solid phase extraction coupled to liquid chromatography with UV detection." *Talanta* 168: 291-297.

Schettler, T. 2006. "Human exposure to phthalates via consumer products." *International Journal of Andrology* 29 (1): 134-139.

Sendón, R., Sanches-Silva, A., Bustos, J., Martín, P., Martínez, N. and Cirugeda, M.E. 2012. "Detection of migration of phthalates from agglomerated cork stoppers using HPLC-MS/MS." *Journal of Separation Science* 35: 1319-1326.

Sener, G., Ozgur, E., Yılmaz, E., Uzun, L., Say, R. and Denizli, A. 2010. "Quartz crystal microbalance based nanosensor for lysozyme detection with lysozyme imprinted nanoparticles." *Biosensors and Bioelectronics* 26: 815-821.

Seyoum, A. and Pradhan, A. 2019. "Effect of phthalates on development, reproduction, fat metabolism and lifespan in Daphnia magna." *Science of The Total Environment* 654: 969-977.

Shen, H. Y., Jiang, H. L., Mao, H. L., Pan, G., Zhou, L. and Cao, Y. F. 2007. "Simultaneous determination of seven phthalates and four parabens in cosmetic products using HPLC-DAD and GC-MS methods." *Journal of Separation Science* 30: 48-54.

Srivastava, K. R., Awasthi, S., Mishra, P. K. and Srivastava, P. K. 2020. "Biosensors/ molecular tools for detection of waterborne pathogens." In M. N. V. Prasad & A. Grobelak (Eds.), *Waterborne Pathogens Detection and Treatment* (pp. 237–277). Elsevier.

Staples, C. A., Peterson, D. R., Parkerton, T. F. and Adams, W. J. 1997. "The environmental fate of phthalate esters: A literature review." *Chemosphere* 35(4): 667-749.

Sun, G. and Liu, K. 2017. "Developmental toxicity and cardiac effects of butyl benzyl phthalate in zebrafish embryos." *Aquatic Toxicology* 192: 165-170.

Tang, M., Wu, Y., Deng, D., Wei, J., Zhang, J., Yang, D. and Li, G. 2018. "Development of an optical fiber immunosensor for the rapid and sensitive detection of phthalate esters." *Sensors and Actuators B: Chemical* 258: 304-312.

Tichý, J., Erhart, J., Kittinger, E. and Přívratská, J. 2010. "Principles of Piezoelectricity." In: *Fundamentals of Piezoelectric Sensorics*. Springer, Berlin, Heidelberg.

Trasande, L., Spanier, A. J., Sathyanarayana, S., Attina, T. M. and Blustein, J. 2013. "Urinary phthalates and increased insulin resistance in adolescents." *Pediatrics* 132 (3): e646-e655.

Tsopela, A., Laborde, A., Salvagnac, L., Ventalon, V., Bedel-Pereira, E., Séguy, I., Temple-Boyer, P., Juneau, P., Izquierdo, R. and Launay, J. 2016. "Development of a lab-on-chip electrochemical biosensor for water quality analysis based on microalgal photosynthesis." *Biosensors and Bioelectronics* 79: 568-573.

Türkoğlu, E. A. 2021. "Molecularly-imprinted nanomaterial-based surface plasmon resonance biosensors in molecular diagnosis." In Mohd Amin Bhat, et al. *Applications of Nanomaterials in Agriculture, Food Science, and Medicine* (pp. 1-28), IGI Global.

United States Consumer Product Safety Commission. 2008. *United States Consumer Product Safety Commission, Consumer Product Safety Improvement Act of 2008, Public Law 110-314-Aug. 14, 2008.* Available from: https://www.everycrsreport .com/.

Villalonga, A., Sánchez, A., Mayol, B., Reviejo, J. and Villalonga, R. 2022. "Electrochemical biosensors for food bioprocess monitoring." *Current Opinion in Food Science* 43: 18-26.

Wang, J. 2005. "Nanomaterial-based electrochemical biosensors." *Analyst* 130: 421-426.

Wang, X., Okoffo, E. D., Banks, A. P., Li, Y., Thomas, K. V., Rauert, C., Aylward, L. L. and Mueller, J. F. 2022. "Phthalate esters in face masks and associated inhalation exposure risk." *Journal of Hazardous Materials* 423: 127001.

Wang, Y., Ding, P., Hu, R., Zhang, J., Ma, X., Luo, Z. and Li, G. 2013. "A dibutyl phthalate sensor based on a nanofiber polyaniline coated quartz crystal monitor." *Sensors* 13: 3765-3775.

Wang, Y., Zhu, H. and Kannan, K. 2019. "A review of biomonitoring of phthalate exposures." *Toxics* 7(2): 21.

Weng, T. I., Chen, M. H., Lien, G. W., Chen, P. S., Lin, J., Fang, C. C. and Chen, P. C. 2017. "Effects of gender on the association of urinary phthalate metabolites with thyroid hormones in children: a prospective cohort study in Taiwan." *International Journal of Environmental Research and Public Health* 14(2): 123.

Wofford, H. W., Wilsey, C. D., Neff, G. S., Giam, C. S. and Neff, J. M. 1981. "Bioaccumulation and metabolism of phthalate esters by oysters, brown shrimp, and sheepshead minnows." *Ecotoxicology and Environmental Safety 5(2): 202-210.*

Wormuth, M., Scheringer, M., Vollenweider, M. and Hungerbuhler, K. 2006. "What are the sources of exposure to eight frequently used phthalic acid esters in Europeans?" *Risk Analysis* 26(3): 803-824.

Xie, H., Han, W., Xie, Q., Xu, T., Zhu, M. and Chen, J. 2022. "Face mask-A potential source of phthalate exposure for human." *Journal of Hazardous Materials* 422: 126848.

Xie, Q., Sun, D., Han, Y., Jia, L., Hou, B., Liu, S. and Li, D. 2016. "Determination of total phthalates in edible oils by high-performance liquid chromatography coupled with photodiode array detection." *Journal of Separation Science* 39: 857-863.

Xu, Q., Gao, X., Zhao, S., Liu, Y-N., Zhang, D., Zhou, K., Khanbareh, H., Chen, W., Zhang, Y. and Bowen, C. 2021. "Construction of Bio-Piezoelectric Platforms: From Structures and Synthesis to Applications." *Advanced Materials* 33: 2008452.

Yang, G. C. C., Yen, C-H. and Wang, C-L. 2014. "Monitoring and removal of residual phthalate esters and pharmaceuticals in the drinking water of Kaohsiung City, Taiwan." *Journal of Hazardous Materials* 277: 53-61.

Yılmaz, E., Özgür, E., Bereli, N., Türkmen, D. and Denizli, A. 2017. "Plastic antibody based surface plasmon resonance nanosensors for selective atrazine detection." *Materials Science and Engineering: C* 73: 603-610.

Zaater, M. F., Tahboub, Y. R. and Al Sayyed, A. N. 2014. "Determination of phthalates in Jordanian bottled water using GS-MS and HPLC-UV: environmental study." *Journal of Chromatographic Science* 52: 447-452.

Zhang, K., Fan, G., Hu, R. and Li, G. 2015. "enhanced dibutyl phthalate sensing performance of a quartz crystal microbalance coated with au-decorated zno porous microspheres." *Sensors* 15: 21153-21168.

Zhang, Y. J., Guo, J. L., Xue, J., Bai, C. L. and Guo, Y. 2021. "Phthalate metabolites: Characterization, toxicities, global distribution, and exposure assessment." *Environmental Pollution* 291: 118106.

Zhang, Z., Luo, L., Cai, R. and Chen, H. 2013. "A sensitive and selective molecularly imprinted sensor combined with magnetic molecularly imprinted solid phase extraction for determination of dibutyl phthalate." *Biosensors and Bioelectronics* 49: 367-373.

Zhao, J. F., Hsiao, S. H., Hsu, M. H., Pao, K. C., Kou, Y. R., Shyue, S. K., and Lee, T. S. 2014. "Di-(2-ethylhexyl) phthalate accelerates atherosclerosis in apolipoprotein E-deficient mice." *Archives of Toxicology* 90(1): 181-190.

Zhao, Z. and Jiang, H. 2010. "Enzyme-based electrochemical biosensors." In P. A. Serra, *Biosensors*, IntechOpen, London. Available from: https://www.intechopen.com/chapters/6911.

Zhou, Z., Li, T., Xu, W., Huang, W., Wang, N. and Yang, W. 2017. "Synthesis and characterization of fluorescence molecularly imprinted polymers as sensor for highly sensitive detection of dibutyl phthalate from tap water samples." *Sensors and Actuators B: Chemical* 240: 1114-1122.

Zhu, J., Liu, X., Shi, Q., He, T., Sun, Z., Guo, X., Liu, W., Sulaiman, O. B. Dong, B. and Lee, C. 2020. "Development trends and perspectives of future sensors and MEMS/NEMS." *Micromachines* 11(1): 7.

Zhu, N., Zou, Y., Huang, M., Dong, S., Wu, X., Liang, G., Han, Z. and Zhang, Z. 2018. "A sensitive, colorimetric immunosensor based on Cu-MOFs and HRP for detection of dibutyl phthalate in environmental and food samples." *Talanta* 186: 104-109.

Zia, A. I., Abdul Rahman, M. S., Mukhopadhyay, S. C., Yu, P. L., Al-Bahadly, I. H., Gooneratne, C. P., Kosel, J. and Liao, T. S. 2013. "Technique for rapid detection of phthalates in water and beverages." *Journal of Food Engineering* 116: 515-523.

Zia, A. I., Mukhopadhyay, S. C., Yu, P. L., Al-Bahadly, I. H., Gooneratne, C. P. and Kosel, J. 2015. "Rapid and molecular selective electrochemical sensing of phthalates in aqueous solution." *Biosensors and Bioelectronics* 67: 342-349.

Editors' Contact Information

Müfide Aydoğan Ahbab
Assoc. Professor,
University of Health Sciences Turkey,
Vocational School of Health Services,
Uskudar, Turkey
mufideaydogan.ahbab@sbu.edu.tr

Nurhayat Barlas
Professor,
Hacettepe University,
Science Faculty, Department of Biology,
Ankara, Turkey
barlas@hacettepe.edu.tr

Index

#

A

B

H

N

O

P

Q

R

S

T

U